Histopathology
A Color Atlas and Textbook

Histopathology
A Color Atlas and Textbook

Ivan Damjanov, M.D., Ph.D.

Professor and Chairman
Department of Pathology
The University of Kansas School of Medicine
Kansas City, Kansas

In collaboration with

Peter A. McCue, M.D.

Associate Professor
Department of Pathology and Cell Biology
Jefferson Medical College
Thomas Jefferson University
Philadelphia, Pennsylvania

Illustrations by
Matthew Chansky

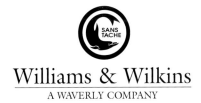

Williams & Wilkins
A WAVERLY COMPANY

BALTIMORE • PHILADELPHIA • LONDON • PARIS • BANGKOK
BUENOS AIRES • HONG KONG • MUNICH • SYDNEY • TOKYO • WROCLAW

Editor: Jane Velker
Managing Editor: Nancy Evans
Development Editor: Kathleen Scogna
Production Coordinator: Barbara J. Felton
Copy Editor: John M. Daniel
Designer: Dan Pfisterer
Illustration Planner: Wayne Hubbel
Cover Designer: Tom Scheuerman
Typesetter: Maryland Composition
Printer/Binder: R. R. Donnelley & Sons
Digitized Illustrations: Prestige Color

Copyright © 1996

Williams & Wilkins
351 West Camden Street
Baltimore, Maryland 21201-2436 USA

Rose Tree Corporate Center
1400 North Providence Road
Building II, Suite 5025
Media, Pennsylvania 19063-2043 USA

Accurate indications, adverse reactions, and dosage schedules for drugs are provided in this book, but it is possible that they may change. The reader is urged to review the package information data of the manufacturers of the medications mentioned.

Printed in the United States of America

Library of Congress Cataloging-in-Publication Data
Damjanov, Ivan.
    Color atlas of histopathology / Ivan Damjanov,
        p.   cm.
    Includes index.
    ISBN 0-683-02334-9
    1. Histology, Pathological—Atlases, I. Title.
RB33.D36   94-47026
611′.018—dc20   CIP

The publishers have made every effort to trace the copyright holders for borrowed material. If they have inadvertently overlooked any, they will be pleased to make the necessary arrangements at the first opportunity.

To purchase additional copies of this book, call our customer service department at **(800) 638-0672** or fax orders to **(800) 447-8438**. For other book services, including chapter reprints and large quantity sales, ask for the Special Sales department.

Canadian customers should call **(800) 268-4178**, or fax **(905) 470-6780**. For all other calls originating outside of the United States, please call **(410) 528-4223** or fax us at **(410) 528-8550**.

Visit Williams & Wilkins on the Internet: **http://www.wwilkins.com** or contact our customer service department at **custserv@wwilkins.com**. Williams & Wilkins customer service representatives are available from 8:30 am to 6:00 pm, EST, Monday through Friday, for telephone access.

96 97 98 99 00
1 2 3 4 5 6 7 8 9 10

To Nevena, a dozen years too late, maybe. But as Henry James said, "We do what we can, we give what we have and the rest is madness of the art."

Preface

The historian Arthur Schlesinger, Jr., when asked why we should study history, responded unapologetically, "First of all, because it's a lot of fun." I could give the same answer for studying histopathology. Unfortunately, in today's compressed medical curriculum students cannot choose courses or study something for the sake of fun only. To make my case I must, therefore, go on record and state that I still consider histopathology essential for the understanding of pathology. Because pathology is the basis of our medical practice, or, in the words of Sir William Osler, "As is our pathology, so is our practice," I compiled this Atlas for students to help them prepare for the clinics. Secretly, I also hoped that the Atlas would show them that the study of histopathology could also be a lot of fun.

The Atlas has two parts: A brief *general pathology* section, comprising the first four chapters, which deal with pathologic processes, and a *systemic pathology* section, organized into 15 chapters, each of which is devoted to the pathology of a given organ system. In every chapter the emphasis is on histopathology, and the Atlas is profusely illustrated with more than 1000 color photographs. To facilitate learning, the photographs are accompanied by a brief but comprehensive text and more than 100 diagrams, which allow the students to interconnect different concepts and place them into the context of pathophysiology and their clinical significance. Diagrammatic summaries of normal histology, essential for the understanding of the abnormalities in the same tissues, are found at the beginning of each chapter.

I envision several possible uses for this Atlas:

> The Atlas could be used as an aid for teaching histopathology in the microscopy room. The book is handy enough to be laid open next to the microscope and could therefore serve as a guide to students studying the microscopic slides. The text is brief so that it could be used as background reading or for review of facts that are essential for the understanding of histopathology. The diagrams have the same purpose and could help the student integrate the facts horizontally as well as vertically, primarily with the pathophysiologic and clinical facts.

> The Atlas could be used in lieu of a histopathology course. In medical schools that do not have histopathology laboratories, this Atlas could serve as a substitute for the microscopic study of glass slides. It illustrates all the essential diseases typically taught in a histopathology course. Because it contains photographs of all major tissue changes that are useful for understanding important principles, I believe that it could also supplement lectures and standard textbooks.

> The Atlas could be used for review of pathology and could help students prepare for examinations during their sophomore pathol-

ogy course or for the examinations of the National Board of Medical Examiners (NBME). Many bare or abstract facts remain longer in our memory when linked to images. Visual memory is closely linked to verbal memory, and a review of pathology through pictures has been shown to help elicit the recall of other facts, even those initially assimilated in other contexts. Also, it should be mentioned here that the NBME examination booklets contain color microphotographs. The students are required not only to recognize such images but also to interpret them together with relevant clinical and pathophysiologic principles. It is my hope that this Atlas could be useful to students preparing for such exams. I also hope that the students would keep the Atlas on their shelves and reuse it while preparing for their clinical examinations and specialty boards many years after their sophomore pathology course.

I. DAMJANOV

Acknowledgments

A project of this size would not have been possible without the help of my colleagues, my students, my secretaries, my technical assistants, artists, and the editorial staff of William & Wilkins, who all contributed to the completion of this Atlas.

First of all, I must acknowledge the contribution of Peter A. McCue, MD, who provided many photographs and read and edited the first draft of several chapters. Matthew Chansky translated my abstract sketches into most comprehensive line drawings. Dennis Nielsen and Bodil Tuma helped me with photography. Sandra Dixon-Ross, Kathy Gordon, Carla Aldi, and Cyndi Van Derbur helped me by patiently typing and retyping the text. Kathleen H. Scogna helped me edit the text and formulate the final format of the book. Nancy Evans guided me through the project. Timothy S. Satterfield, who signed me up, and Pat Coryell, who inherited the project from him, were always there whenever I needed them. I owe them my gratitude.

Most of the photographs used in this Atlas were taken from the histopathologic slides that I have been collecting since my halcyon days. In addition, I had the opportunity to review and photograph the teaching slide collections of my colleagues and friends: James R. Newland, MD, University of Nebraska; Robert E. Lee, MD, University of Pittsburgh; Howard J. Igel, MD, and Ludwig Deppisch, MD, Northeastern Ohio University School of Medicine. Ana Sotrel, MD, University of Illinois, John J. Kepes, MD, and Michael Handler, MD, University of Kansas, allowed me to photograph some of their neuropathology slides. Peter B. Hukill, MD, Torrance, Connecticut, donated his dermatopathology collection. Bong H. Hyun, MD, and Karen van Hoeven, MD, Thomas Jefferson University, gave me several hematopathologic and cytologic slides. Individual color diapositive slides were contributed by William M. Thurlbeck, MD, University of British Columbia; Robert M. Genta, MD, Baylor University; William D. Edwards, MD, Mayo Clinic; F. Steven Vogel, MD, USCAP, Augusta; James M. Powers, University of Rochester; James Fishback, MD, and H. Clarke Anderson, MD, University of Kansas.

Some glass slides in my collection come from my teachers, residents, and friends. Unfortunately, I did not keep good records of the provenance of these slides. I hope that these "unacknowledged contributors" will remain my friends even if they recognize their own material in some of my photographs.

Diagram of Normal Cells and Tissue Components

This diagram contains the symbols for the most important normal tissue elements. Whenever possible, the artist has used these schematic renditions to illustrate the participation of normal cells in various pathologic processes.

⬤	Erythrocyte	⠿	Platelets
⬤	Plasma cell	⬤	Multinucleated giant cell
⬤	Lymphocyte	⬤	Fibroblast
⬤	Neutrophil	⬤	Angioblasts (neovascularization)
⬤	Eosinophil	▨	Fibrin
⬤	Macrophage	〜	Collagen fibers

Key to the diagrams

All the microphotographs were prepared from standard hematoxylin and eosin stained histologic slides unless specified otherwise. Other stains include periodic acid-Schiff for complex carbohydrate, oil red O or osmium tetroxide for lipids, and Trichrome stain for connective tissue. Prussian blue reaction was used for demonstration of iron. Some neuropathology slides were stained with Luxol fast blue or impregnated with silver. Amyloid was demonstrated with Congo red stain.

Immunoperoxidase and immunofluorescence microscopy (with fluoresceinated antibodies) were used for immunohistochemical reactions. Papanicolaou stain was used for cytologic specimens. Hematologic smears were stained by the May-Grünwald-Giemsa technique. Electron microscopy specimens were fixed in glutaraldehyde, post-fixed in osmium tetroxide, and stained with uranyl acetate.

Contents

CHAPTER 4

NEOPLASIA

CHAPTER 5

CARDIOVASCULAR SYSTEM

CHAPTER 6

RESPIRATORY SYSTEM

CHAPTER 7

HEMATOPOIETIC SYSTEM

CHAPTER 8

DIGESTIVE SYSTEM

CHAPTER 9

HEPATOBILIARY SYSTEM

CHAPTER 13
FEMALE GENITAL SYSTEM

CHAPTER 14
BREAST

CHAPTER 15
ENDOCRINE GLANDS

CHAPTER 16

SKIN

CHAPTER 17

BONES AND JOINTS

CHAPTER 18

SKELETAL MUSCLES

CHAPTER 19

NERVOUS SYSTEM

CHAPTER 1

Cell Pathology

INTRODUCTION

The cell is the smallest living unit of the human body. In multicellular living organisms, such as the human body, the cells are in close contact with other cells and are surrounded by body fluids and an extracellular matrix that provide the *internal milieu* essential for the maintenance of cell functions. The cells are normally in *homeostasis*, i.e., a metabolic equilibrium with other cells and extracellular fluids that make up their microenvironment.

Cells respond to metabolic demands of the body, energy supply, and various physiological and pathological stimuli by **adaptation.** Adaption is a reversible adjustment to environmental conditions that includes changes in cell function, morphology, or both (Diagram 1.1). If the stimulus is removed, the cells revert to their normal state. Under certain circumstances, such as prolonged stimulation with carcinogenic chemicals, reversible cellular changes may become irreversible and even progress to dysplasia and neoplasia.

If the external stimuli exceed the capacity of the cell to adapt, irreversible cell injury occurs, and ultimately the cell dies. Pathological cell death is called **necrosis**.

Necrosis is an irreversible change that occurs in response to irreparable cell injury. Although in this textbook we consider adaptation and necrosis as distinct from one another, in real life the dividing line between reversible and irreversible cell injury is not always sharp. The differences between reparable and irreparable cell injury are to a certain extent quantitative rather than qualitative. The spectrum of cytoplasmic changes that may occur in both conditions, as revealed by electron microscopy, is shown in Diagram 1.2.

ADAPTATION

Normal cells can respond to a number of physiological and/or pathological stimuli by changing their functions. Functional changes are often reflected in an altered cell morphology, which can be recognized with a microscope.

The examples of cell adaptations are:

- Cellular swelling
- Cytoplasmic storage and accumulation of metabolites and other substances
- Atrophy
- Hypertrophy and hyperplasia
- Metaplasia

Diagram 1.1. Response of the cell to physiologic and pathologic stimuli.

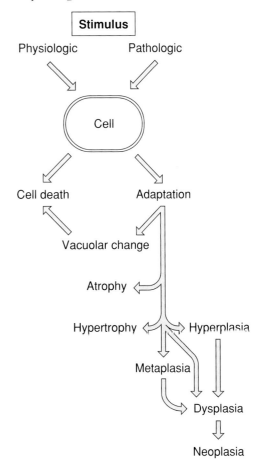

Cellular Swelling and Vacuolization

Cellular swelling and vacuolization are common forms of cell reaction to various physiologic and pathologic stimuli (Diagram 1.3). For example, vacuolar change of the proximal tubules of the kidney occurs during osmotic diuresis, reflecting an excessive passage of fluids through the kidney (Fig. 1.1). Viral hepatitis may cause vacuolization of liver cells (Fig. 1.2). Electron microscopy may reveal swollen cells showing dilatation of the rough endoplasmic reticulum (Fig. 1.3) and enlarged, vacuolated mitochondria (Fig. 1.4).

Storage of Metabolites

Storage of metabolites in the cytoplasm occurs in many metabolic disorders. Several inborn errors of intermediate metabolism of carbohydrates, mucopolysaccharides, lipids, or proteins typically fall into the category of genetic storage disorders. For example, *Tay-Sachs disease*, a congenital deficiency of hexosaminidase A, is characterized by an accu-

Diagram 1.2. Reaction of the cell to injury. Ultrastructure of the normal cell is presented in the right half and the reaction of the cell to injury in the left half of this schematic drawing. **Right. Normal cell.** 1. The cell membrane is a selectively permeable bilayer composed of lipids, proteins, and carbohydrates. Its integrity ensures the maintenance of equilibrium between the internal and external milieu. The *ATP-dependent sodium potassium pump* (ATPase) maintains the water-salt gradients across the membrane, keeping the intracellular potassium high and sodium low. 2. Absorptive vacuoles are formed from the invaginated cell membrane. They are called phagocytic vacuoles if filled with particulate material, and pinocytotic if filled with solutes. 3. Absorptive vacuoles fuse with primary lysosomes, membrane-bound vesicles rich in hydrolytic enzymes, which are derived from the Golgi apparatus. Primary lysosomes fused with absorptive vacuoles form secondary lysosomes. The hydrolytic enzymes, active at low pH, are activated in the secondary lysosomes and metabolize the ingested material. The residual bodies containing undigested material are expelled from the cell. 4. Rough endoplasmic reticulum consists of parallel membranes studded with attached ribosomes. Proteins synthesized for export in the rough endoplasmic reticulum are translocated into the lumen of the cisternae and excreted. 5. Mitochondria are organelles surrounded by a double membrane that invaginates to form cristae. Mitochondria are rich in oxidative enzymes, which generate the energy for most of the cell processes. 6. Smooth endoplasmic reticulum consists of small vesicles. Its primary function is metabolism of hormones and drugs and synthesis of steroid hormones. 7. The cytoskeleton consists of microtubules, intermediate filaments, and microfilaments that maintain the shape of the cell, participate in the movement of organelles in the cytoplasm, and enable cell locomotion and phagocytosis. 8. Metabolites such as proteins, glycogen, and lipids are stored in the hyaloplasm. Proteins cannot be visualized by electron microscopy. A few lipid droplets and glycogen granules are present in most cells. 9. The nucleus has a bilayered membrane that separates it from the cytoplasm. DNA, RNA, and nucleoproteins form finely granular aggregates of euchromatin and coarser heterochromatin, which is often attached to the nuclear membrane. The nucleolus is rich in RNA and consists of closely intertwined fibrillar and granular material. **Left. Reaction of the cell to injury.** 1. Acute injury causes influx of water into the cell and the appearance of fluid-filled hypoxic vacuoles that form from the cell membrane. 2. The microvilli are edematous and swollen. 3. Water and solutes accumulate in the cisternae of rough endoplasmic reticulum, which also undergo degranulation of ribosomes. This results in reduced protein synthesis. 4. Accumulation of water causes swelling and rupture of mitochondria. Ruptured mitochondria may be calcified. Mitochondrial remnants may be included into autophagosomes. Undigested material in heterophagosomes or autophagosomes is compacted into residual bodies (RB) or lipofuscin pigment granules. Since the expulsion of residual bodies requires energy, which is unavailable in adequate amounts in the injured cell, lipofuscin accumulates in the cytoplasm. 5. Autophagosomes form from lysosomes. These digestive vacuoles contain fragments of endoplasmic reticulum or mitochondria and other organelles. 6. The smooth endoplasmic reticulum may enlarge to meet the increased metabolic demands, as in drug overload. 7. Cytoskeletal fibrils may aggregate and form cytoplasmic bodies, as typically seen in liver cells of alcoholics (Mallory hyaline). 8. Glycogen is depleted in injured cells, whereas the cytoplasm may contain more lipid droplets than usual. 9. Cell injury may cause nuclear changes such as dissociation of the fibrillar and granular components of the nucleolus or the disappearance of nucleolus. These changes, together with the degranulation of rough endoplasmic reticulum, result in decreased synthesis of proteins for export.

mulation of gangliosides in the cytoplasm of neurons. Such cells appear swollen and have a vacuolated cytoplasm (Fig. 1.5). Electron microscopy reveals that the cytoplasm of these cells contains numerous lysosomes, which are filled with concentric whorls composed of undegradable metabolites. Tay-Sachs disease and related disorders are examples of lysosomal storage diseases.

Other examples of genetic storage disorders characterized by accumulation of metabolites in the cytoplasm are **Gaucher disease** and **glycogenoses**.

Gaucher disease is characterized by an accumulation of glucocerebrosides in the phagocytic cells of the spleen and the bone marrow (Fig. 1.6). Glycogenoses are characterized by an accumulation of glycogen in the cytoplasm of several organs. The liver, kidney, or muscles can be involved (Fig. 1.7).

Fatty Change

Fatty change occurs in many organs following ischemia, chemical or physical injury, or metabolic disturbances caused by

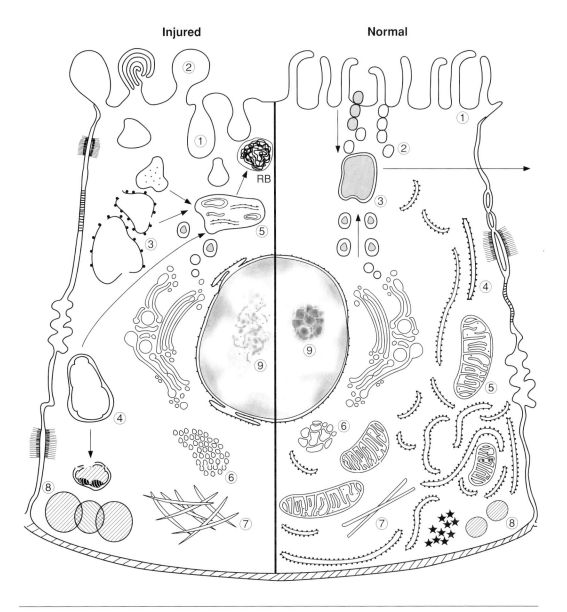

infections and other systemic diseases. Fat typically accumulates in liver cells exposed to alcohol (Fig. 1.8). Fat is stored in the cytoplasm in the form of triglyceride-rich droplets. Small droplets ultimately coalesce into large vacuoles, which fill the entire cytoplasm and peripherally displace the nucleus.

Accumulation of Pigmented Material

Accumulation of pigmented material is a form of cell adaptation that usually results when there is an oversupply of such pigments. Pigments are endogenous or exogenous colored substances. For example, carbon particles that accumulate in lungs exposed to polluted air are exogenous pigments (see Fig. 1.17). Hemoglobin, the red pigment of erythrocytes, is an endogenous pigment. Hemolysis of red blood cells results in a release of hemoglobin, which is then phagocytized by macrophages of the liver and spleen and stored in their cytoplasm as the brown pigment **hemosiderin** (Fig. 1.9). Hemosiderin contains ferric iron, which can be detected by the Prussian blue reaction. This histochemical test is used to distinguish hemosiderin from other non–iron-containing brown pigments, such as bilirubin, melanin, or lipofuscin.

Atrophy

Atrophy is a form of adaptation characterized by a reduction of cell size (Diagram 1.4). Atrophy of individual cells combined with increased cell loss or inadequate replenishment of lost cells ultimately results in a reduced size of organs and thinning of tissues (e.g., atrophy of skin). Atrophy is often associated with accumulation of lipofuscin, a brown lipid-rich pigment derived from material accumulated in lysosomes.

Hypertrophy

Hypertrophy is characterized by increased cell size. This adaptation typically occurs in skeletal, heart, and smooth muscle, but may occur in other organs and tissues as well.

Hyperplasia

Hyperplasia is an increased number of cells. Hyperplasia can only occur in organs composed of facultatively mitotic cells that divide and multiply in response to stimuli, such as the liver, kidney, or endometrium. Hyperplasia cannot occur in the heart, brain, or other organs composed of postmitotic, nondividing cells.

Complex Adaptations

Hypertrophy and hyperplasia sometimes occur concomitantly. The thickening of the muscularis of the urinary bladder due to chronic obstruction by an enlarged prostate is a typical example of simultaneous hypertrophy and hyperplasia. Cell atrophy is often associated with compensatory hypertrophy of adjacent cells. Various forms of atrophy, hypertrophy, and hyperplasia are illustrated in Figures 1.10 to 1.13.

Metaplasia

Metaplasia occurs when cells typical of one differentiated tissue change into cells of another differentiated tissue (Diagram 1.5). It may involve epithelial or mesenchymal cells. For example, apocrine cells similar to those in sweat glands may appear in the breast (Fig. 1.13D). Endocervical *columnar epithelium* may change into stratified *squamous epithelium* in chronic cervicitis (Fig. 1.14). Intestinal metaplasia of esophageal epithelium seen in Barrett esophagus is characterized by replacement of squamous epithelium with columnar epithelium typical of the lining of the small intestine (Fig. 1.15). Osseous metaplasia of the fibrous stroma of muscle in *myositis ossificans* is an example of mesenchymal metaplasia (Fig. 1.16). Heterotopic ossification may occur in scar tissue in various organs, e.g., lung (Fig. 1.17).

CELL DEATH

If limited in extent, almost all the cytoplasmic changes shown in Diagram 1.2 are reversible. However, if many organelles are damaged simultaneously or the injury is so extensive that it cannot be repaired, cell death occurs. Death of a group of cells caused by irreversible injury is called **necrosis**. Dying cells initially show the same ultrastructural alterations as reversibly injured cells do, but at a "point of no return," which is morphologically recog-

---

nized as changes in nuclear morphology or disruption of the cell membrane, cell death is imminent.

The irreversibly damaged nuclei are characterized by one of the following three features: nuclear membrane rupture and fragmentation of the nucleus (*karyorrhexis*), lysis of the chromatin (*karyolysis*), or clumping of the nuclear contents (*pyknosis*) (Diagram 1.6 and Figs. 1.18 and 1.19).

Necrosis is caused by anoxia, lack of energy supply, or the effects of noxious agents that disrupt cell functions. This pathological cell death should be distinguished from natural cell death that occurs for intrinsic reasons and is often programmed or predetermined. This form of cell death, called **apoptosis**, occurs normally in most tissues. It is most prominent in tissues that undergo constant renewal, such as the intestinal mucosa. Apoptosis requires active RNA and protein synthesis and is an energy-dependent process. Morphologically, it is recognized by condensation of chromatin along the nuclear membrane, which typically shows irregular blebbing (Fig. 1.20).

MORPHOLOGIC TYPES
OF TISSUE NECROSIS

Several forms of necrosis can be recognized by the naked eye and by microscopic examination of affected tissues. These include:

- Coagulation necrosis
- Liquefactive necrosis
- Caseous necrosis

Coagulation necrosis is associated with inhibition of lytic enzymes. The cells do not lyse; thus, their outlines are relatively preserved. Nuclei disappear and the acidified cytoplasm becomes eosinophilic (Fig. 1.21).

Liquefactive necrosis is marked by dissolution of tissue due to enzymatic lysis of dead cells. Typically, it takes place in the brain when autocatalytic enzymes are released from dead cells (Fig. 1.22). Liquefactive necrosis occurs also in purulent inflammation due to the heterolytic action of polymorphonuclear leukocytes in pus. Liquefied tissue is soft, diffluent, and composed of disintegrated cells and fluid.

Fat necrosis is a consequence of lipolytic action of enzymes on fat tissue. Typically, it occurs in acute pancreatic necrosis (Fig. 1.23) and is a consequence of the release of pancreatic lipase into the peripancreatic tissues. Lipolysis is marked by loss of the contours of fat cells. Free fatty acids released from fat cells undergo saponification by binding sodium, potassium, or calcium. The soaps formed from fatty acids are deposited in tissues as amorphous or finely granular material, which appears bluish in slides stained with hematoxylin and eosin.

Caseous necrosis has features of both coagulation and liquefactive necrosis. Typically, it occurs in the center of tuberculous granulomas, which contain a white or yellow "cheesy" material (Latin *caseum* = cheese) that accounts for the name of this lesion. Histologically, the outlines of necrotic cells are not preserved, but the tissue has not been liquefied either. The remnants of the cells appear as finely granular, amorphous material (Fig. 1.24).

PLATE 1.1. VACUOLAR CHANGE

Figure 1.1. Vacuolar change of renal tubules in osmotic diuresis, induced by mannitol. This hyperosmotic substance given intravenously to increase diuresis is accumulated in the absorptive cytoplasmic vacuoles of the proximal tubules. The cytoplasm of the proximal renal tubules contains an increased amount of water. It appears vacuolated and clear, in contrast to normal renal tubular epithelial cells, which are eosinophilic.

Figure 1.3. Vacuolar change. This electron microphotograph shows prominent cytoplasmic vacuoles filled with finely granular material. Some of the vacuoles are derived from degranulated endoplasmic reticulum or plasma membrane and swollen mitochondria.

Figure 1.2. Viral hepatitis. The hepatocytes infected with hepatitis virus B appear enlarged and have vacuolated cytoplasm ("ballooning degeneration").

Figure 1.4. Mitochondrial swelling. The mitochondria of the myocardial cells appear swollen and have disrupted cristae. There are also foci of intramitochondrial calcification.

Diagram 1.3. Cell swelling, vacuolization, and cytoplasmic storage. A. Normal cell. **B.** Hydropic change (vacuolar degeneration). The cytoplasm contains fluid-filled vacuoles derived from the invaginated cell membrane (hypoxic vacuoles), dilated rough endoplasmic reticulum (RER), and swollen mitochondria. **C.** Lysosomal storage disease. The lysosomes contain undigested metabolites. **D.** Glycogen storage disease. Granular glycogen accumulates in the hyaloplasm between the mitochondria, lysosomes, and other formed organelles. **E.** Lipid accumulation. Lipid droplets coalesce and displace the nucleus peripherally.

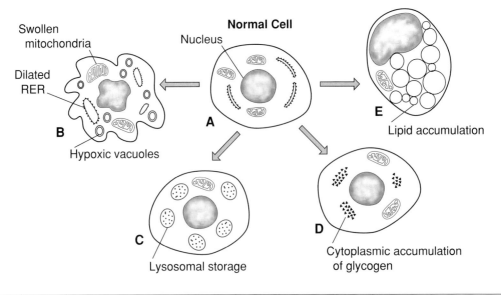

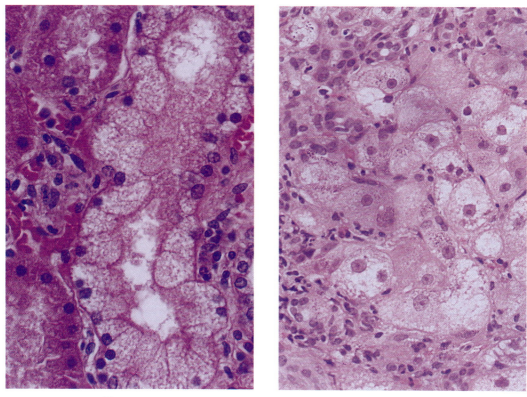

Figure 1.1

Figure 1.2

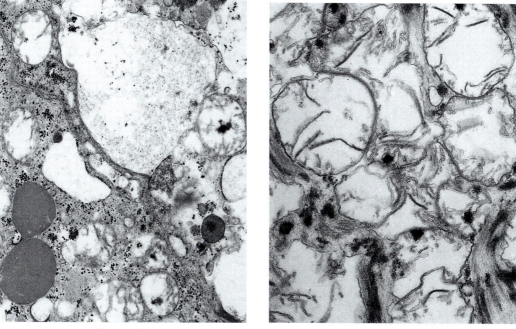

Figure 1.3

Figure 1.4

PLATE 1.2. GENETIC STORAGE DISEASES

Figure 1.5. Tay-Sachs disease. A. The brain cells appear enlarged and vacuolated because of the accumulation of gangliosides in the lysosomes. **B.** This electron microphotograph shows lysosomes filled with whorls of membranes.

Figure 1.6. Gaucher disease. A. Gaucher cells from the bone marrow have abundant cytoplasm that appears fibrillar (like "wrinkled tissue paper"). **B.** Electron microscopy shows twisted fibrils. These fibrils are composed of glucocerebroside.

Figure 1.7. Glycogenosis type I. A. The cytoplasm of liver cells appears pale and clear because the cells are filled with glycogen. **B.** Electron microscopy shows numerous granules of glycogen in the cytoplasm.

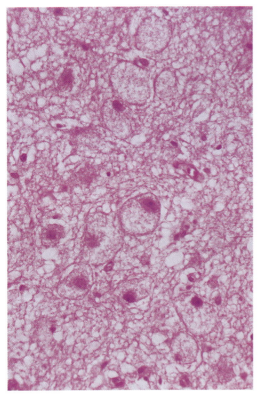
Figure 1.5A

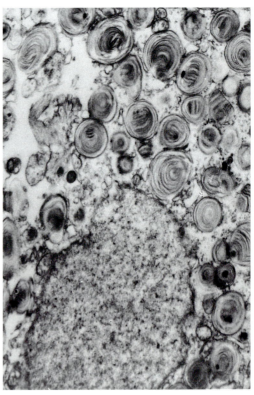
Figure 1.5B

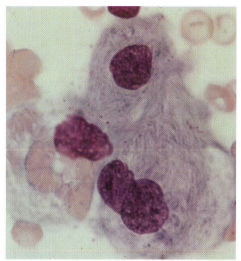

Figure 1.6A

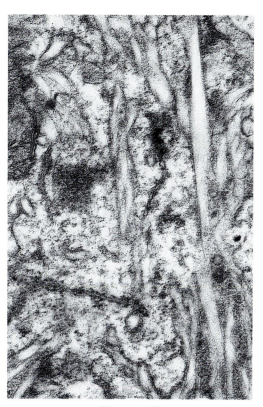

Figure 1.6B

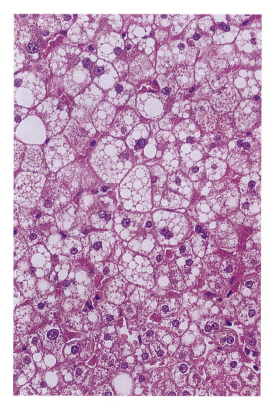

Figure 1.7A

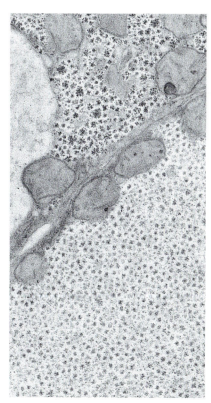

Figure 1.7B

PLATE 1.3. CYTOPLASMIC STORAGE

Figure 1.8.   **Fatty liver induced by alcohol. A.** The liver cells contain large vacuoles. These vacuoles represent the cytoplasmic spaces from which the fat was removed during tissue processing. **B.** Osmium fixation preserves the fat droplets, which appear as black round bodies in the cytoplasm. **C.** Fat can be demonstrated in freshly frozen cryostat-sectioned tissue stained with special stains such as Oil red.

Figure 1.9.   **Hemosiderosis. A.** Liver from a patient who received numerous blood transfusions shows brown cytoplasmic granules of hemosiderin in liver and Kupffer cells. **B.** In this slide stained with Prussian blue, hemosiderin appears as blue cytoplasmic granules.

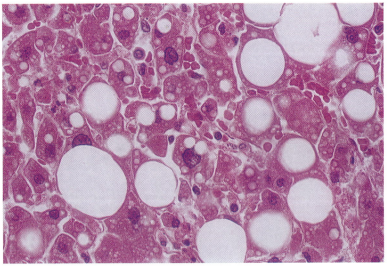

Figure 1.8A

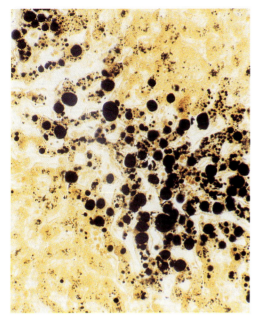

Figure 1.8B

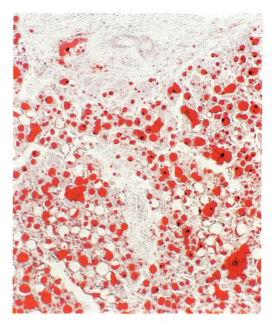

Figure 1.8C

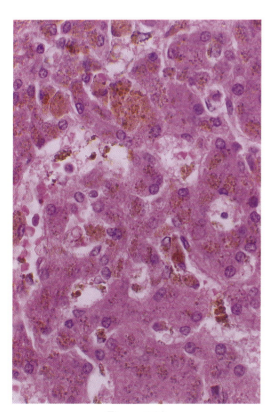

Figure 1.9A

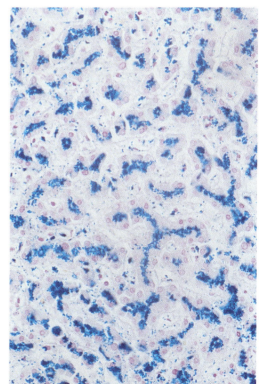

Figure 1.9B

PLATE 1.4. CELLULAR ADAPTATIONS

Figure 1.10. Neurogenic atrophy of skeletal muscle. A. Transection of the nerve caused the atrophy of the entire muscle fascicle that was innervated by this particular nerve (*arrow*). **B.** Focal atrophy with compensatory hypertrophy of skeletal muscle. Atrophic (*A*) and hypertrophic (*H*) fibers are indicated with arrows.

Figure 1.11. Atrophy of the heart. This heart is from a person debilitated by chronic disease. The muscle fibers appear thin, vacuolated, and paler than normal because they contain fewer myofilaments. Compare this photo with Figure 1.12, which shows hypertrophic heart cells.

Figure 1.12. Hypertrophy of the heart. A. The muscle fibers, sectioned longitudinally, appear thick and eosinophilic, reflecting the abundance of actin and myosin filaments in the cytoplasm. Nuclei are also enlarged. **B.** On cross-sectioning, the nuclei of muscle fibers appear enlarged and irregularly shaped.

Diagram 1.4. Adaptive changes induced by cell injury. A. Atrophy is marked by decreased size of individual cells or a decreased number of cells within the tissue. **B.** Hypertrophy is marked by an increased size of individual cells. Both the cytoplasm and the nucleus are increased in size. **C.** Hyperplasia is marked by an increased number of cells and always entails cell proliferation. **D.** Metaplasia is characterized by changes in cell morphology and acquisition of new features that are normally not present.

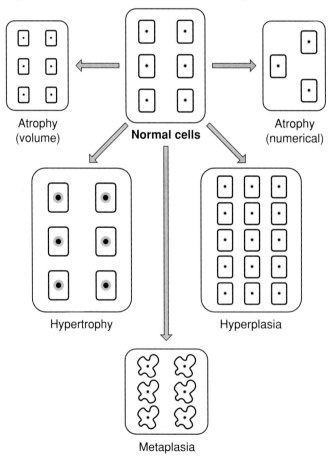

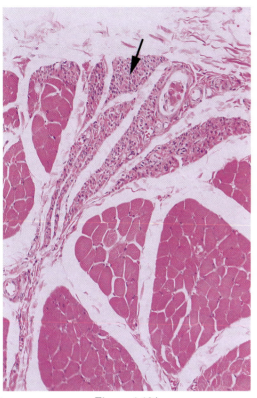

Figure 1.10A

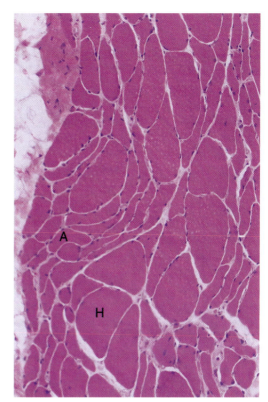

Figure 1.10B

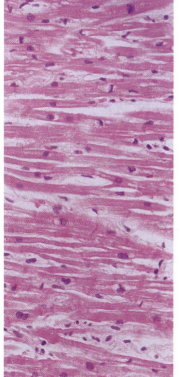

Figure 1.11

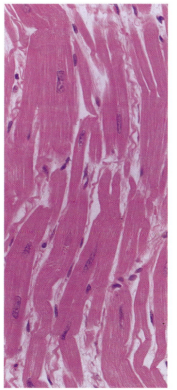

Figure 1.12A

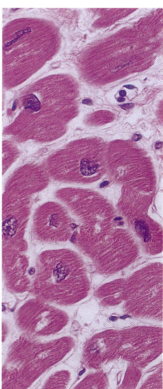

Figure 1.12B

PLATE 1.5. CELLULAR ADAPTATIONS IN THE BREAST

Figure 1.13.   Cellular adaptations in the breast. A. Normal breast from a young woman. The well developed racemose ducts are surrounded by loose intralobular connective tissue. **B.** Atrophy of the breast. With advancing age, the breast atrophies and the normal parenchyma is replaced with fibrous tissue or fat. In this slide, the atrophic ducts are surrounded by dense collagenous stroma. **C.** Lactating breast. Hormonally induced hyperplasia of the breast is marked by an increased number of ducts and acinar cells that produce milk. **D.** Apocrine metaplasia in fibrocystic disease of breast. The ducts are lined with columnar cells that resemble those in apocrine sweat glands. Normal breast does not contain apocrine cells.

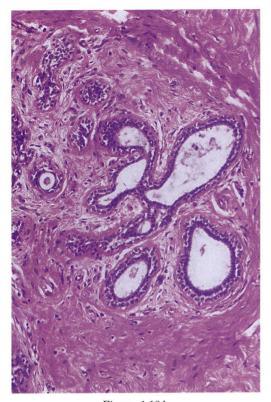

Figure 1.13A

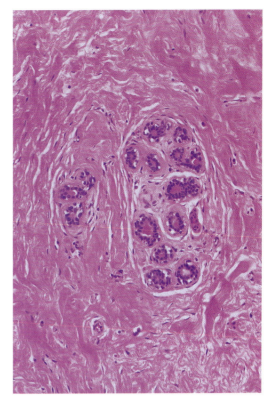

Figure 1.13B

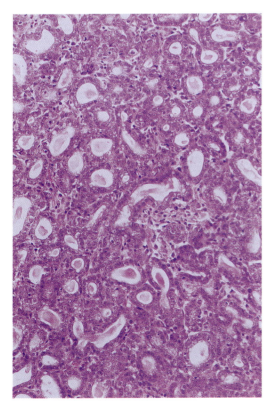

Figure 1.13C

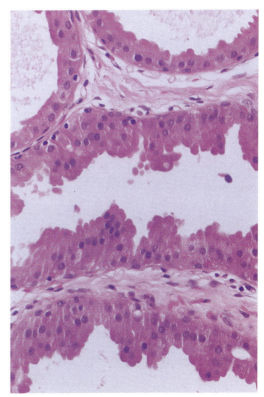

Figure 1.13D

PLATE 1.6. METAPLASIA

Figure 1.14. Chronic cervicitis. Squamous metaplasia of endocervical glands is caused by chronic inflammation. Normal glands are lined by columnar epithelium (*C*), and the foci of metaplasia appear as multilayered squamous epithelium (*arrows*).

Figure 1.16. Myositis ossificans. The striated muscle has been replaced by fibrous tissue that contains trabeculae of bone.

Figure 1.15. Intestinal metaplasia of the esophagus. In this lesion, caused by reflux of gastric juice (called Barrett esophagus), the normal squamous epithelium of the esophagus is replaced with intestinal epithelium.

Figure 1.17. Ossification in pulmonary scar. The fibrous tissue contains black pigment (carbon) and a focus of bone formation.

Diagram 1.5. Metaplasia. Examples of metaplasia include: A. Transformation of columnar into squamous epithelium. **B.** Transformation of squamous into columnar intestinal epithelium. **C.** Transformation of striated muscle into bone.

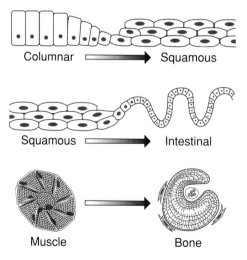

Columnar ⟶ Squamous

Squamous ⟶ Intestinal

Muscle ⟶ Bone

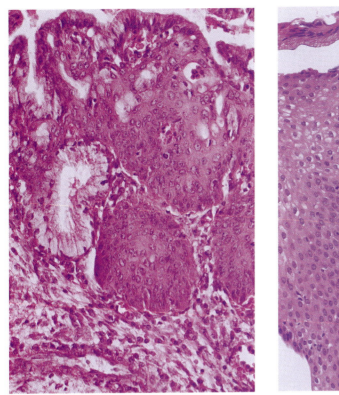

Figure 1.14

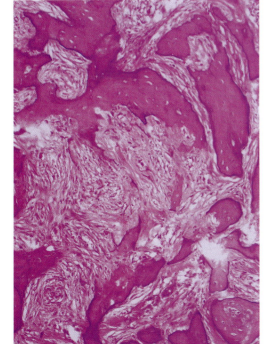

Figure 1.15

Figure 1.16

Figure 1.17

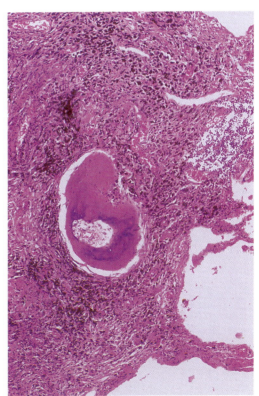

PLATE 1.7. CELL DEATH

Figure 1.18. Coagulation necrosis of the liver caused by herpesvirus infection. Viral infection causes various forms of necrosis. Nuclei that appear "washed-out" have undergone karyolysis; those that are fragmented into "nuclear dust" have undergone karyorrhexis; and those that appear condensed are pyknotic. Note the relative preservation of the eosinophilic cytoplasm. Viable liver cells infected with the virus contain eosinophilic or slightly basophilic nuclear inclusions.

Figure 1.19. Electron microscopy of necrotic cells. A. Pyknosis. The chromatin is condensed. **B.** Karyolysis. The chromatin has been dissolved and the nucleus appears washed out.

Figure 1.20. Apoptosis. Semilunar condensation of chromatin and irregularities of the nuclear membrane are accompanied by the formation of round apoptotic bodies composed of dark chromatin.

Diagram 1.6. Cell death. Cell death is characterized by typical nuclear changes or by a loss of cell integrity due to rupture of the cell membrane. **A.** Pyknosis is marked by compaction of chromatin. **B.** Karyorrhexis is marked by fragmentation of the nucleus. **C.** Karyolysis is marked by dissolution of chromatin in the nucleus. **D.** Cell membrane rupture is another sign of irreversible cell injury. **E.** Apoptosis is marked by condensation of chromatin along the nuclear membrane, which also shows blebbing.

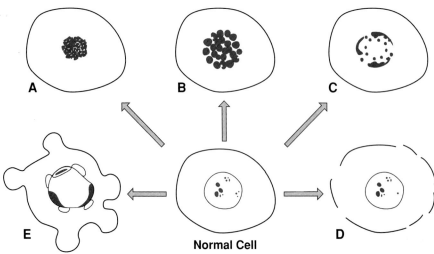

COLOR ATLAS OF HISTOPATHOLOGY

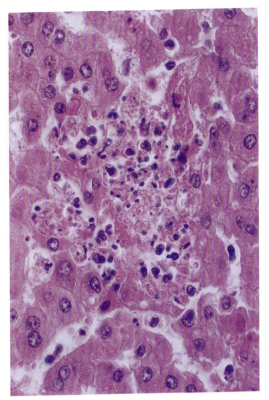

Figure 1.18

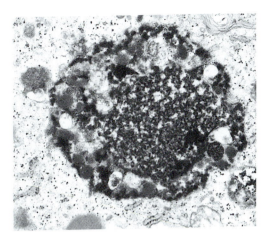

Figure 1.19A

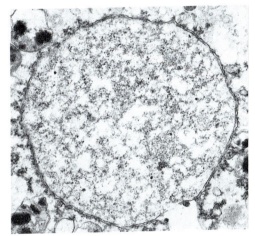

Figure 1.19B

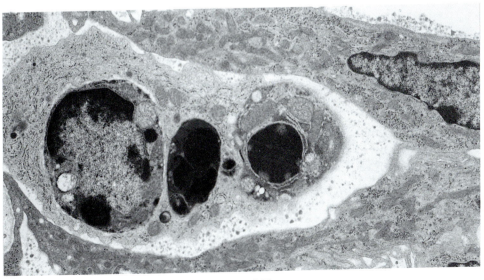

Figure 1.20

PLATE 1.8. NECROSIS

Figure 1.21. Coagulation necrosis of the kidney. The necrotic cells have no nuclei and the remaining cytoplasm is red (eosinophilic).

Figure 1.23. Fat necrosis of the pancreas. This enzymatically induced necrosis of fat tissue results in a blurring of the cell outlines. The normal fat tissue has been focally replaced by saponified homogeneous material, which has a bluish tinge imparted by calcium. An acute inflammatory reaction is seen at the margins of necrotic fat tissue and in the pancreatic parenchyma.

Figure 1.22. Liquefactive necrosis of the brain. The normal structure of the tissue is lost and the outlines of cells or their nuclei have been lost.

Figure 1.24. Caseous necrosis of tuberculosis. Granulomas of tuberculosis contain central caseous necrosis, which appears as amorphous granular material. The area of necrosis is surrounded by granuloma that contains multinucleated giant cells.

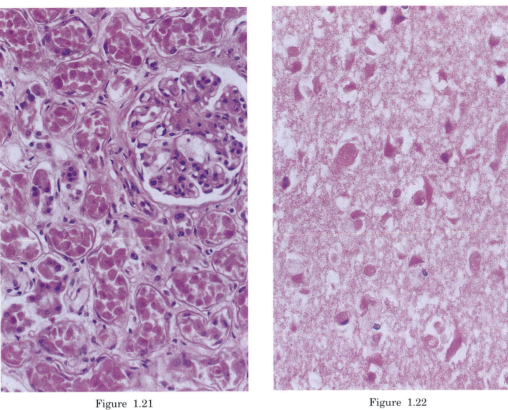

Figure 1.21

Figure 1.22

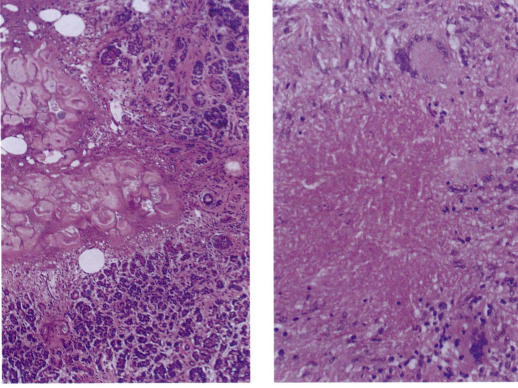

Figure 1.23

Figure 1.24

NOTES

CHAPTER 2

Inflammation and Repair

INTRODUCTION

Inflammation is a complex response of tissue to injury involving cellular, humoral, vascular, and cellular changes. **Acute inflammation** involves changes that occur within minutes and last several hours or days. Acute inflammation is a simple stereotypic response to a variety of stimuli, such as bacteria, chemicals, or allergens. It may resolve spontaneously or with treatment. **Chronic inflammation** is more variable and includes several forms of tissue reaction of longer duration. Chronic inflammation is the result of unresolved or recurrent acute inflammation, various chronic diseases, and/or persistent irritation.

Repair of damaged tissues may occur by *regeneration* or by replacement of damaged parenchymal cells with fibrous tissue. Regeneration takes place in organs composed of mitotic or facultative mitotic cells. Replacement of destroyed parenchymal cells with connective tissue cells and collagenous extracellular matrix leads to *scarring*.

INFLAMMATORY CELLS

Acute inflammation is mediated mostly by *polymorphonuclear granulocytes,* also called *neutrophils.* Chronic inflammation is dominated by *macrophages*, *lymphocytes,* and *plasma cells.* Allergic reactions also involve *basophils* and *eosinophils. Epithelioid cells* and *multinucleated giant cells,* seen in granulomas and in foreign body reactions, are derived from macrophages. Typical electron microscopic features of inflammatory cells are illustrated in Figures 2.1 to 2.5 and in Diagram 2.1.

Neutrophils account for 70% of leukocytes in circulating blood and are the most prominent cells in acute inflammation. The name "neutrophil" is derived from the "neutral" granules in their cytoplasm, which are neither acidophilic or basophilic. These granules are of two types: *azurophilic granules,* which are lysosomes; and *specific granules,* which contain alkaline phosphatase, lactoferrin, lysozyme, and collagenases. Neutrophils are also called polymorphonuclear or segmented leukocytes because their nuclei are divided into 3–5 segments (Fig. 2.1).

Eosinophils account for 2–3% of all circulating white blood cells but are more numerous in tissues. The ratio of circulating and tissue eosinophils is 1:300; hence, they are more numerous in tissues than in circulation. Eosinophils have a bilobed nucleus and abundant cytoplasm filled with granules (Fig. 2.2). These granules stain red with eosin in standard histology slides and contain characteristic crystalloids that can be seen by electron microscopy. Eosinophil granules contain various mediators of inflammation. Eosinophils are most prominent in allergic reactions and parasitic infections.

Basophils account for 1% of circulating white blood cells. Tissue basophils, called **mast cells,** are more numerous. Basophils/mast cells have a bean-shaped nucleus and well developed cytoplasm rich in specific granules. These granules can be seen only upon special staining and are not evident in routine histology slides. The granules contain histamine, heparin, and various mediators of inflammation. Basophils/mast cells have cell surface receptors for IgE that enables them to participate in atopic (type I) immune reactions, such as hay fever and bronchial asthma.

Lymphocytes account for 20–30% of circulating white blood cells. They are small cells with round nuclei, little cytoplasm, and few organelles (Fig. 2.3). Lymphocytes belong to two cell lineages and are classified as either T or B cells. Various T and B lymphocytes have the same cytological features but can be distinguished one from another functionally and cytochemically with labeled antibodies to their specific surface markers. Lymphocytes mediate immune reactions.

Macrophages are tissue cells derived

from circulating monocytes. They have bean-shaped or vesicular nuclei and abundant cytoplasm (Fig. 2.4). The cytoplasm contains lysosomes and various secretory granules. Macrophages are precursors of epithelioid cells and multinucleated giant cells in granulomas. The primary functions of macrophages are:

- Phagocytosis—in this respect they resemble neutrophils
- Antigen processing and presentation to lymphocytes
- Secretion of mediators of inflammation (e.g., prostaglandins and leukotrienes) and cytokines that regulate the function of other cells and act as growth factors (e.g., interleukin-1)

Plasma cells are found only in tissues and are not present in circulating blood. They are derived from B lymphocytes. Plasma cells have a round, excentrically located nucleus and abundant cytoplasm. The cytoplasm is rich in rough endoplasmic reticulum (Fig. 2.5). Plasma cells secrete antibodies. They participate in chronic inflammation and various immune reactions.

ACUTE INFLAMMATION

Acute inflammation evolves through several phases, which include both vascular and cellular events (Diagram 2.2). Major **mediators** of vascular and cellular events of acute inflammation are: *vasoactive amines* (e.g., histamine), *kinins* (e.g., bradykinin), *complement proteins*, and *arachidonic acid derivatives* (e.g., prostaglandins, leukotrienes)

Vascular events of acute inflammation include: neurogenic vasodilatation of the precapillary sphincter in arterioles resulting in active hyperemia and increased permeability of the venules and capillaries, resulting in transudation and exudation.

Cellular events include: margination of leukocytes in the circulating blood, adhesion of leukocytes to the endothelium ("pavementing"), emigration of leukocytes across the blood vessel wall into the tissue spaces, and active migration toward the source of chemotactic stimuli, which attract the inflammatory cells toward the causative agent.

Acute inflammation is dominated by edema and exudation of neutrophils (Fig. 2.6). Accumulation of neutrophils results in formation of a yellow viscid fluid known as **pus**. Histologically, pus consists of neutrophils, many of which have died or are in the process of disintegrating. Pus may accumulate in the tissue (Fig. 2.7) or inside the lumen of organs (Fig. 2.8). Severe acute inflammation is characterized by a mixture of pus and fibrin and is called fibrinopurulent inflammation (Fig. 2.9).

CHRONIC INFLAMMATION

Chronic inflammation may present in three histological forms: as mononuclear cell infiltrates that may be diffuse or focal, as granulation tissue, or as granulomas (Diagram 2.3). These reaction patterns are often interrelated and may coexist.

Infiltrates of chronic inflammation are composed of lymphocytes, plasma cells, and macrophages in various proportions (Fig. 2.10). Persistent tissue damage is repaired continuously by fibroblasts and related connective tissue cells (Fig. 2.11). Eosinophils may be prominent in inflammation caused by parasites (Fig. 2.12). Retained foreign bodies elicit a giant cell reaction (Fig. 2.13).

Chronic inflammation occurs under several circumstances. For example, chronic inflammation may result from poor resolution of an acute infection or from recurrent acute infections as in *chronic pelvic inflammatory disease* (PID). PID most often involves the fallopian tubes, which become diffusely infiltrated with plasma cells and lymphocytes (Fig. 2.14).

Cell-mediated immune reactions to transplanted organs also present histologically as chronic inflammation (Fig. 2.15).

Persistence of the causative organism or infection with viruses that are intracellular or pathogens that cannot be eradicated, such as *Mycobacterium tuberculosis* and *Treponema pallidum* (Fig. 2.16), also results in chronic inflammation. Tuberculosis is characterized by the formation of granulomas. Such granulomas are composed of macrophages, epithelioid cells, multinucleated giant cells, and lymphocytes (Diagram 2.3). In the central area, granulomas of tuberculosis undergo caseous necrosis.

Chronic diseases of unknown etiology such as *sarcoidosis* may also produce granulomas (Fig. 2.17). In contrast to tuberculosis, these granulomas are noncaseating.

HISTOLOGICAL FEATURES OF MACROSCOPICALLY DISTINCT FORMS OF INFLAMMATION

Several forms of inflammation can be recognized with the naked eye. The histological features of common morphologically distinct forms of inflammation are shown in Figures 2.18 to 2.21.

Serous inflammation is marked by extravasation of protein-rich fluid containing sparse cells. Most acute inflammations begin in serous form. However, serous inflammation may also be a unique manifestation of tissue injury that heals on its own, as in skin burns (Fig. 2.18).

Fibrinous inflammation is marked by exudation of fibrinogen-rich plasma. Fibrinogen is a high-molecular-weight plasma protein, and its exudation indicates increased vascular permeability, usually due to disruption of the vessel wall. Fibrinogen polymerizes into fibrin upon exudation from the blood vessel. Fibrinous pericarditis is an example of fibrinous inflammation (Fig. 2.19).

Purulent inflammation is marked by exudation of neutrophils and formation of pus. Pus is a yellow, viscous fluid that contains polymorphonuclear leukocytes in various stages of disintegration as well as tissue debris from the liquefactive necrosis of tissue. An **abscess** is a typical example of a localized purulent inflammation (Fig. 2.20).

Pseudomembranous inflammation is a form of fibrinopurulent inflammation of mucosal surfaces, in which the exudate is intermixed with necrotic tissue and mucus or other contents of that organ (e.g., fecal material in the large intestine). Pseudomembranous colitis is an example of pseudomembranous inflammation (Fig. 2.21).

HEALING AND REPAIR

The outcome of inflammation depends on the type, extent, and duration of the injury; the body's response to injury; and the ability of the tissue to heal.

Three major forms of healing of inflammation are:

- **Resolution** with complete restoration of normal structure and function. Resolution is typical of mild infections without tissue destruction.
- **Regeneration** of destroyed cells from remaining cells that are capable of replication.
- **Repair by scarring** in tissues that are composed of postmitotic cells unable to regenerate or extensive loss of tissue that cannot be repaired by other means.

Granulation tissue is the hallmark of repair by connective tissue (Diagram 2.4). It occurs in all wounds, during the repair of bone fractures, and in many forms of chronic inflammation such as ulcers.

Granulation tissue consists primarily of a connective tissue network and sprouts of new blood vessels. The composition of granulation tissues varies over time (Figs. 2.22 and 2.23). Initially, granulation tissue is infiltrated with scavenger cells engaged in removing the damaged and dead cells. After the debris is cleared, granulation tissue is predominantly composed of fibroblasts and myofibroblasts. The later stages are characterized by scarring, i.e., deposition of extracellular matrix (Fig. 2.24). As healing continues, the scar tissue becomes less cellular and more collagenous (Fig. 2.25).

PLATE 2.1. INFLAMMATORY CELLS—ELECTRON MICROSCOPY

Figure 2.1. Neutrophil or polymorphonuclear leukocyte. This cell has a trilobed, segmented nucleus and numerous cytoplasmic granules.

Figure 2.2. Eosinophil. This cell has a bilobed nucleus and crystalloid-containing cytoplasmic granules.

Figure 2.3. Lymphocyte. The round nucleus contains prominent clumped heterochromatin. The cytoplasm is scant and contains only free ribosomes.

Figure 2.4. Macrophage. The bean-shaped nucleus and well developed cytoplasm that contains numerous absorptive vacuoles and prominent dark lysosomes.

Figure 2.5. Plasma cell. The round nucleus with heterochromatin is condensed along the nuclear membrane. A well developed cytoplasm is rich in rough endoplasmic reticulum.

Diagram 2.1. Inflammatory cells.

Polymorphonuclear leukocyte
- Segmented nucleus
- Primary granules
- Secondary granules

Eosinophil
- Bilobed nucleus
- Nucleolus
- Granules with crystalloids

Mast cell (basophil)
- Nucleus
- Inhomogeneous granules of irregular shape

Lymphocyte
- Nucleus
- Free ribosomes

Macrophage
- Mitochondria
- Lysosomes
- Nucleus
- Absorptive and phagocytic vacuoles

Plasma cell
- Nucleus
- Rough endoplasm reticulum
- Mitochondria

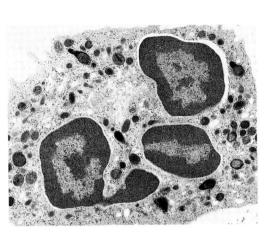

Figure 2.1

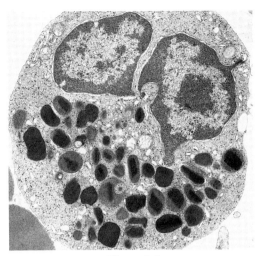

Figure 2.2

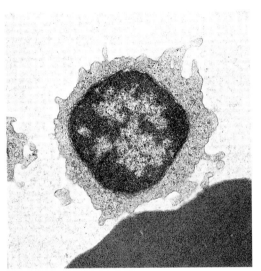

Figure 2.3

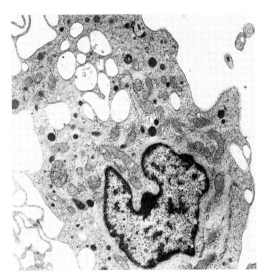

Figure 2.4

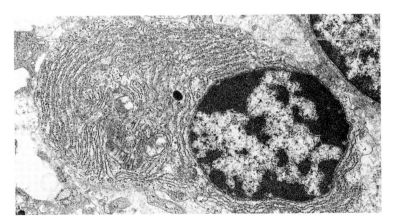

Figure 2.5

PLATE 2.2. ACUTE INFLAMMATION

Figure 2.6. Acute salpingitis. The mucosal folds of the fallopian tube are edematous and infiltrated with neutrophils. Some protein-rich edema fluid is seen in the lumen.

Figure 2.7. Pustule of the skin. The epidermis is separated from the dermis, and the newly formed space is filled with inflammatory cells, most of which are neutrophils.

Figure 2.8. Purulent inflammation. The infiltrate consists predominantly of neutrophils.

Figure 2.9. Fibrinopurulent and hemorrhagic inflammation. This exudate contains neutrophils, blood (bright red), and fibrin (dull red).

Diagram 2.2. Schematic presentation of acute inflammation. A. Increased permeability of the vessel is accompanied by transudation of fluid through the intercellular gaps and the cytoplasm of endothelial cells. **B.** The polymorphonuclear leukocytes that are normally mixed with the red blood cells in the circulating blood attach to the endothelium (pavementing). **C.** The leukocytes emigrate through the intercellular gaps between the endothelial cells and continue to migrate toward the chemotactic stimuli in the interstitial space. **D.** Severe injury causes necrosis of endothelial cells. These defects allow unimpeded passage of intravascular fluid and white and red blood cells into the interstitial spaces.

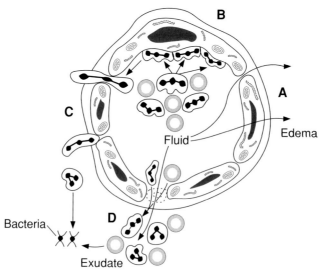

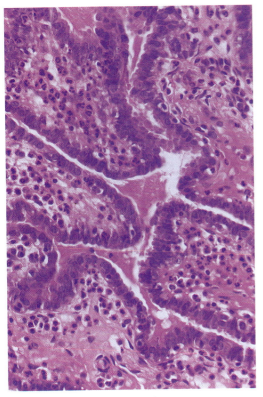

Figure 2.6

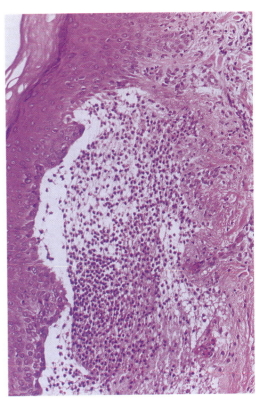

Figure 2.7

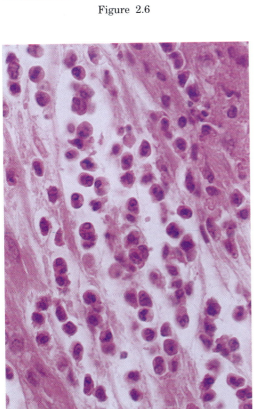

Figure 2.8

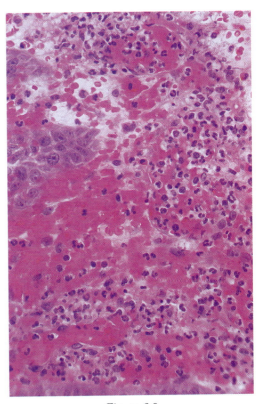

Figure 2.9

PLATE 2.3. CHRONIC INFLAMMATION

Figure 2.10.   Chronic inflammation. A. The parotid gland contains infiltrates of mononuclear cells and shows a loss of glandular tissue. **B.** Most of the cells are lymphocytes, plasma cells, and macrophages.

Figure 2.11.   Chronic inflammation and fibrosis. In addition to lymphocytes (L), plasma cells (P), and macrophages (M), there are prominent fibroblasts (F) surrounded by fibrous extracellular matrix (Ex).

Figure 2.12.   Reaction to parasites. A. This chronic inflammation is evoked by filaria. The parasite can be seen in the middle of the field. **B.** The tissue around the parasite contains chronic inflammatory cells and numerous eosinophils.

Figure 2.13.   Foreign body giant cell reaction. The giant cell is multinucleated and contains a large phagocytic vacuole filled with some unidentified foreign material.

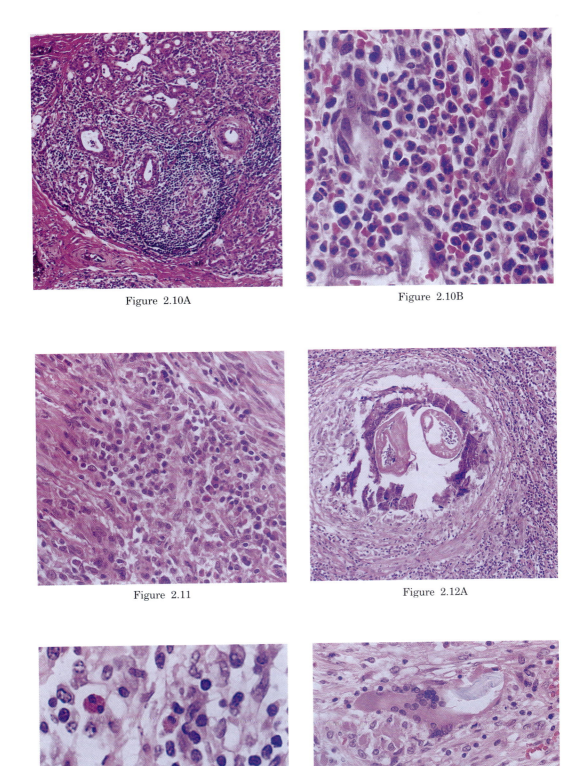

Figure 2.10A

Figure 2.10B

Figure 2.11

Figure 2.12A

Figure 2.12B

Figure 2.13

PLATE 2.4. CHRONIC INFLAMMATION

Figure 2.14. Chronic salpingitis. The wall of the fallopian tube is densely infiltrated with lymphocytes, macrophages, and plasma cells. There are, however, also neutrophils accounting for the suppurative nature of this disease.

Figure 2.16. Tuberculosis of the lung. An early lesion devoid of caseous necrosis. Even so, it is marked by an infiltrate of epithelioid cells, multinucleated giant cells, and lymphocytes.

Figure 2.15. Renal transplant rejection. Kidney transplant from an unrelated donor elicits an immune reaction including both B and T lymphocytes. Plasma cells and lymphocytes infiltrate the interstitial spaces of the graft and actively destroy nephrons.

Figure 2.17. Sarcoidosis. The tissue is infiltrated with epithelioid cells that form a granuloma.

Diagram 2.3. Granuloma. Several forms of granulomas are recognized, but all of them have the same basic features. Typically, granulomas consist of macrophages (transformed into so-called epithelioid cells and multinucleated giant cells) and lymphocytes, which are more prominent at the periphery. **Left.** Sarcoidosis is characterized by noncaseating granulomas. **Middle.** Granulomas of tuberculosis and fungal infections contain central necrosis. **Right.** Foreign body granulomas contain multinucleated foreign body giant cells, which have foreign particles in their cytoplasm.

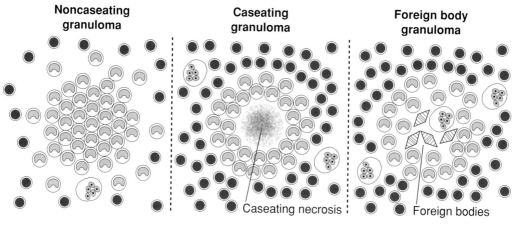

Noncaseating granuloma · Caseating granuloma · Foreign body granuloma

Caseating necrosis · Foreign bodies

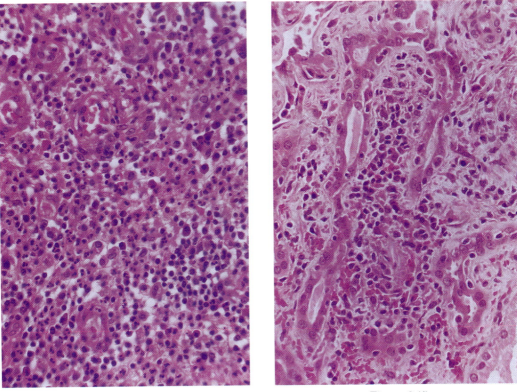

Figure 2.14 Figure 2.15

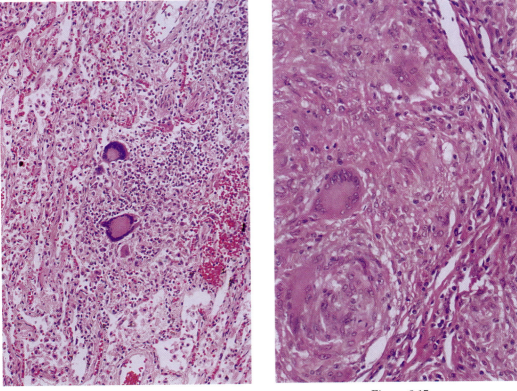

Figure 2.16 Figure 2.17

PLATE 2.5. HISTOLOGICAL FEATURES OF VARIOUS MACROSCOPICALLY DISTINCT FORMS OF INFLAMMATION

Figure 2.18.   Blister due to burns. This serous inflammation is marked by transudation of serous fluid into the skin between the cells of the skin. This transudation results in the cleavage of cell layers of the epidermis or the separation of epidermis from dermis.

Figure 2.20.   Abscess. An abscess is a localized purulent inflammation. The center of the abscess contains pus composed of dead and dying polymorphonuclear leukocytes and destroyed tissue. Histologically, pus is composed of pyknotic and karyorrhectic leukocytic nuclei ("nuclear dust"). The normal tissue architecture has been lost.

Figure 2.19.   Fibrinous pericarditis. The epicardium is covered with an exudate composed predominantly of fibrin (*F*), scattered inflammatory cells, and newly formed blood vessels that have grown into the exudate in an attempt to organize it.

Figure 2.21.   Pseudomembranous colitis. The pseudomembrane (*P*) consists of remnants of the necrotic intestinal epithelium and mucus intermixed with fibrin and inflammatory cells

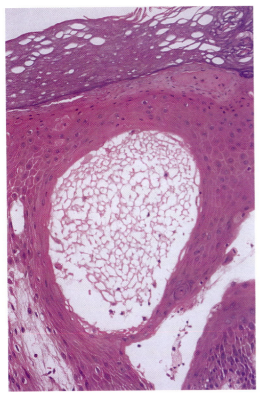

Figure 2.18

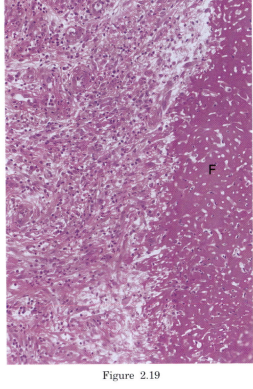

Figure 2.19

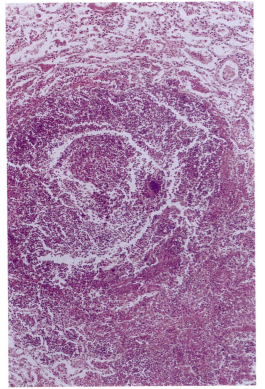

Figure 2.20

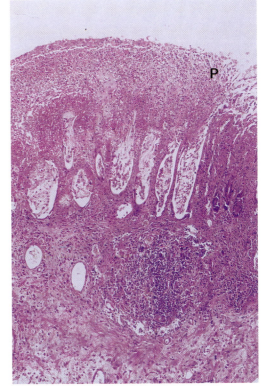

Figure 2.21

PLATE 2.6.   REPAIR AND HEALING

Figure 2.22.   Vascular granulation tissue. In early stages of repair, granulation tissue is highly vascular and consists predominantly of small blood vessels lined by angioblasts, scattered fibroblasts, lymphocytes, and macrophages.

Figure 2.24.   Scarring. Repair is characterized by proliferation of fibroblasts and deposition of collagen.

Figure 2.23.   Granulation tissue composed predominantly of myofibroblasts. Myofibroblasts are elongated cells with hybrid features of fibroblasts and smooth muscle cells.

Figure 2.25.   Scar. Older scars are composed predominantly of interstitial connective tissue matrix and sparse fibroblasts and blood vessels.

Diagram 2.4.   Granulation tissue. Left. Early granulation tissue contains many scavenger cells, extravasated blood, and tissue debris. **Middle.** Granulation tissue in the stage of healing consists of newly formed blood vessels, fibroblasts, and myofibroblasts. **Right.** Scarring is the ultimate result of granulation tissue. Scarring is relatively cellular and consists predominantly of collagenous connective tissue.

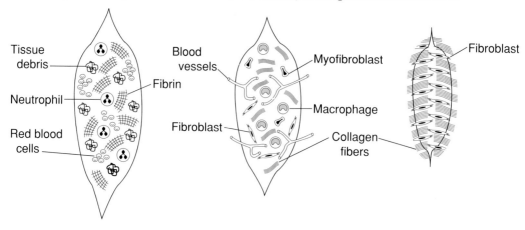

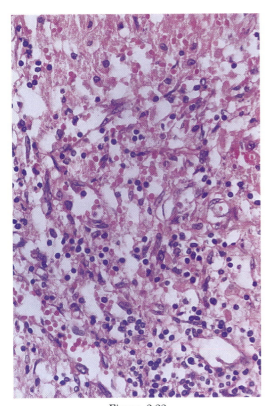

Figure 2.22

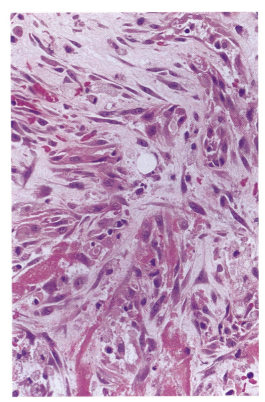

Figure 2.23

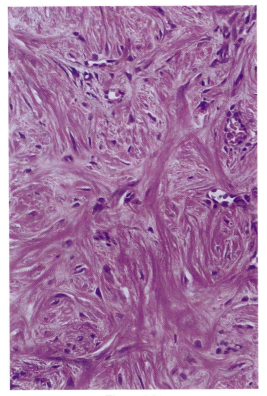

Figure 2.24

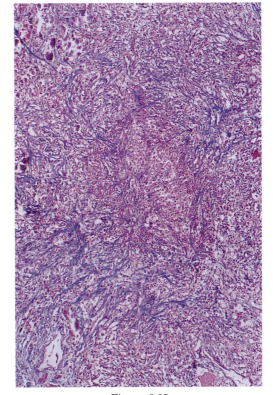

Figure 2.25

NOTES

CHAPTER 3

Circulatory Disturbances

INTRODUCTION

Disturbances in the circulation of blood, lymph, and extravascular intercellular fluids occur in many systemic diseases. They may be also a consequence of dysfunction of a single organ, such as the heart or lungs.

Circulatory disturbances may be generalized or localized to an anatomical region (Diagram 3.1). The main causes of circulatory disturbances are:

- **Heart failure,** due to damage of the myocardium (pump failure) or obstruction of blood flow by valvular disease.
- **Vascular changes**, both functional and anatomic, involving any part or the arterial, capillary or venous circulation. Vascular changes include: constrictions caused by vascular spasm, dilatations of vascular lumen; obstructions of vessel, abnormal arteriovenous communications (A-V anastomosis), rupture of vessel wall, and increased vascular permeability.
- **Blood disturbances**, such as changes in the volume, composition, viscosity, or coagulability of blood.
- **Multisystemic organ failure**, as in shock or sepsis.

EDEMA

Edema is excessive accumulation of fluids inside cells, in extracellular interstitial spaces, or in body cavities. It may be localized to an anatomical region or generalized (*anasarca*). The various clinical forms of edema are shown in Diagram 3.2. The various clinical forms of edema are shown in Diagram 3.2.

Edema is pathogenetically classified into three groups:

- Hydrostatic edema (as in pulmonary edema in left-sided heart failure) or pedal edema in right-sided heart failure
- *Oncotic edema* due to hypoproteinemia caused by proteinuria (as in nephrotic syndrome) or inadequate protein synthesis (as in chronic liver disease)

Diagram 3.1.   Circulatory disturbances. Heart failure and brain pathogenetic mechanisms include vascular changes, blood disturbances, and multisystemic organ failure (shock).

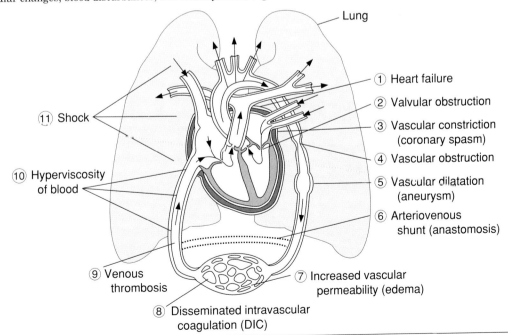

Lung

1 Heart failure
2 Valvular obstruction
3 Vascular constriction (coronary spasm)
4 Vascular obstruction
5 Vascular dilatation (aneurysm)
6 Arteriovenous shunt (anastomosis)
7 Increased vascular permeability (edema)
8 Disseminated intravascular coagulation (DIC)
9 Venous thrombosis
10 Hyperviscosity of blood
11 Shock

- *Edema related to increased vascular permeability* (as in the early stages of inflammation or in toxic shock)

Typical pathological changes caused by edema in various organs and body parts are best appreciated by the naked eye. Histological features of edema vary and depend on the organ involved and the protein content of edema fluid. *Transudates,* which have low protein content and do not contain cells, may not be visible histologically, but are recognized by the widening of intercellular spaces or the lumina of organs (e.g., alveolar spaces of the lung). *Exudates* contain more protein and inflammatory cells. The protein-rich extracellular fluid is eosinophilic. Examples of edema are shown in Figures 3.1 to 3.4.

HEMORRHAGE

Hemorrhage is the escape of blood from the blood vessels or heart. The major clinically important forms of hemorrhage are presented schematically in Diagram 3.3. Hemorrhages are classified by site of origin as:

- **Cardiac,** as following a penetrating heart wound
- **Arterial,** due to trauma and rupture of a dissecting aneurysm
- **Capillary,** which is usually due to trauma, inherent vessel wall weakness, or a coagulation defect
- **Venous,** which is usually caused by trauma or surgical operations

Small mucosal or dermal hemorrhage is called **petechia** (Fig. 3.5) if smaller than 1 mm in diameter, **purpura** if 1 mm to 1 cm in diameter, and **ecchymoses** in cases of confluent hemorrhage larger than 1 cm. **Hematoma** is a grossly visible localized collection of blood in tissue (Fig. 3.6). Hemorrhage can also occur into preexisting tissue spaces. For example, pulmonary hemorrhage into the alveoli, which are filled with blood, may occur (Fig. 3.7). In hematuria caused by glomerular diseases, blood enters the urinary space of the glomerulus, from which it passes into the tubules (Fig. 3.8) and urine.

HYPEREMIA AND CONGESTION

Hyperemia is marked by increased amounts of blood in the blood vessels. **Active hyperemia**, which entails dilatation of arteries and arterioles, typically occurs in inflammation, but may be caused by neurogenic stimuli (e.g., blushing), hyperactivity (e.g., exercise), or heat (e.g., sunbathing).

Histologically, the blood vessels appear dilated and filled with blood (Fig. 3.9). It is usually temporary and reversible; there is usually no extravasation of blood. Prolonged hyperemia caused by inflammation may cause diapedesis of red blood cells into interstitial tissues.

Passive hyperemia, or congestion, may be *acute or chronic.* It usually reflects some disturbance of venous outflow.

Congestive heart failure dominated by right ventricular failure leads to congestion of the liver, which may be acute (Figs. 3.10 and 3.11) or chronic (*nutmeg liver*) (Fig. 3.7).

Left ventricular heart failure causes chronic passive congestion of the lungs (Fig. 3.12). Hemoglobin from intra-alveolar blood is transformed into *hemosiderin,* which is then phagocytized by macrophages. These macrophages are known as *heart failure cells*. Hemosiderin contains ferric iron, which can be histochemically detected by the Prussian blue reaction.

THROMBOSIS

Thrombosis is the formation of *thrombi,* i.e., blood clots, inside the blood vessels or heart of a living organism. Three principal causes of thrombosis known as the *Virchow triad* are: Endothelial injury, circulatory disturbances, and the hypercoagulability of the blood.

The pathogenesis of thrombosis and the secondary changes that occur in the formed thrombus and lead to its dissolution or restructuring are shown in Diagram 3.4.

Histologically, thrombi consist of clotted blood, i.e., red blood cells, white blood cells, and platelets, enmeshed in strands of fibrin (Fig. 3.13A). The fibrin strands may be distinct from the cellular elements, forming the so-called *lines of Zahn* (Fig. 3.13B). Thrombi elicit a response in the vessel wall composed of the angioblasts and fibroblasts, which grow into the thrombus. This process is called *organization of the thrombus* because the ingrown cells "*organize*" the thrombus into granulation tissue (Fig. 3.14). Organized thrombi are anchored to the vessel wall with granulation tissue. Blood vessels in the granulation tissue fuse into larger channels that cross the thrombus so that the blood may flow again through the vessel. The reestablishment of the vascular lumen through the occluding thrombus is called *recanalization of the thrombus* (Fig. 3.15).

EMBOLISM

Embolism denotes vascular occlusion by a mass or any particulate intravascular material transferred from one place to another by the blood stream.

Thromboemboli. These emboli are formed from thrombi. According to the route of embolization, they can be classified as *venous* if carried by venous blood, *arterial* if carried through arteries, or *paradoxical* if they cross from the venous circulation into the arterial, as through a cardiac septal defect. Venous thromboemboli most often lodge in the lungs (Fig. 3.16). Arterial emboli localize in many organs (e.g., brain or kidney) and major body parts (e.g., the foot).

Fat emboli. These emboli originate from fat that has entered into circulation. Fat particles reach venous blood typically after a fracture of long bones. Small fat particles may occlude lung vessels, but are usually filtered through the lungs and thus reach system arterial circulation. The most important lesions induced by fat emboli are in the brain, where they cause microscopic infarcts and hemorrhages (Fig. 3.17).

Amniotic fluid emboli. Entry of amniotic fluid into the venous circulation during birth is associated with embolization of lung vessels with fetal squames, lanugo hair, and vernix as well as other particular material from the amniotic fluid. The foreign material in the circulation triggers disseminated intravascular coagulation (DIC) and formation of numerous small microthrombi (Fig. 3.18).

Cholesterol emboli. Cholesterol crystals from atherosclerotic plaques of the aorta may occlude peripheral arteries (Fig. 3.19).

Bone marrow emboli. These emboli are composed of hematopoietic and fat cells that are normally found in the bone marrow. Most bone marrow emboli are of no clinical significance because they occur in terminally ill patients in whom they are a consequence of rib fractures sustained during cardiopulmonary resuscitation.

INFARCTS

An **infarct** is a localized area of necrosis due to the interruption of the blood supply. In most instances, infarcts are caused by thrombi or emboli. Infarcts may be *anemic (white)* or *hemorrhagic (red)*.

Anemic infarcts usually occur in solid tissue that has a terminal arterial supply and no collaterals. Typically, such infarcts occur in the heart, the kidneys, or the spleen (Figs. 3.20 and 3.21).

Hemorrhagic infarcts occur upon venous occlusion and in organs that have a dual (functional and nutritional) blood supply, such as the lung and liver (Fig. 3.22). In the brain or intestines—organs with extensive collateral circulation and well developed arterial anastomoses between major arteries—white infarcts become hemorrhagic when blood from the anastomoses reaches the necrotic area (Fig. 3.23).

SHOCK

Shock is defined as multiorgan failure characterized by a disproportion between the volume of blood in circulation and the vascular space. It leads to hypoperfusion of tissues and widespread cellular dysfunction (Diagram 3.5). Pathogenetically, shock can be classified as *cardiogenic, hypovolemic* (reduced blood volume), or *hypotonic* (loss of tonus of blood vessels with pooling of blood in dilated vessels). However, all forms of shock show the same nonspecific histological features.

Most organs show signs of hypoxia during shock. The brain shows signs of *cellular hypoxia* most prominently in the hippocampus and cerebellum (Fig. 3.24). Kidneys show acute *tubular necrosis* (Fig. 3.25). "Shock lung," a typical feature of adult respiratory distress syndrome (*ARDS*) that develops in shock, is characterized by an increased permeability of alveolar capillaries, edema and formation of intra-alveolar hyaline membranes (Fig. 3.26). DIC with widespread capillary microthrombi and mucosal hemorrhages (Fig. 3.27) develops in almost all patients dying in shock.

PLATE 3.1. EDEMA

Figure 3.1. Hydrostatic pulmonary edema caused by left ventricular heart failure. The alveoli contain eosinophilic proteinaceous fluid.

Figure 3.3. Edema of the brain in encephalitis. The perivascular spaces (Virchow-Robin spaces) are widened and contain edema fluid. Since this edema fluid contains little protein, it cannot be seen in routine histology slides. A few inflammatory cells responding to viral infection are seen around the larger vessel.

Figure 3.2. Inflammatory pulmonary edema. The fluid is rich in protein, which accounts for the eosinophilic staining of alveolar content and scattered inflammatory cells.

Figure 3.4. Edema of the skin caused by sun exposure. The epidermal cells appear separated one from another because the intercellular spaces are filled with fluid. The fluid cannot be seen because most of it has leaked out during tissue processing, and the remaining transudate contains little stainable protein.

Diagram 3.2. Clinically important forms of edema.

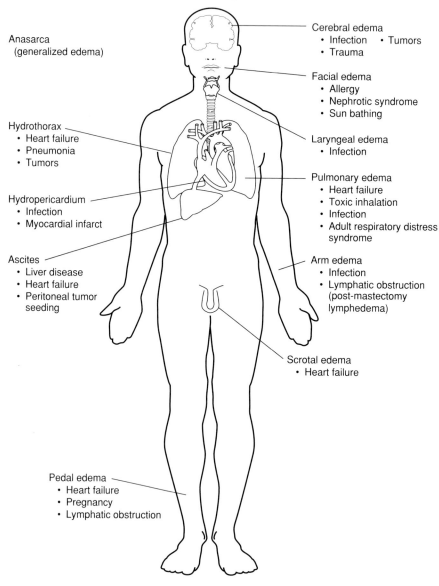

Anasarca
(generalized edema)

Hydrothorax
• Heart failure
• Pneumonia
• Tumors

Hydropericardium
• Infection
• Myocardial infarct

Ascites
• Liver disease
• Heart failure
• Peritoneal tumor
  seeding

Pedal edema
• Heart failure
• Pregnancy
• Lymphatic obstruction

Cerebral edema
• Infection   • Tumors
• Trauma

Facial edema
• Allergy
• Nephrotic syndrome
• Sun bathing

Laryngeal edema
• Infection

Pulmonary edema
• Heart failure
• Toxic inhalation
• Infection
• Adult respiratory distress
  syndrome

Arm edema
• Infection
• Lymphatic obstruction
  (post-mastectomy
  lymphedema)

Scrotal edema
• Heart failure

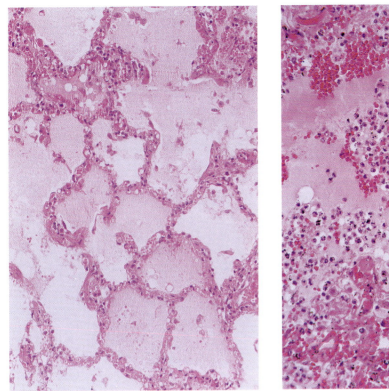

Figure 3.1

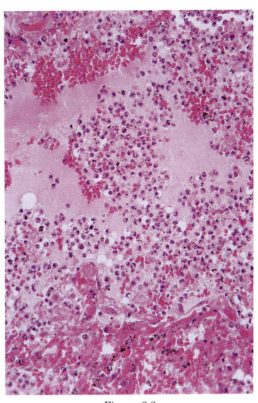

Figure 3.2

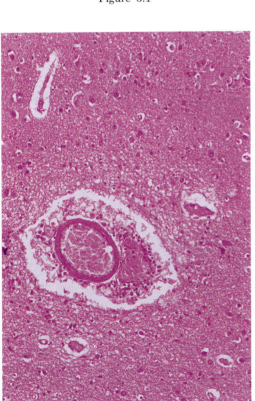

Figure 3.3

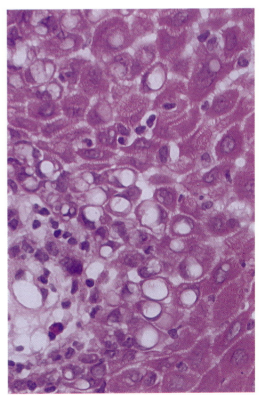

Figure 3.4

PLATE 3.2. HEMORRHAGE

Figure 3.5.   Petechia of the skin. Extravasated blood is found in the dermis.

Figure 3.7.   Pulmonary hemorrhage. Alveoli are filled with extravasated blood. Some blood may be seen in the subpleural interstitial tissue as well.

Figure 3.6.   Hematoma. The extravasated blood has obliterated the normal tissue architecture.

Figure 3.8.   Glomerular hematuria. Red blood cell casts are seen in the lumen of the renal tubules.

Diagram 3.3.   Major clinically important forms of hemorrhage.

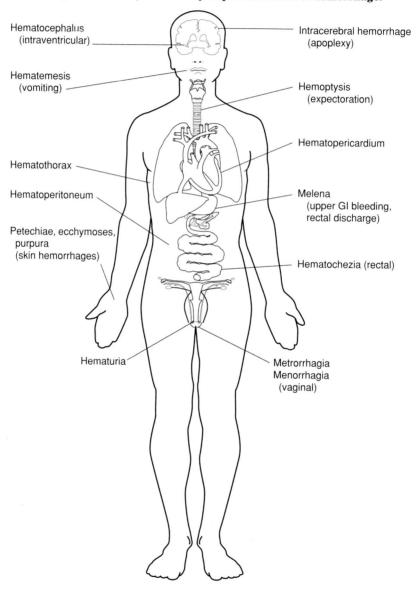

Hematocephalus (intraventricular)

Hematemesis (vomiting)

Hematothorax

Hematoperitoneum

Petechiae, ecchymoses, purpura (skin hemorrhages)

Hematuria

Intracerebral hemorrhage (apoplexy)

Hemoptysis (expectoration)

Hematopericardium

Melena (upper GI bleeding, rectal discharge)

Hematochezia (rectal)

Metrorrhagia Menorrhagia (vaginal)

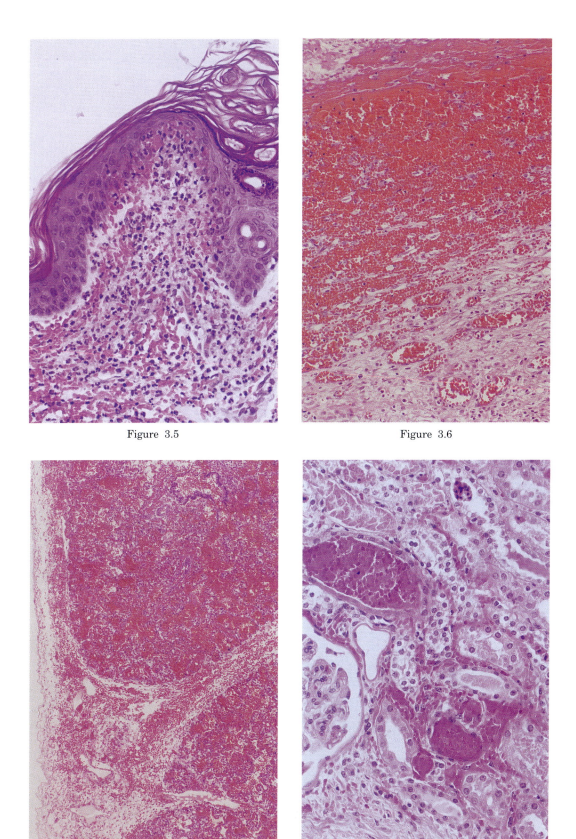

Figure 3.5

Figure 3.6

Figure 3.7

Figure 3.8

PLATE 3.3. HYPEREMIA AND CONGESTION

Figure 3.9. **Active hyperemia of the skin.** All blood vessels appear filled with blood.

Figure 3.10. **Congestion of the liver.** In the centrolobular areas, the sinusoids are dilated and engorged with blood.

Figure 3.11. **Chronic passive congestion of liver.** Centrolobular zones appear collapsed and consist of fibrous tissue that has replaced the liver cells. The central veins appear dilated and contain blood.

Figure 3.12. **Chronic passive congestion of the lung. A.** Alveolar septa are thickened, and the alveoli contain macrophages laden with hemosiderin granules. These are known as *"heart failure cells."* **B.** Heart failure cells stain blue with the Prussian blue reaction that reduce the ferric iron in hemosiderin to a bluish pigment. **C.** Expectorated heart failure cells can be found in sputum. This cytological smear shows brown discoloration of cytoplasm of pulmonary macrophages (heart failure cells)

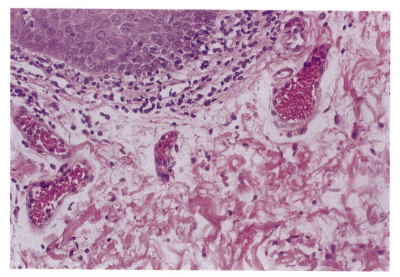

Figure 3.9

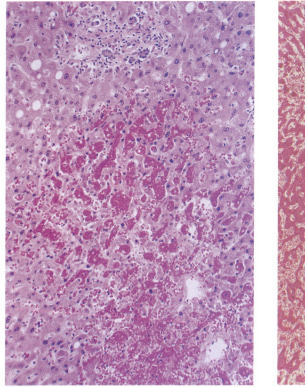

Figure 3.10

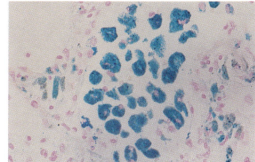

Figure 3.11

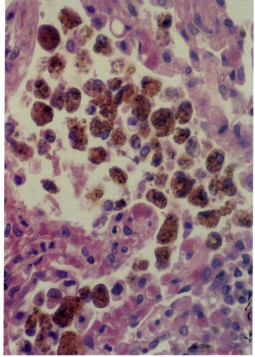

Figure 3.12A

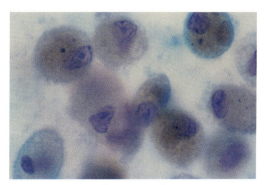

Figure 3.12B

Figure 3.12C

PLATE 3.4. THROMBOSIS

Figure 3.13.   Thrombosis. A. The larger vessel contains a thrombus of variegated appearance composed of layers of red blood cells, white blood cells, and fibrin. The empty spaces in the thrombus in the smaller vessel are newly formed vascular channels indicating that the thrombus is recanalized. **B.** The thrombus is seen to consist of layers of fibrin and red blood cells corresponding to the lines of Zahn, which are visible to the naked eye.

Figure 3.14.   Organizing thrombus. Strands of fibrin within the granulation tissue, which is composed predominantly of angioblasts and fibroblasts.

Figure 3.15.   Recanalized thrombus. The thrombus occluding the wall of the artery has been recanalized by newly formed smaller blood vessels.

Diagram 3.4.   Thrombosis. A. Endothelial injury exposes collagen in vessel wall to circulating blood. **B.** Turbulent blood flow facilitates adhesion of platelets. **C.** Fibrin is deposited and thrombus is formed. **D.** Thrombus is organized. **E.** Thrombus is remodeled (or organized). **F.** Thrombus is recanalized. **G.** Thrombus forms a tail through orthograde retrograde propagation. **H.** Thrombus gives rise to emboli. **I.** Bacteria invade the thrombus and infect it.

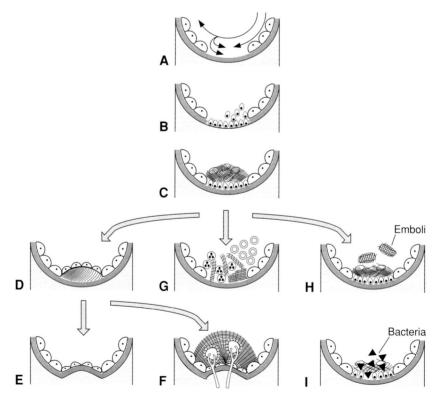

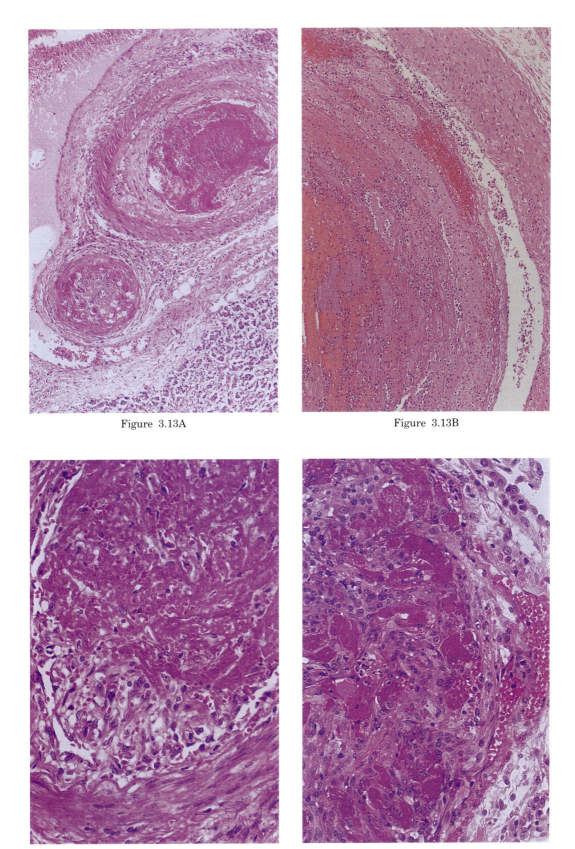

Figure 3.13A

Figure 3.13B

Figure 3.14

Figure 3.15

PLATE 3.5. EMBOLISM

Figure 3.16.   Pulmonary embolus. This pulmonary artery branch is occluded with a thromboembolus (T). Attached to this thromboembolus is a bone marrow embolus (*BM*), composed of hematopoietic cells and fat cells, i.e., the normal components of the bone marrow. This secondary embolus probably was superimposed on the first thromboembolus and resulted from ribs broken during terminal cardiopulmonary resuscitation. The lower part of the pulmonary artery contains blood, indicating that the occlusion of the blood vessel was not complete.

Figure 3.18.   Disseminated intravascular coagulation (DIC). A. Glomerular capillaries are occluded with fibrin thrombi. **B.** Small cardiac vessels contain thrombi that appear red because they are composed of fibrin and platelets.

Figure 3.17.   Fat embolism of the brain. A. The brain capillary is filled with fat, stained orange-red. The pericapillary space is filled with blood. This slide was from a frozen section. Because processing of tissues for paraffin embedding dissolves the fat, it would not have been visible in routinely prepared histologic slides. **B.** Occlusion of small cerebral vessels results in subsequent multiple small perivascular hemorrhages.

Figure 3.19.   Cholesterol emboli. The blood vessel is occluded with cholesterol crystals. Cholesterol crystals are dissolved in alcohol and xylene during tissue processing and slide preparation. Thus, only empty clefts previously occupied by these crystals remain.

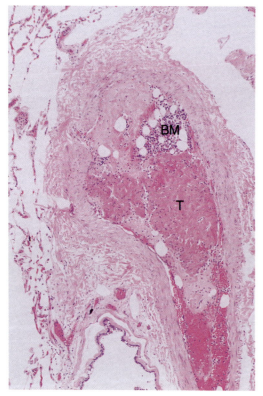

Figure 3.16

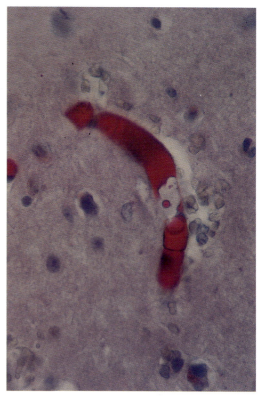

Figure 3.17A

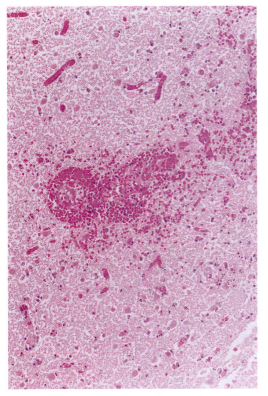

Figure 3.17B

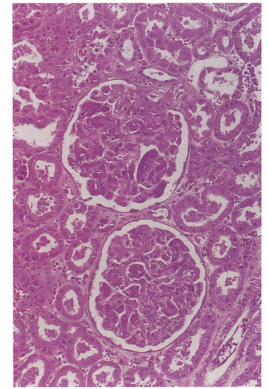

Figure 3.18A

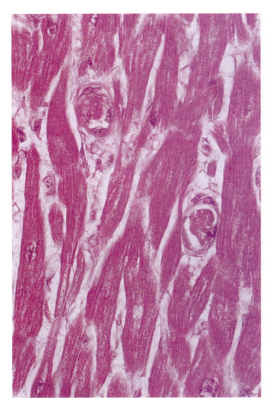

Figure 3.18B

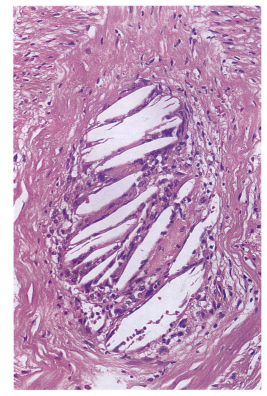

Figure 3.19

PLATE 3.6. INFARCT

Figure 3.20. Myocardial infarct. This 2-day-old infarct shows coagulation necrosis of myocardial cells. Almost no blood is seen in the vessels. The peripheral portion of the infarct has been invaded by acute inflammatory cells (lower part of the photograph), which act as scavengers and remove the dead cells.

Figure 3.22. Lung infarct. The pulmonary artery contains a thromboembolus. The alveoli are filled with blood. Alveolar septa have indistinct outlines due to ischemic necrosis.

Figure 3.21. Renal infarct. Central zone of ischemia is characterized by coagulation necrosis of nephrons (N). The margins of the infarct are infiltrated by extravasated blood.

Figure 3.23. Liver infarct. This red infarct is marked by necrosis of liver cells and parenchymal hemorrhage. Only a rim of remaining normal liver is seen adjacent to the portal tract (P).

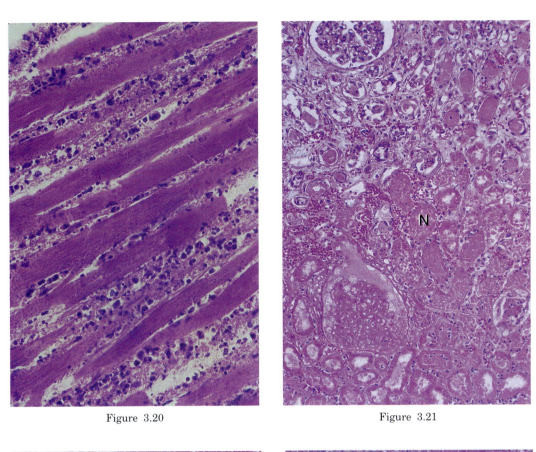

Figure 3.20

Figure 3.21

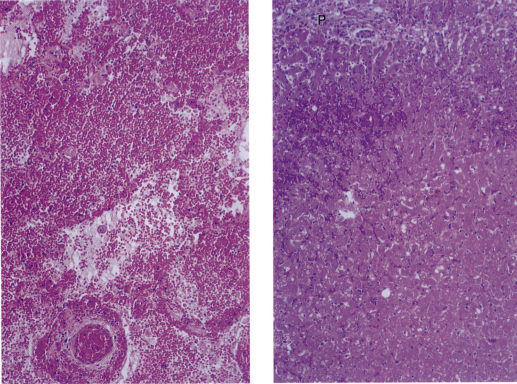

Figure 3.22

Figure 3.23

PLATE 3.7. SHOCK

Figure 3.24. Hypoxic changes in the brain. Ischemic neurons appear shrunken and have eosinophilic cytoplasm. The pericellular and perivascular spaces are dilated because of edema.

Figure 3.26. Shock lung. The alveoli are dilated because of edema fluid, which is low in protein and is therefore not visible in histological slides. Hyaline membranes (arrows) line the alveolar walls.

Figure 3.25. Focal renal tubular necrosis. A. The tubules appear dilated and contain amorphous cellular debris. The tubules are lined with flattened nonspecific cells that have lost part of their cytoplasm. **B.** The medullary junction contains congested blood vessels. At autopsy, this corresponds to the dark appearance of medulla, with pale, hypoperfused renal cortex.

Figure 3.27. Gastric mucosal hemorrhage.

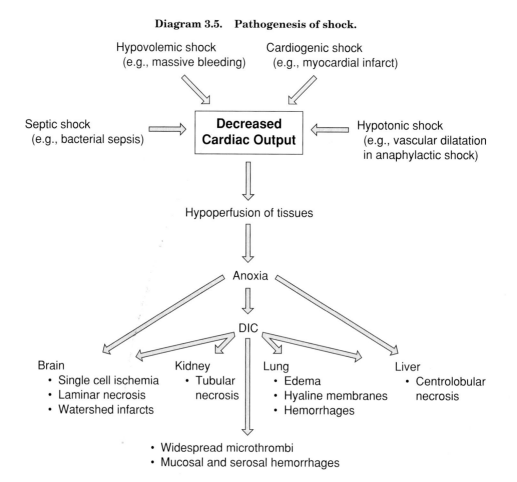

Diagram 3.5. Pathogenesis of shock.

Hypovolemic shock (e.g., massive bleeding)

Cardiogenic shock (e.g., myocardial infarct)

Septic shock (e.g., bacterial sepsis)

Decreased Cardiac Output

Hypotonic shock (e.g., vascular dilatation in anaphylactic shock)

Hypoperfusion of tissues

Anoxia

DIC

Brain
• Single cell ischemia
• Laminar necrosis
• Watershed infarcts

Kidney
• Tubular necrosis

Lung
• Edema
• Hyaline membranes
• Hemorrhages

Liver
• Centrolobular necrosis

• Widespread microthrombi
• Mucosal and serosal hemorrhages

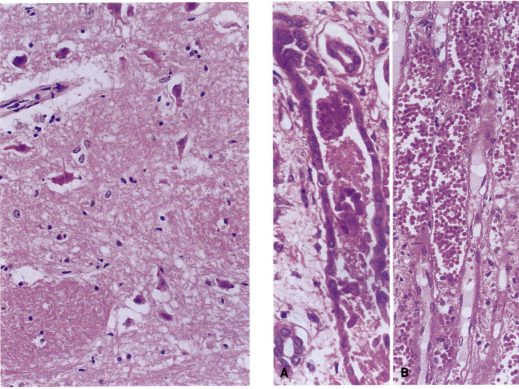

Figure 3.24

Figure 3.25

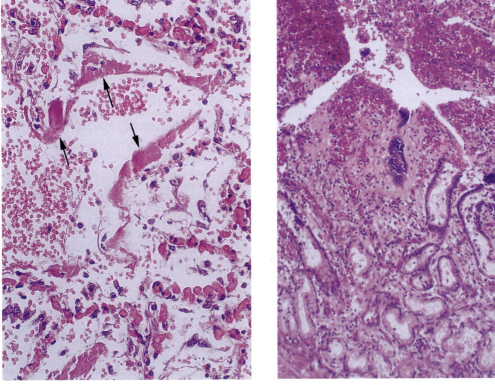

Figure 3.26

Figure 3.27

NOTES

CHAPTER 4

Neoplasia

INTRODUCTION

Neoplasms or *tumors* are lesions resulting from abnormal growth of cells, whose replication cannot be controlled by mechanisms that operate in normal tissues.

Tumor cells that resemble their normal predecessors and counterparts are called *well differentiated.* Such tumors grow slowly and form tumors that are clinically called *benign.* In contrast, tumor cells that bear little resemblance to the tissue of origin are called *poorly differentiated,* and those that do not resemble normal cells at all are called *undifferentiated* or *anaplastic.* Anaplastic cells form rapidly growing tumors, which tend to spread, kill the host, and are clinically *malignant.* Typical microscopic differences between benign and malignant tumors are listed in Table 4.1.

By electron microscopy, cells of benign tumors have a well developed cytoplasm that contains organelles typically found in the corresponding normal tissue (Fig. 4.1). Malignant tumors consist of cells that little resemble normal cells (Fig. 4.2). Their nuclei are pleomorphic and vary in size, shape, and the distribution of chromatin. The cytoplasm of malignant tumors usually contains fewer organelles than the cytoplasm of benign cells.

CYTOLOGY OF TUMORS

The differences between normal and neoplastic cells are easily recognized cytologically (Diagram 4.1). For example, vaginal smears taken from women with cervical neoplasia contain normal cells as well as cells that show mild nuclear atypia (*dysplastic cells*) and overtly malignant cells (Figs. 4.3 to 4.5). In contrast to normal squamous cells that have a small nucleus with evenly distributed chromatin and abundant cytoplasm, dysplastic cells have enlarged nuclei and a higher nuclear-to-cytoplasmic ratio. In malignant cells, the enlarged nuclei are not only hyperchromatic but also con-tain irregularly clumped chromatin. Such nuclei are surrounded by scant cytoplasm, and the nuclear-to-cytoplasmic ratio is therefore high.

Malignant tumor cells appear atypical in histological sections as well and often do not resemble the normal tissue of their origin. Sometimes, these malignant cells are extremely large or even multinucleated (Fig. 4.6). Malignant cells can also be small and reminiscent of undifferentiated embryonic cells (Fig. 4.7). The rapid proliferation rate of tumor cells is reflected in the frequent occurrence of mitoses, many of which are abnormal—tripolar, multipolar, or irregular (Fig. 4.8).

HISTOLOGY OF TUMORS

Malignant tumors differ from benign tumors in their histological (tissue) organization. For example, benign liver tumors may form cords with sinusoidal blood vessels, an arrangement resembling normal hepatic microscopic architecture, whereas cells of malignant tumors are arranged into unstructured groups unlike anything in the normal liver (Figs. 4.9 and 4.10).

The degree of differentiation of malignant tumors can be assessed histologically, and the tumors can be graded into well differentiated (*grade I*), moderately differentiated (*grade II*), or poorly differentiated (*grade III*) (Diagram 4.2). For example, well differentiated adenocarcinomas form glands that are regular (Fig. 4.11). In moderately differentiated adenocarcinomas (*grade II*), the glands are less regular (Fig. 4.12), and in the poorly differentiated tumors (*grade III*), the glands are barely recognizable (Fig. 4.13).

Along the same lines, squamous cell carcinomas are graded on the basis of their resemblance to normal squamous epithelium and the ability of tumor cells to undergo keratinization. Systems for histological grading of transitional cell tumors, gliomas, neuroblastomas, and other tumors are also in use.

Table 4.1
Principal Microscopic Differences Between Benign and Malignant Tumors

Morphologic Features	Benign	Malignant
Tissue	Organized	Disorganized
• Architecture	Resembles tissues of origin	Resembles less or not at all tissue of origin
• Secondary changes	None or rare	Necrosis, hemorrhage
Cells	Well differentiated	Poorly differentiated
• Size, shape	Uniform	Pleomorphic
Nuclei	Similar to normal	Atypical
• Size, shape	Regular	Irregular
• Chromatin	Uniformly distributed	
• Nucleolus	Inconspicuous	Prominent, multiple
• Mitoses	Few	Many Irregular

HISTOLOGICAL CLASSIFICATION OF TUMORS

Histological classification is the most widely used approach to classifying tumors. The approach correlates well with the clinical classification of tumors and is therefore most useful in clinical oncology. Keep in mind, however, that histological classification, like any other classification, cannot be always consistent. It has limitations because of the methods used for tumor examination, but the precision of histological diagnosis can be improved by ancillary techniques such as histochemistry, electron microscopy, and molecular biology.

This atlas uses a simplified approach to tumor classification. Thus, tumors are considered either *benign* or *malignant* and only in exceptional instances as *borderline malignant* or *intermediate*. Tumors are classified according to their constituent cells or tissues into the following categories:

- Epithelial tumors
- Mesenchymal (connective tissue) tumors
- Mixed epithelial and mesenchymal tumors
- Tumors of blood-forming and lymphoid cells
- Tumors of neural cells
- Tumors of glial and cells and neural supporting structures
- Embryonal tumors (blastomas), germ cell tumors, placental tumors, and teratomas

A comprehensive classification of human tumors, supplemented with salient examples, is given in Table 4.2.

Epithelial Tumors

Epithelial tumors originate from transformed cells in squamous, transitional, ductal, and glandular epithelia, as well as in organs such as the gastrointestinal tract, liver, kidney, thyroid, skin, or genitourinary tract. Benign epithelial tumors of the skin and mucosae are called **epitheliomas** or **papillomas** if they project from the surface (Figs. 4.14 and 4.15 and Diagram 4.3). Papillomas of the skin are composed of basal cells (*basal cell papilloma*, also known as seborrheic keratosis) or squamous cells (*squamous cell papilloma*). In the urinary tract, papillomas are lined by transitional epithelium (*transitional cell papilloma*).

Benign tumors composed of ductal, glandular, or follicular cells are called **adenomas** (Fig. 4.16). This term is often expanded with qualifiers to specify the site of origin and gross features of the tumor or the cell type forming it. For example, *papillary cystadenoma of the ovary* indicates that the tumor forms cavities (cysts), that the epithelium within these cysts projects into papillae, and that the tumor originated in the ovary. **Oncocytic adenoma** of the thyroid or salivary glands is composed of oncocytes, i.e., cells that have finely granular eosinophilic cytoplasm. *Liver cell adenoma* and *renal cell adenoma* are terms used for benign tumors in these organs. Histologically, they are compact and are also called *solid adenomas*. Most benign tumors of endocrine glands are also

Table 4.2
Classification of Human Tumors

Tumor Type	Cell Type	Benign	Malignant
Tumors of epithelial cells	Squamous epithelium	Epithelioma (papilloma)	Squamous cell carcinoma
	Transitional	Transitional cell papilloma	Transitional cell carcinoma
	Glandular/ductal	Adenoma	Adenocarcinoma
	Neuroendocrine	Carcinoid	Oat cell carcinoma
	Organ-specific: Liver cell	Liver cell adenoma	Hepatocellular carcinoma
	Kidney cell	Renal cell adenoma	Renal cell carcinoma
Tumors of mesenchymal cells	Fibroblast	Fibroma	Fibrosarcoma
			Malignant fibrous histiocytoma
	Fat cell	Lipoma	Liposarcoma
	Endothelial cell	Hemangioma	Angiosarcoma
	Smooth muscle cell	Leiomyoma	Leiomyosarcoma
	Striated muscle cell	Rhabdomyoma	Rhabdomyosarcoma
	Cartilage cell	Chondroma	Chondrosarcoma
	Bone cell	Osteoma	Osteosarcoma
Mixed tumor composed of epithelial and mesenchymal cells	Epithelial and connective tissue cells		
	Breast	Fibroadenoma	Cystosarcoma phyllodes
	Salivary gland	Mixed tumor	Malignant mixed tumor
Tumors of hematopoietic-lymphoid cells	Blood stem cell	—	Leukemia
	Lymphocyte	—	Lymphoma
	Plasma cell	MGUS	Myeloma
Tumors of neural cells	Neuroblast	Ganglioneuroma	Neuroblastoma
			Medulloblastoma
Tumors of glial and neural supporting cells	Glia cells	—	Glioma
	Meninges	Meningioma	Malignant meningioma
	Schwann cell	Schwannoma (neurilemoma)	Malignant schwannoma
Tumors of melanocytes	Melanocyte	Nevus	Malignant melanoma
Tumors of blastemal embryonal cells	Blastema of various organs	—	Nephroblastoma
	Early embryonic cells	—	Embryonal carcinoma
Tumors of germ cells, placental cells, and teratomas	Germ cell	—	Seminoma, dysgerminoma
	Trophoblast	—	Choriocarcinoma
	Derivatives of primordial germ layers	Teratoma	Teratocarcinoma

MGUS, monoclonal gammopathy of unknown significance.

solid adenomas, and are called by the name of the organ from which they originate, such as *pituitary adenoma* or **adrenal cortical adenoma** (Fig 4.17).

Malignant epithelial tumors are called **carcinomas**. **Squamous cell carcinoma** is composed of squamous epithelial cells that often undergo overt keratinization (Fig. 4.18). The tumor cells are interconnected with desmosomes seen on light microscopy as intercellular bridges. The center of the tumor nests may contain concentrically layered aggregates of keratin called *keratin pearls*. **Transitional cell carcinomas** typically originate in the urinary tract (Fig. 14.19). Carcinomas of specialized organs such as the liver or kidney or those originating from endocrine glands are called by their anatomical site of origin (e.g., *liver cell carcinoma, renal carcinoma,* or *islet cell carcinoma*).

Tumors of low-grade malignancy derived from gastrointestinal and respiratory tract neuroendocrine cells (Fig. 4.20) are called **carcinoids** for historical reasons. These tumors were named "carcinoids" (or carcinoma-like) by pioneers in histopathology who noticed a discrepancy between the histological invasiveness of these tumors on the one hand, and the uniformity of the nuclei of tumor cells and their slow growth on the other. Carcinoids have a good clinical prognosis if removed while the tumor is small. Highly malignant neuroendocrine tumors, most often found in the lungs, are called **oat cell carcinomas** (Fig. 14.21).

Adenocarcinomas are malignant tumors composed of cells that are arranged into gland-like structures (*adeno* is derived from the Greek word for glands). These tumors originate from gastrointestinal and respiratory tracts, breast, accessory skin glands, and parts of the reproductive system.

Various terms are used to describe variants of adenocarcinoma more precisely (Diagram 4.4). **Papillary adenocarcinoma** forms projections known as papillae (Fig. 4.22), and **mucinous adenocarcinomas** produce mucin (Fig. 4.23). In the ovary, such a tumor is usually cystic. If the cyst contains mucinous fluid, it may be called **mucinous cystadenocarcinoma**. Adenocarcinoma that evokes a strong connective tissue stromal reaction (*desmoplastic reaction*) is called **scirrhous adenocarcinoma** (Fig. 4.24). Such tumor masses contain abundant fibrous stroma and are firm to palpation and gritty on sectioning. Carcinomas of the breast composed of tumor cells with little intervening stroma are soft, like marrow, and are therefore called **medullary carcinomas** or **solid carcinomas** (Fig. 4.25). Note that some of these terms are not used consistently. For example, medullary carcinoma of the thyroid has a prominent stroma rich in amyloid and is not soft!

Tumors of Mesenchymal Cells

The names for benign tumors of mesenchymal cells (i.e., connective tissue, muscle, and skeletal cells) are constructed by combining the term for the cell type with a suffix *-oma*.

For example, **fibroma** is a tumor composed of fibroblasts (Fig. 4.26), **lipoma** of fat cells (Fig. 4.27), **leiomyoma** of smooth muscle cells, and **rhabdomyoma** of striated muscle cells (Fig. 4.28). **Hemangiomas** are tumors composed of blood vessels (Fig. 4.29).

The names for malignant mesenchymal or connective tissue tumors are constructed by combining the term for the cell type with the suffix *-sarcoma*. **Fibrosarcoma** is the term used for malignant tumors composed of fibroblasts (Fig. 4.30). **Liposarcomas** (Fig. 4.31) are malignant fat cell tumors. **Rhabdomyosarcoma** is a malignant tumor of striated muscle cells (Fig. 4.32). **Angiosarcoma** is a malignant tumor of blood vessels (Fig. 4.33).

Mixed Epithelial Mesenchymal Tumors

Mixed tumors are composed of neoplastic epithelial and mesenchymal stromal cells. All malignant epithelial tumors (carcinomas) have a stromal component, which in some cases, as in scirrhous carcinomas, may be extremely prominent. In carcinomas, these stromal cells (usually fibroblasts, myofibroblasts, and blood vessels) are normal host-derived cells responding to the tumor. However, in mixed tumors, the stromal cells are neoplastic, i.e., an integral part of the tumor growth. Mixed tumors may be composed of benign epithelial and mesenchymal cells (e.g., **fibroadenoma** of the breast) (Fig. 4.34), benign epithelial and malignant mesenchymal cells (e.g., **adenosarcoma** of the uterus) (Fig. 4.35), or malignant epithelial and mesenchymal cells (e.g., *carcinosarcoma or mixed mullerian tumor of the uterus*) (Fig. 4.36). Mixed tumors of the salivary glands, called **pleomorphic adenomas**, are composed of proliferating epithelial and myoepithelial cells. Myoepithelial cells in these tumors may give rise to cartilage or loose myxoid stroma. This variegated appearance of stroma accounts for the name of the tumor (Fig. 4.37). Most mixed tumors of the salivary glands are benign, but malignant mixed tumors occur as well. Such malignant tumors may be composed of malignant epithelium and benign stroma, or malignant epithelium and stroma.

Other Tumors

Tumors of hematopoietic, lymphoid, neural, and glial cels are described in Chapters 7 and 18.

Tumors composed of embryonic cells resembling those seen in the primordia ("anlage") of adult organs are classified as embryonic or developmental neoplasms. Such tumors are also called **blastomas** and are classified according to their organ of origin or predominant cell type, and as *nephroblastoma* (kidney), *hepatoblastoma* (liver), or *neuroblastoma* (neuroblasts).

Retinoblastoma (Fig. 4.38) is a tumor of the eye composed neoplastic cells resembling immature retinal cells. These cells resemble primitive neural cells found in the fetal retina as well as in other parts of the nervous system. These cells have a high nucleocytoplasmic ratio, which accounts for the "small blue cell" pattern seen histologically. Abortive differentiation of tumor cells leads to formation of wreath-like structures, called *rosettes* (Fig. 4.39).

Teratomas are tumors composed of mature tissues developmentally derived from the three embryonic germ layers: ectoderm, mesoderm, and endoderm (Diagram 4.5). The tissues are intermixed at random and without any regularity (Fig. 4.40).

Malignant teratomas, also known as **teratocarcinomas,** contain developmentally pluripotent stem cells resembling undifferentiated embryonic cells called **embryonal carcinomas**. Like the equivalent normal embryonic cells, embryonal carcinoma cells can differentiate into ectodermal, mesodermal, and endodermal derivatives. These cells can also give rise to the cells resembling those in extraembryonic membranes such as trophectoderm and the yolk sac, which are not found in adult organisms. Occasionally, embryonal carcinoma cells form even embryo-like structures called embryoid bodies.

Finally, one should mention those tumors that are difficult to classify unequivocally even though they have distinct morphological characteristics.

The best example is **malignant melanoma**, a pigmented tumor that originates most often in the skin and eye but may arise in other organs as well (Fig. 4.41). This tumor is presumably of neural crest origin, but has no neural features. Histologically, it may show the cohesiveness and the nesting pattern of epithelial tumors, but it is not a carcinoma. Biochemically and immunochemically, it does not have epithelial characteristics and is more akin to sarcomas, even though it is not classified as sarcoma. It is best to consider it as an entity unto itself.

Synovial sarcoma is yet another example of the difficulties in classifying tumors. These tumors originate in soft tissues and are thus classified as sarcomas. However, the tumors are composed of spindle-shaped sarcomatous cells and gland-like structures lined by cuboidal epithelial cells (Fig. 4.42) and look like carcinosarcomas. Furthermore, classification is confused by the fact that there are monophasic sarcomatous variants devoid of the biphasic epithelial pattern. Also, the term synovial sarcoma is inappropriate because synovial sarcomas do not originate from cells in synovial joints.

The uncertainty about the proper taxonomy of certain tumors is reflected in the usage of *eponyms* for such lesions. Best known examples are *Hodgkin lymphoma, Kaposi sarcoma,* and *Ewing sarcoma.* Even though Thomas Hodgkin described the disease known by his name more than 150 years ago, we still do not understand it and do not know whether **Hodgkin lymphoma** is one entity that presents in several forms, or a group of disorders that share some common clinical features. It is illustrated in Chapter 7. **Kaposi sarcoma** is probably an angiosarcoma, but the exact nature of cells that form the typical dermal hemorrhagic lesions remains elusive (Fig. 4.43). *Ewing sarcoma* is a malignant bone tumor, composed of cells of undetermined nature and uncertain origin. It is illustrated in Chapter 17.

Merkel cell tumor, a skin tumor identified in the 1970s, was named for its resemblance to cells found in the Merkel corpuscle of the skin. Although the evidence that Merkel cell tumors originate from Merkel cells is not overwhelming, this eponym has been used for neuroendocrine skin tumors that have distinct histological features (Fig. 4.44).

ANCILLARY TECHNIQUES OF HISTOPATHOLOGY OF TUMORS

If a tumor cannot be precisely diagnosed by gross and microscopic examination, additional studies may be required. These include techniques of tissue examination such as immunohistochemistry, electron microscopy, cytogenetics, and molecular biology.

Immunohistochemistry is based on the application of specific antisera to tissue sections. Typically, an antibody is layered over the tissue section and allowed to bind to the antigen under investigation. Subsequently, the bound antibody is visualized by a chromogen reaction, making it possible to recognize those cells expressing the given antigen (Diagram 4.6).

Application of immunohistochemistry to pathology is based on the fact that most tumors retain some characteristics of their parental or embryonic origin. These cell components or secretory products can be used as markers for identifying the tumor cells.

Cell type–specific markers. Many tumor cells retain some of the characteristics of normal cells from the organ in which they arose. For example, adenocarcinomas of the prostate usually contain prostatic acid phosphatase or express prostate-specific antigen (Fig. 4.45).

Embryonic and oncofetal antigens. Tumors composed of immature cells may resemble the cells forming that organ during embryogenesis. For example, hepatocellular carcinoma cells secrete alpha fetoprotein, the major protein produced by fetal liver cells.

Cell lineage–specific markers. To date, the most useful markers for cell lineages are the proteins forming the intermediate filaments of the cytoskeleton. Epithelial cell intermediate filaments are composed of keratin, and this protein is also expressed in epithelial malignancies, i.e., carcinomas (Fig. 4.46). On the other hand, sarcomas express vimentin, the intermediate filament protein of mesenchymal cells (Fig. 4.47). In carcinomas, the antibody to vimentin stains only the connective tissue cells and blood vessels.

Electron microscopy is also useful for tumor diagnosis. Benign and malignant tumor cells differ ultrastructurally from one another as shown in Figure 4.1. However, these differences are not always evident and, therefore, electron microscopy should not be used as an ultimate proof of malignancy. Nevertheless, electron microscopy allows one to identify many cytoplasmic organelles that are specific for certain tumors. For example, carcinoids and related tumors contain neuroendocrine granules (Fig. 4.48). Melanomas contain melanosomes (Fig. 4.49). Squamous cell carcinomas contain tonofilaments and desmosomes, which connect one cell with another (Fig. 4.50). Rhabdomyosarcomas contain myofilaments arranged into abortive contractile units with Z bands (Fig. 4.51).

NOTES

PLATE 4.1. MORPHOLOGY OF TUMOR CELLS

Figure 4.1. **Benign tumor cell. A.** The electron microscopic photograph of this salivary gland tumor shows that cells have abundant cytoplasm, which contains numerous mitochondria and secretory granules. **B.** Cytological imprint preparation of a similar benign tumor shows that the cells have small round nuclei and abundant cytoplasm.

Figure 4.2. **Malignant tumor. A.** The electron microscopic photograph shows that the tumor cells have cytoplasm devoid of organelles. In contrast to well differentiated cells of benign tumor, which contain numerous organelles in their cytoplasm, these poorly differentiated cells have few organelles. There are only a few mitochondria (essential for generating energy) and numerous free ribosomes (for synthesis of proteins for endogenous use). Note the prominent nucleoli. **B.** Cytological imprint of a malignant tumor. The tumor cells have large, irregularly shaped nuclei with prominent nucleoli and scant cytoplasm.

Diagram 4.1. **Cytological differences between normal and neoplastic cells. A.** Normal cell. **B.** Benign tumor cell. **C.** Malignant tumor cell.

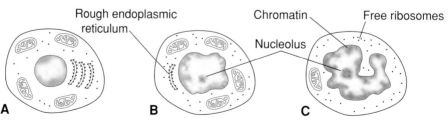

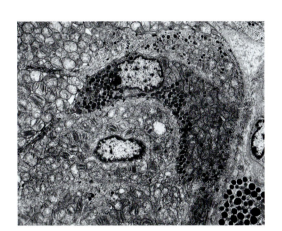

Figure 4.1A

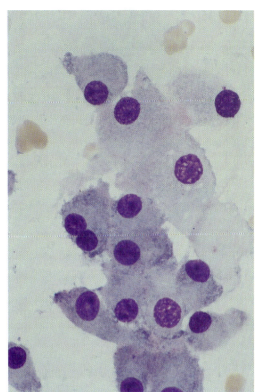

Figure 4.1B

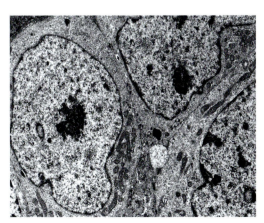

Figure 4.2A

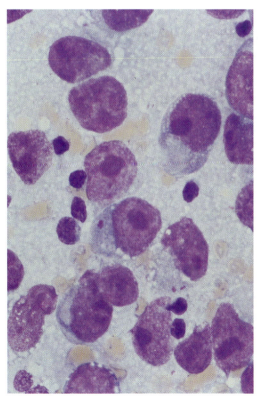

Figure 4.2B

PLATE 4.2. CYTOLOGY OF NEOPLASIA

Figure 4.3. Normal cervical smear. The normal squamous cell has a small clumped nucleus and abundant cytoplasm.

Figure 4.5. Carcinoma in situ. This smear contains cells with irregular hyperchromatic nuclei and scant cytoplasm.

Figure 4.7. Neuroblastoma. The tumor is composed of small undifferentiated cells that have little cytoplasm surrounding the hyperchromatic (blue) nuclei.

Figure 4.4. Dysplasia. The cells have enlarged nuclei. However, the nuclei have a regular shape and show only slight hyperchromasia.

Figure 4.6. Sarcoma. The tumor cells vary in size and shape and are loosely arranged.

Figure 4.8. Squamous cell carcinoma. A. The tumor cells form compact sheets. The nuclei show marked pleomorphism. **B.** Abnormal, tripolar mitosis.

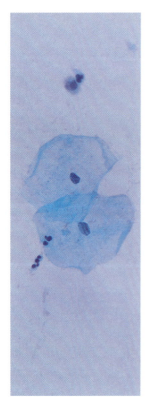

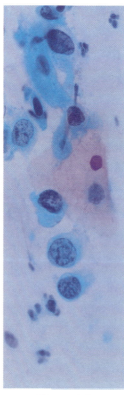

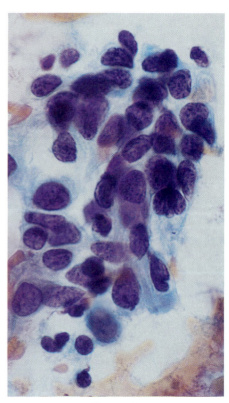

Figure 4.3   Figure 4.4   Figure 4.5

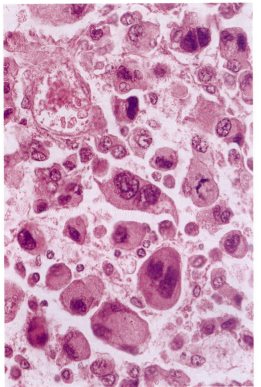

Figure 4.6

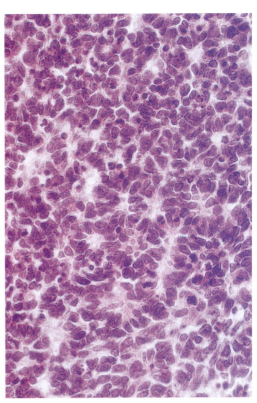

Figure 4.7

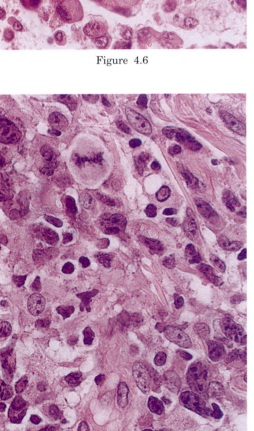

Figure 4.8A

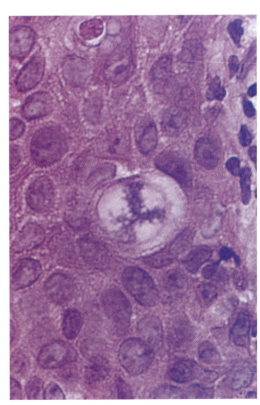

Figure 4.8B

PLATE 4.3. GRADING OF TUMORS

Figure 4.9. Liver cell adenomas. The tumor cells resemble normal liver cells, which are compressed by the tumor in the lower portion of the photograph.

Figure 4.11. Adenocarcinoma grade I. Tumor cells form well developed glands.

Figure 4.13. Adenocarcinoma grade III. The tumor is composed of cells arranged into solid nests with only occasional lumen formation.

Figure 4.10. Liver cell carcinoma. The tumor shows more pleomorphism and only superficial resemblance to normal liver tissue.

Figure 4.12. Adenocarcinoma grade II. Tumor cells form irregularly shaped glands and solid areas.

Diagram 4.2. Grading of adenocarcinomas. Grade I tumor is composed of well formed regular glands. Grade II tumor is composed of highly irregular glands, showing deep invaginations ("glands within glands"), back-to-back arrangement, and focal solid areas. Grade III tumors consist predominantly of solid areas and form only occasional glands.

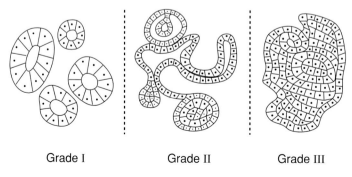

Grade I   Grade II   Grade III

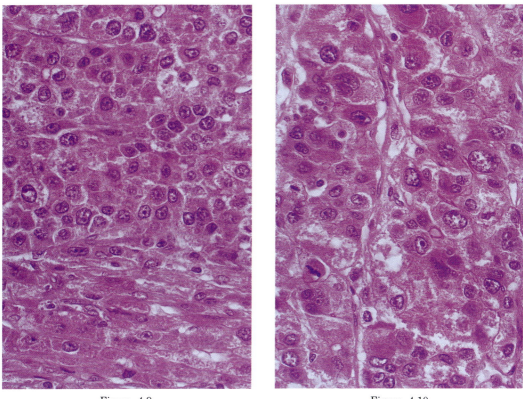

Figure 4.9   Figure 4.10

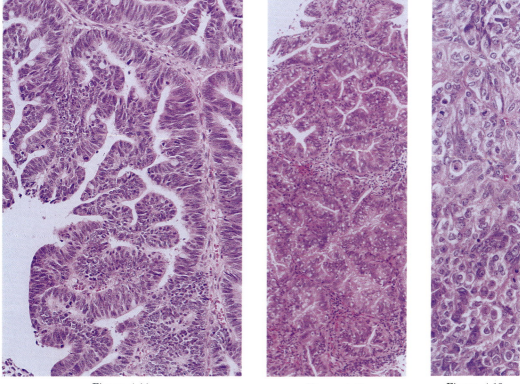

Figure 4.11   Figure 4.12   Figure 4.13

PLATE 4.4. BENIGN EPITHELIAL TUMORS

Figure 4.14. Basal cell papilloma of the skin. The tumor is composed of cells resembling those in the basal layer of the epidermis. The exophytic tumor forms papillae projecting above the surface of the skin.

Figure 4.16. Follicular adenoma of the thyroid. This tumor is composed of uniform cells forming follicles filled with colloid as in a normal thyroid. The tumor compresses normal thyroid follicles in the lower part of the photograph.

Figure 4.15. Transitional cell papilloma. The tumor consists of fronds lined with regular transitional epithelium and a central vascular core.

Figure 4.17. Adrenal cortical adenoma. The tumor is composed of cells that have uniform round nuclei surrounded by clear cytoplasm. The cells are arranged in solid nests.

Diagram 4.3. Epithelial tumors of epidermis and mucosal surfaces. A. Epithelioma, endophytic. **B.** Epithelioma, exophytic. **C.** Papilloma. **D.** Carcinoma. **E.** Intraepithelial neoplasia.

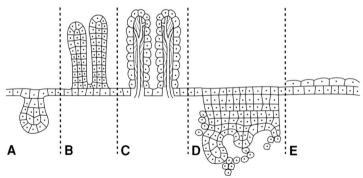

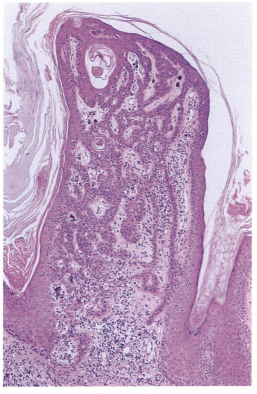

Figure 4.14

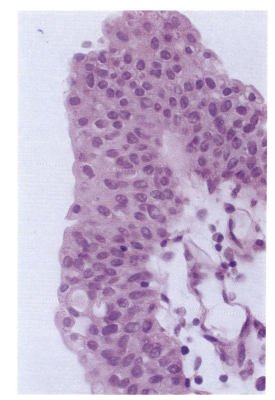

Figure 4.15

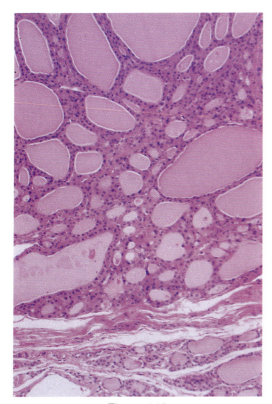

Figure 4.16

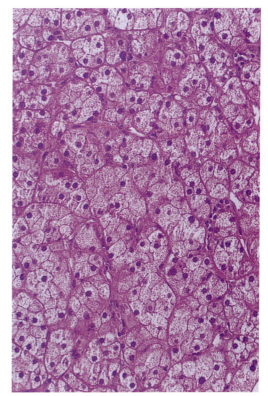

Figure 4.17

PLATE 4.5. MALIGNANT EPITHELIAL TUMORS

Figure 4.18. Squamous cell carcinoma. The surface of the tumor shows extensive keratinization.

Figure 4.20. Carcinoid. The tumor is composed of nest of cells located in the lamina propria mucosae. The tumor cells have round nuclei and appear relatively uniform. However, the tumor cells extend into the wall of the intestine, indicating that this is an invasive neoplasm.

Figure 4.19. Transitional cell carcinoma. The tumor is composed of sheets of cells resembling normal transitional epithelium. However, these cells form thick layers and nests of irregular shape.

Figure 4.21. Oat cell carcinoma of the lung. The tumor is composed of small hyperchromatic cells.

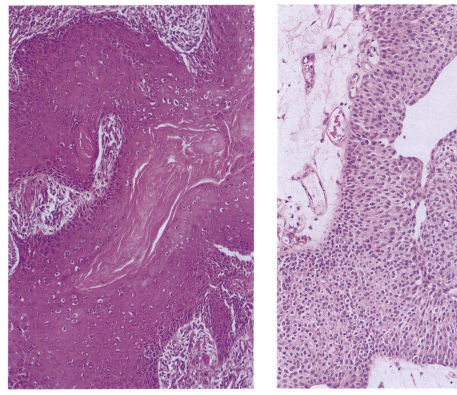

Figure 4.18

Figure 4.19

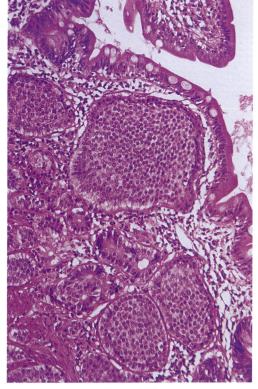

Figure 4.20

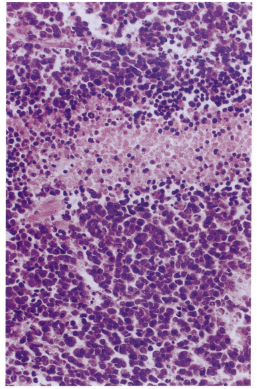

Figure 4.21

PLATE 4.6. MALIGNANT EPITHELIAL TUMORS

Figure 4.22.   Papillary adenocarcinoma. The tumor cell line papillae have a central vascular core. Papillae project into the lumina lined by the same malignant tumor cells, which shows that the tumor is an adenocarcinoma.

Figure 4.24.   Scirrhous adenocarcinoma of the breast. The tumor cells form irregular glands surrounded by abundant dense connective tissue.

Figure 4.23.   Mucinous adenocarcinoma. The tumor is composed of cuboidal cells that contain clear material in their cytoplasm. This material is biochemically mucin.

Figure 4.25.   Medullary carcinoma of the breast. The tumor cells are closely packed and the stroma is scant. Histologically, this tumor could be also classified as "solid" since it consists of solid masses of tumor cells. The term medullary is derived from the softness of tumor on gross examination.

Diagram 4.4.   Adenocarcinoma. A. Well differentiated adenocarcinoma composed of regular glands. **B.** Cystadenocarcinoma is composed of cystic spaces lined by glandular epithelium. **C.** Papillary carcinoma forms papillae that project into the lumen of glands. **D.** Mucinous carcinoma contains mucin in the cells, around them, and in the lumen of glands. **E.** Solid carcinoma is composed of solid masses of tumor cells. **F.** Scirrhous carcinoma contains abundant collagenous stroma between the infiltrating tumor cells.

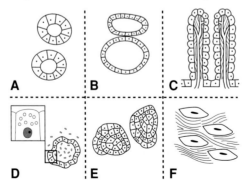

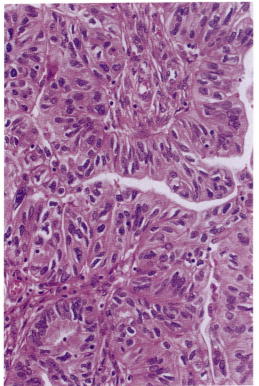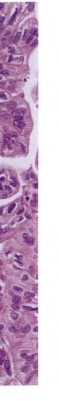

Figure 4.22

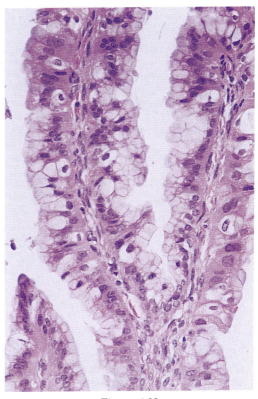

Figure 4.23

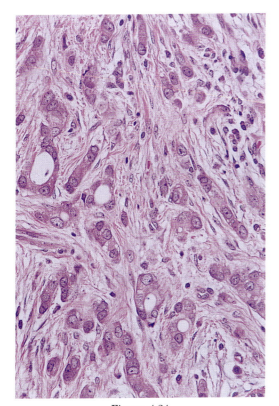

Figure 4.24

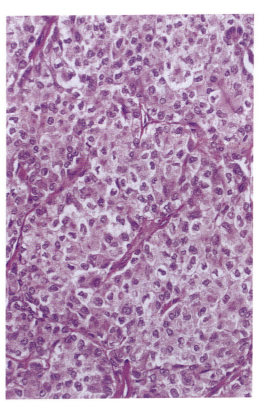

Figure 4.25

PLATE 4.7. BENIGN MESENCHYMAL TUMORS

Figure 4.26. Fibroma of the maxilla. The tumor is composed of spindle-shaped elongated cells that are indistinguishable from normal fibroblasts.

Figure 4.28. Rhabdomyoma of the pharynx. The tumor is composed of large cells that have abundant cytoplasm. These cells resemble striated muscle cells.

Figure 4.27. Lipoma of subcutaneous tissue. The tumor is composed of fat cells, some fibroblasts, and blood vessels. The fat has been dissolved during processing of tissue, and the cytoplasm of fat cells therefore appears clear.

Figure 4.29. Hemangioma. The tumor is composed of endothelial cells that line spaces filled with blood.

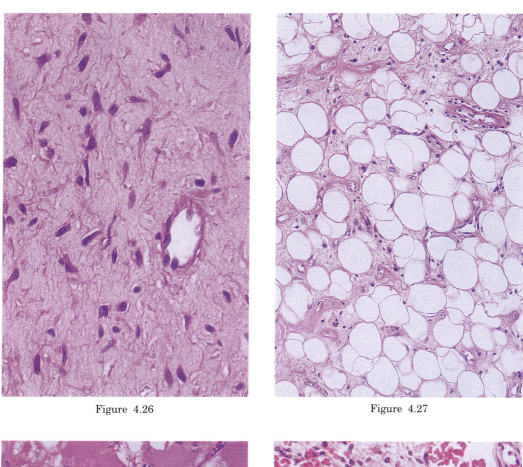

Figure 4.26

Figure 4.27

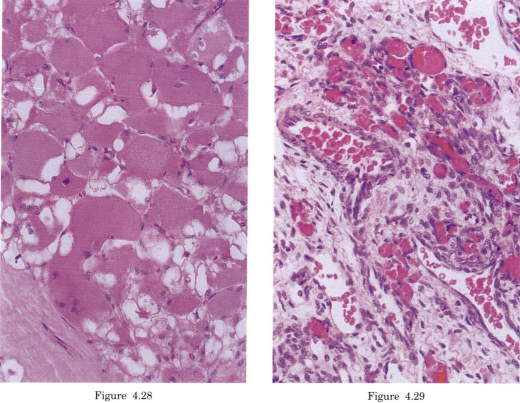

Figure 4.28

Figure 4.29

PLATE 4.8. MALIGNANT MESENCHYMAL TUMORS

Figure 4.30.   Fibrosarcoma. The tumor is composed of elongated fibroblastic cells and large cells that do not have normal equivalents, i.e., they are anaplastic.

Figure 4.32.   Rhabdomyosarcoma. The tumor consists of cells with irregularly shaped nuclei that vary in size and shape. Many cells have prominent eosinophilic cytoplasm resembling rhabdomyoblasts. The cytoplasm of these cells shows cross-striations.

Figure 4.31.   Liposarcoma. The tumor is composed of atypical vacuolated cells (malignant lipoblasts).

Figure 4.33.   Angiosarcoma. The tumor cells line vascular spaces, partially filled with red blood cells.

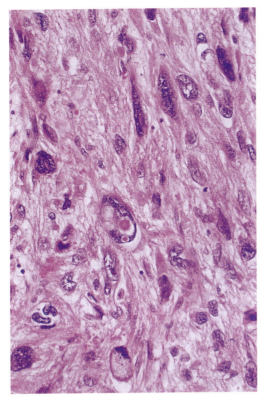

Figure 4.30

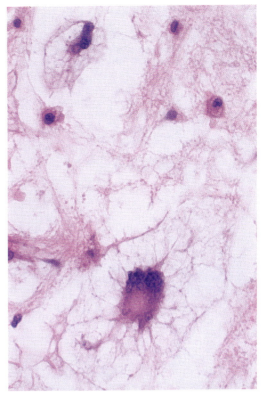

Figure 4.31

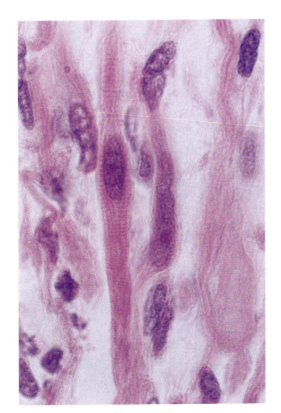

Figure 4.32

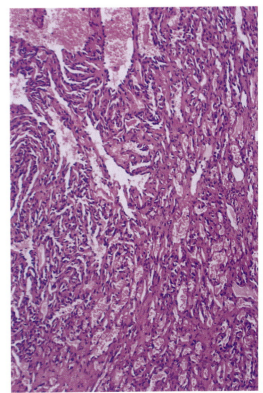

Figure 4.33

PLATE 4.9. MIXED TUMORS

Figure 4.34.   Fibroadenoma of the breast. The tumor is composed of ducts made of epithelial cells surrounded by mesenchymal cells.

Figure 4.36.   Carcinosarcoma (mixed mullerian tumor) of the uterus. The tumor consists of malignant epithelial (carcinoma—C) and mesenchymal (sarcomatous—S) components.

Figure 4.35.   Adenosarcoma of the uterus. The mesenchymal cells in the stroma show atypia and pleomorphism, whereas the epithelial lining cells are benign.

Figure 4.37.   Mixed tumor of salivary glands. This benign tumor is composed of epithelial (E) and stromal (S) elements.

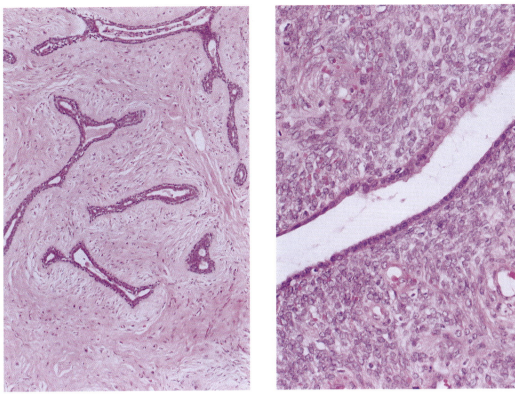

Figure 4.34

Figure 4.35

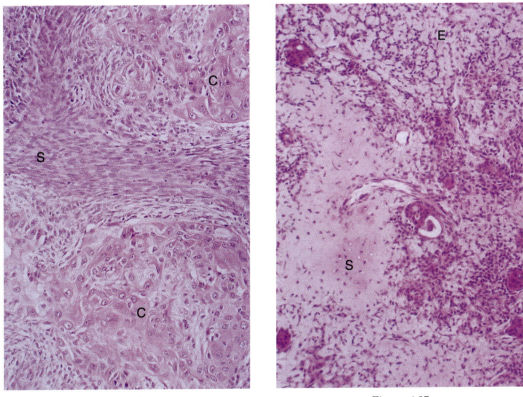

Figure 4.36

Figure 4.37

PLATE 4.10. EMBRYONAL TUMORS

Figure 4.38.   Retinoblastoma. The bulbus of the eye contains a large mass of small blue cells.

Figure 4.39.   Retinoblastoma. Higher-power view of tumor cells that are focally arranged into rosettes.

Figure 4.40.   Teratoma. Tumor consists of haphazardly arranged mature adult tissues. **A.** Tumor contains skin, primordium of the tooth (pale area), and neural tissue. **B.** Another part of the tumor contains glands, neural tissue, fat cells, and pigmented epithelium.

Diagram 4.5.   Histogenesis of teratomas. Teratoma consists of derivatives of three germ layers found in the early embryo: ectoderm, mesoderm, and endoderm.

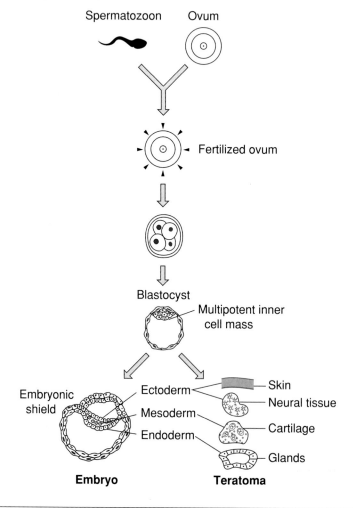

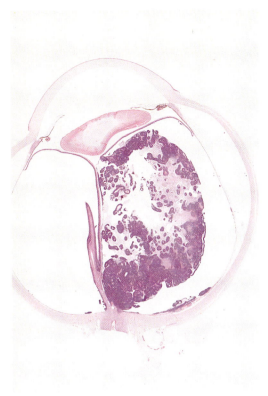

Figure 4.38

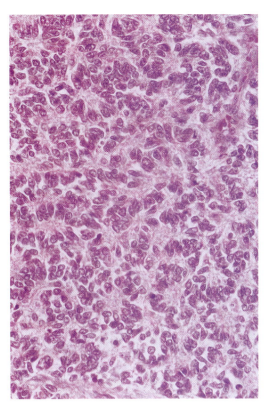

Figure 4.39

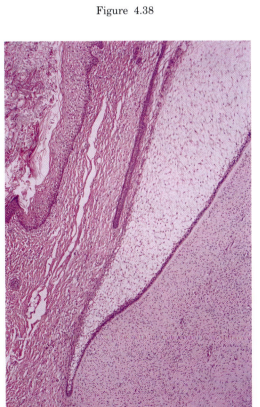

Figure 4.40A

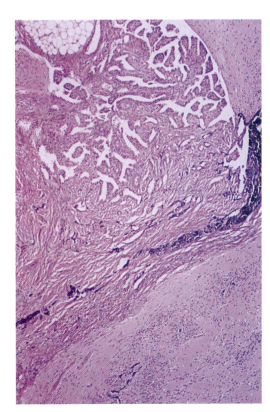

Figure 4.40B

PLATE 4.11. OTHER TUMORS

Figure 4.41. **Melanoma.** The tumor is composed of atypical polygonal cells that focally contain brown pigment (*melanin*).

Figure 4.42. **Synovial cell sarcoma.** The tumor consists of spindle-shaped sarcomatoid cells and gland-like structures lined by epithelial cells.

Figure 4.43. **Kaposi sarcoma.** The tumor is composed of spindle-shaped cells that are separated from one another by slits that contain blood.

Figure 4.44. **Merkel cell tumor.** The tumor is composed of a mass of densely compacted blue cells.

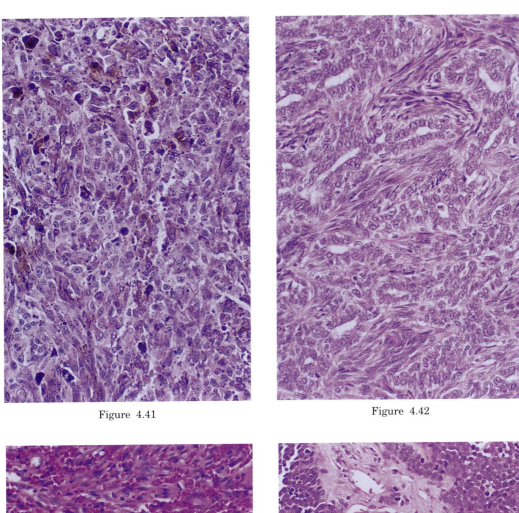

Figure 4.41

Figure 4.42

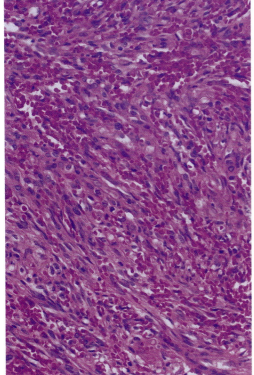

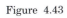

Figure 4.43

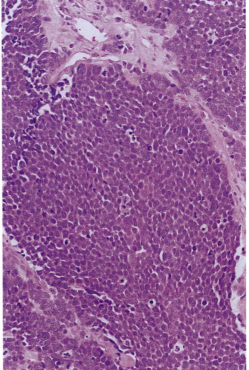

Figure 4.44

PLATE 4.12. SPECIAL TECHNIQUES—IMMUNOHISTOCHEMISTRY

Figure 4.45.   Adenocarcinoma of the prostate reacted with antibody to prostate specific antigen. The immunoreactive cells are recognized by the brown pigment generated by the immunoperoxidase reaction.

Figure 4.47.   Sarcoma. Tumor cells are positively stained with the antibody to vimentin, the mesenchymal cell marker.

Figure 4.46.   Carcinoma. A. Tumor cells were cultured in vitro and stained with a fluorescein-tagged antibody to keratin. By fluorescence microscopy, one may see the cytoplasmic immunoreactive intermediate filaments. **B.** Histological sections stained by immunoperoxidase technique contain keratin-positive carcinoma cells, which appear brown.

Diagram 4.6.   Principles of immunohistochemistry. The tissue is covered with a fluorescent antibody (F) that is allowed to bind to the specific antigen. The unbound antibody is washed away. The bound antibody can be recognized also with a secondary tagged antibody. This antibody carries an enzyme (horseradish peroxidase, P). The bound secondary antibody may be visualized by incubating the slide in a fluid solution containing the appropriate substrate for the enzyme in the presence of a die that changes color during the enzymatic reaction. In the most commonly used immunoperoxidase method the substrate for horseradish peroxidase is hydrogen peroxide, and the chromogen is diaminobenzidine. The enzyme reaction thus forms a brown pigment at the site of the antigen antibody reaction in the tissue. The reaction can be amplified by using several additional intermediate steps and cross-linking antibodies (peroxidase antiperoxidase [PAP] technique).

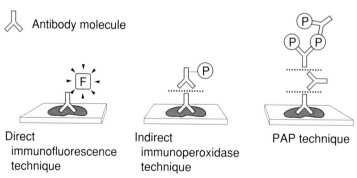

Antibody molecule

Direct
immunofluorescence
technique

Indirect
immunoperoxidase
technique

PAP technique

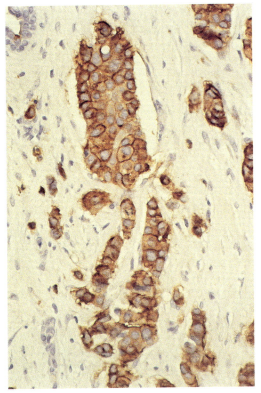

Figure 4.45

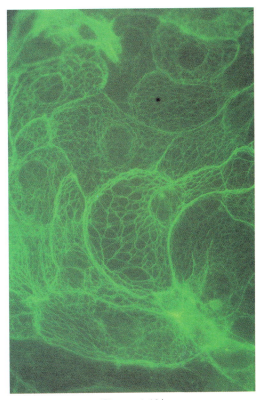

Figure 4.46A

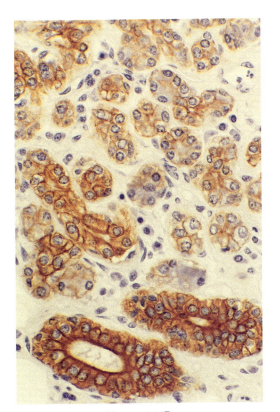

Figure 4.46B

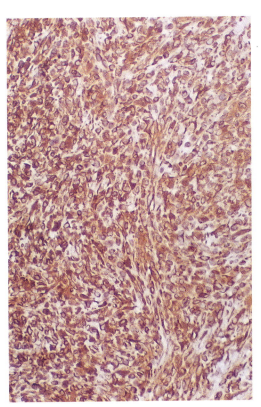

Figure 4.47

PLATE 4.13. ELECTRON MICROSCOPY

Figure 4.48. Electron microscopy of carcinoid. The tumor contains neuroendocrine granules composed of a dense core and a halo that separates it from the limiting membrane.

Figure 4.50. Squamous cell carcinoma. Desmosomes linking two adjacent cells. The cytoplasm contains bundles of keratin filaments called tonofilaments.

Figure 4.49. Electron microscopy of melanoma. The cytoplasm contains melanosomes and premelanosomes. These dark cytoplasmic organelles are recognized by their typical striation.

Figure 4.51. Rhabdomyosarcoma. The tumor cells contains disorganized myofilaments with dense Z bands.

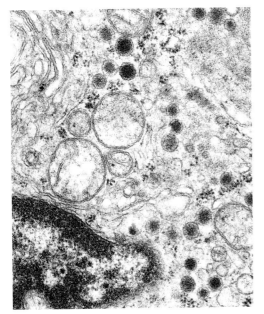

Figure 4.48

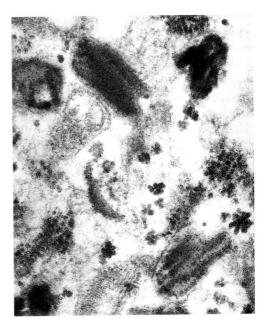

Figure 4.49

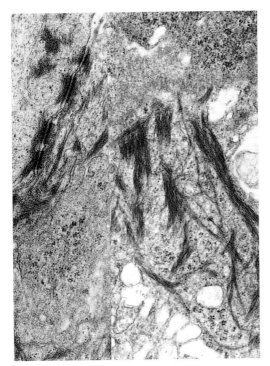

Figure 4.50

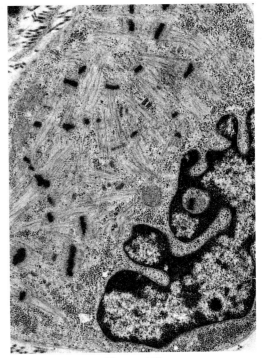

Figure 4.51

NOTES

CHAPTER 5

Cardiovascular System

NORMAL HISTOLOGY

The cardiovascular or circulatory system consists of the heart and blood vessels (Diagram 5.1). The vessels include arteries, capillaries, and veins.

The *heart* has four chambers—two atria and two ventricles. The wall of all chambers has three layers: endocardium, myocardium, and epicardium. The *endocardium* covers the inside of the atria and ventricles and the leaflets of the tricuspid, pulmonary, mitral, and aortic valves. The *myocardium* is composed of striated muscle cells that are interconnected into a syncytium. The *epicardium* forms the external surface of the heart. It extends into the *pericardium*, which forms the outer layer of the pericardial cavity. Both the epicardium and the pericardium are lined on their opposing surfaces with a layer of flat mesothelial cells. Connective tissue, which contains some fat cells, separates the myocardium from the mesothelial surface of the epicardium. All major coronary arteries are located in this portion of the epicardium, from where they extend in the form of smaller branches into the myocardium proper.

Arteries are classified according to their size as large, medium, and small. Histologically, all arteries have three layers (tunicae): *intima*, *media*, and *adventitia*. In larger (elastic) arteries, such as the aorta and its major branches, these layers are separated from one another by an elastic lamina. Coronary arteries are typical of elastic arteries. The smaller, muscular arteries, such as those in internal organs and peripheral tissues, do not show such distinctive layering.

The arteries extend into *arterioles*, which in turn form *capillaries*. The arterioles are composed of endothelium and only one or two layers of smooth muscle cells. Capillaries are lined by an endothelial layer and a basement membrane. Capillaries then extend into *venules,* which in turn form veins.

Large veins resemble arteries, except that they have a thinner wall and do not have elastic laminae separating their wall into three distinct layers.

OVERVIEW OF PATHOLOGY

The most important diseases of the cardiovascular system are:

- Atherosclerosis
- Coronary heart disease
- Rheumatic carditis
- Endocarditis
- Cardiomyopathy
- Tumors of the heart and blood vessels
- Vasculitis

Atherosclerosis

Atherosclerosis is a multifactorial disease that affects the intima of elastic arteries. The disease is characterized by intramural deposits of lipids, proliferation of vascular smooth muscle cells and fibroblasts, and accumulation of macrophages. These changes are accompanied by calcification of arterial wall, loss of elasticity of vessel wall, and narrowing of dilatation of vascular lumen.

According to the *response to injury hypothesis* (Diagram 5.2), the pathogenesis of atherosclerosis begins with an insudation of lipid into the vessel wall (Fig. 5.1). Fatty streaks consist of aggregates of lipid-laden macrophages. Endothelial injury is followed by attachment of monocytes and platelets to the internal surface of the artery and local thrombus formation. These changes alter the *permeability* of the arterial wall, facilitating even more influx of lipids. Scavenger monocytes infiltrate the intima, transforming into macrophages that phagocytize lipid-laden fragments of damaged cells and stroma. Macrophages that have accumulated lipid in their cytoplasm appear histologically as foam cells.

Macrophages secrete growth factors and cytokines, which recruit additional monocytes, macrophages, and other cells. Cy-

Diagram 5.1. The cardiovascular system comprises the heart and blood vessels.

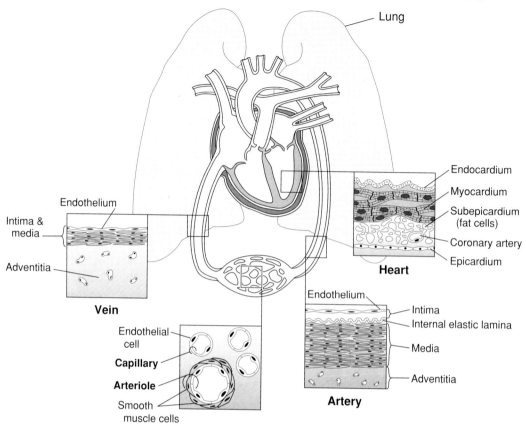

tokines and growth factors also stimulate the proliferation of smooth muscle cells and their ingrowth into the intima from the tunica media. Lipid accumulates not only in macrophages but also in smooth muscle cells. From dead and dying cells, cholesterol is released into interstitial spaces. These events lead to the formation of **fibrofatty plaques** and **atheromas** (Fig. 5.2). Atheromas consist of amorphous, lipid-rich material (Greek *atheros* = porridge) and are soft. On the luminal side, atheromas are typically covered with an intimal **fibrous cap**, consisting of fibroblasts surrounded by collagen, which replaces the normal intimal cells. Many atheromas undergo fibrosis and become hard plaques.

Atheromas are complicated by secondary changes, which include *calcification*, *rupture* of the fibrous cap, and *ulceration* overlying endothelium with secondary *thrombosis*. Thrombosis is the most common complication of ulcerated atheromas (Fig. 5.3). The calcification of vessels leads to hardening of arteries. Atheromas weaken the arteries and predispose to formation of aneurysms.

Coronary Heart Disease

Coronary atherosclerosis is clinically the most important aspect of atherosclerosis. Coronary arteries are relatively narrow, and atherosclerosis could seriously reduce the blood flow through them (Fig. 5.4). Slow, progressive narrowing of the arterial lumen that occurs over an extended period causes myocardial hypoxia and presents clinically either as *angina pectoris* or *congestive heart failure*. Sudden occlusion of a coronary artery by a thrombus formed over an ulcerated atheroma causes *myocardial infarct*.

Myocardial infarct is a localized area of necrosis of myocardial cells. The necrosis is caused by anoxia brought on by the sudden occlusion of one of the main coronary arteries. Such myocardial infarcts are typically *transmural* and localized to an anatomical area that corresponds to the portion of the heart supplied by the occluded coronary artery (Diagram 5.3).

In contrast to transmural myocardial infarcts, which are localized and caused by coronary artery occlusion, *hypotensive infarcts* are multifocal and limited to the subendocardial zones. These infarcts are not associated with occlusion of a major coronary artery.

The first morphological signs of myocardial injury can be seen within the first few hours after onset of anoxia by electron microscopy. These signs include swelling of mitochondria, separation of myofibrils due to the influx of water into the cytoplasm, and formation of calcific granules within the mitochondria. Light-microscopic signs of myocardial necrosis appear 6–12 hours after the onset of infarction (Fig. 5.5). Chemotactic substances are released from necrotic cells, and neutrophils appear 12–24 hours after the onset of infarction (Diagram 5.4). Neutrophils persist for 2–4 days and then disintegrate together with the necrotic myocardial cells. Neutrophils are gradually replaced by macrophages, which predominate in the infarcted area 5–10 days after the onset of anoxia. Macrophages secrete cytokines and growth factors, which stimulate the ingrowth of fibroblasts and angioblasts and the formation of granulation tissue. Over a period of 2–3 weeks, the granulation tissue, in turn, is replaced by fibrous tissue that becomes progressively less cellular, forming a mature collagenous scar. Scar formation occurs with 5–8 weeks from the onset of infarction.

Rheumatic Carditis

Rheumatic fever is an immunologically mediated, multisystemic disease that typically follows an upper respiratory tract infection with certain strains of streptococci. It is believed that the antibodies formed against the streptococcal antigens cross-react with similar antigens on cells of the joints, heart, skin, and central nervous system. Affected patients also develop a cell-mediated immune reaction against their own tissues, most prominently the myocardium. Rheumatic heart disease may present as an **isolated endocarditis, myocarditis, pericarditis,** or more often **pancarditis** that involves the entire heart (Diagram 5.5 and Figure 5.6).

Acute and Subacute Rheumatic Endocarditis. Acute and subacute rheumatic endocarditis is most often found in the valves of the left ventricle, i.e., mitral and aortic valves. The inflammation leads to the formation of excrescences composed of fibrin (**verrucae** or **"vegetations"**) on the surface of damaged leaflets. The valve covered with the thrombus is infiltrated with lymphocytes and macrophages and shows evidence of vascularization. The inflammation stimulates the formation of granulation tissue, which organizes the thrombotic vegetations, incorporating them into the leaflets. These inflammatory changes heal by collagenous scaring, which causes thickening and deformities of the valves and predisposes them to calcification. Valvular changes cause functional changes in blood flow typical of valvular stenosis, insufficiency, or both.

Myocarditis. Myocarditis of rheumatic fever presents in the form of typical **Aschoff bodies**. These inflammatory lesions begin first as infiltrates of histiocytes surrounding foci of fibrinoid necrosis in the interstitial spaces. The fully formed Aschoff bodies consist of aggregates of modified macrophages and scattered lymphocytes around centrally located fibrinoid material. Aschoff bodies persist for an indefinite period before they finally heal and transform into scars.

Epicarditis and Pericarditis. Rheumatic **epicarditis** and **pericarditis** are associated with extensive exudation of fibrin. Underneath the fibrin, which covers the surfaces of the pericardial cavity, the epicardium and pericardium are infiltrated with chronic inflammatory cells.

Endocarditis

Bacterial Endocarditis. Infectious endocarditis is an inflammation typically caused by bacteria. The most common pathogens are *Streptococcus,* which accounts for 50–60%, and *Staphylococcus,* which accounts for 20% of all cases. Various other gram-positive and -negative bacteria and fungi account for the rest (Diagram 5.6).

Endocarditis preferentially involves the valves (**valvulitis**) and less often the mural endocardium (**mural endocarditis**). The mitral and aortic valves are more often involved than the valves of the right ventricle. However, drug addicts show a predisposition for right ventricular valvulitis. Congenital heart defects, e.g., interventricular defects, are common sites of mural endocarditis.

Histologically, endocarditis usually shows surface thrombosis overlying an inflamed and vascularized portion of the valve (Fig. 5.7). Such lesions resemble those of rheumatic valvulitis, except that the latter are bacteriologically sterile and the former often contain bacteria.

Nonbacterial Thrombotic Endocarditis (NBTE). The term *NBTE* is synonymous with *marantic endocarditis*. It develops on normal valves in emaciated patients suffering from chronic diseases, especially those who are dying of cancer and who have hypercoagulability of blood. The sterile vegetations composed of fibrin form on valves showing minimal endothelial defects (Fig. 5.8). Normally, these incidental defects are repaired by regeneration from adjacent endothelium. However, in marantic patients, such repair is inefficient and thrombi form at the site of injury. Increased coagulability of the blood, frequently seen in cancer patients, promotes the growth of valvular thrombi.

Sterile endocarditis similar to NBTE occurs in lupus erythematosus (*Libman-Sacks* endocarditis). It involves both surfaces of mitral or aortic leaflets.

Carcinoid Heart Disease. Carcinoid heart disease occurs in patients with **carcinoid tumors** of the intestine that have metastasized to the liver. Serotonin and other vasoactive substances secreted by such tumors into the hepatic vein escape the inactivation that normally occurs in the liver. These substances reach the heart in venous blood, causing fibrosis of the right ventricular endocardium. Endocardial fibrosis is most prominent in the outflow tract of the right ventricle and the pulmonary valve (Fig. 5.9).

Myocarditis

Myocarditis, or inflammation of the myocardium, may be:

- *Infectious*, caused by bacteria, viruses, protozoa, or other microbial pathogens
- *Toxic*, caused by various bacterial toxins, such as diphtheria toxin, drugs (e.g., certain cytotoxic drugs for cancer), and heavy metals (e.g., cobalt)
- *Immunologically* mediated, as in rheumatic fever or transplant rejection
- *Idiopathic* (e.g., giant cell myocarditis)

Viruses are the most common cause of myocarditis. Among these pathogens, the most prominent are *Coxsackie B virus* and *influenza virus*. **Viral myocarditis** presents histologically as focal myocytolysis accompanied by infiltrates of lymphocytes and macrophages (Fig. 5.10).

Myocarditis of **Chagas disease** is caused by ***Trypanosoma cruzi,*** a protozoon that is endemic in South America. Trypanosoma tends to invade myocardial cells and cause myocarditis (Fig. 5.11).

Myocarditis is a common complication of ***acquired immunodeficiency syndrome (AIDS).*** Approximately 50% of all patients dying of AIDS have myocarditis. This infection may be caused by *Toxoplasma gondii, Sarcosporidia, Mycobacterium avium intracellulare,* and various fungi such as *Histoplasma capsulatum, Coccidioides immitis,* and other opportunistic pathogens. Bacterial abscesses caused by *Staphylococcus* or *Streptococcus* may also be formed (Fig. 5.12).

Immunologically mediated myocarditis is found in cardiac transplants (Fig. 5.13). Transplant rejection is a cell-mediated reaction. It may be mild and present with a few cell infiltrates, or severe, causing diffuse myocarditis.

Idiopathic myocarditis may resemble viral myocarditis. It may be characterized also by eosinophils (eosinophilic myocarditis) or giant cells (giant cell myocarditis) (Fig. 5.14).

Cardiomyopathy

Cardiomyopathy is a term used for a group of noninflammatory diseases of the heart, which can be classified, as shown in Diagram 5.7, into three groups: congestive (dilated), hypertrophic, and constrictive/restrictive.

Congestive Cardiomyopathy. Congestive cardiomyopathy presents with marked dilatation of cardiac chambers. It has no typical histological features. The dilatation of the heart is often associated with prominent subendocardial fibrosis extending into the myocardium (Fig. 5.15). Mural thrombi are a common complication.

Hypertrophic Cardiomyopathy. Hypertrophic cardiomyopathy, also known as *hypertrophic subaortic stenosis*, is inherited as an autosomal dominant trait in approximately 50% of cases. This disease causes hypertrophy of ventricular myocardium, which often produces asymmetrical thickening of the interventricular septum. Histologically, this form of cardiomyopathy is characterized by myocyte hypertrophy and disorganization of myocardial bundles (Fig. 5.16). Nevertheless, similar histologic changes can be found in other hypertrophic hearts and are therefore not pathognomonic of this cardiomyopathy. Inborn errors of metabolism, such as glycogenosis or hemosiderosis, can also cause hypertrophic cardiomyopathy. Glycogenosis type II (Pompe disease) is characterized by infiltration of myocardial cells with glycogen (Fig. 5.17). In hemosiderosis, the myocardial cells contain large amounts of hemosiderin (Fig. 1.18).

Restrictive/Constrictive Cardiomyopathy. Restrictive/constrictive cardiomyopathy is characterized by interstitial infiltrates that cause thickening of the myocardium. Mural thickening prevents the dilatation of the ventricles. The infiltrating material could be fibrous connective tissue as in diffuse endomyocardial fibroelastosis or amyloid (Fig. 5.19).

Pericarditis

Pericarditis is an inflammation of the parietal and visceral layers of the pericardial cavity, i.e., both epicardium and pericardium. The inflammation can be due to infectious (e.g., viruses, bacteria) or noninfectious causes, such as rheumatic fever, systemic lupus erythematosus, uremia, radiation injury, trauma, and surgery ("postcardiotomy pericarditis").

Pericarditis may present as a serous, serofibrinous, fibrinohemorrhagic, or fibrinopurulent exudate. It is usually accompanied by accumulation of fluid in the pericardial cavity, which together with the surface inflammation may restrict the normal diastolic dilatation of the chambers (*constrictive pericarditis*). This may become more prominent during the chronic stages of pericarditis, which typically lead to fibrosis and obliteration of the pericardial cavity.

Histologically, the mesothelial layer of the epicardium, which may be destroyed or partially disrupted, is covered with a fibrin-rich exudate. Underneath the fibrin is an inflammatory infiltrate (Fig. 5.20). Minor inflammation heals without any residual changes. Copious exudate is organized by an ingrowth of granulation tissue. Finally, the granulation tissue transforms into a collagenous scar that may result in formation of dense fibrous adhesions between the epicardium and pericardium (constrictive pericarditis) (Fig. 5.21).

Tuberculous pericarditis, which was common previously but is rare today, presents with broad areas of caseating necrosis and scattered granulomas (Fig. 5.22).

Tumors of the Heart and Blood Vessels

Tumors of the heart are rare. The most common benign tumor is **myxoma**. It typically occurs in the left atrium, and grows as a pedunculated mass from the mural or valvular endocardium into the chamber. On gross examination, myxomas appear gelatinous and are either yellowish-white or blood-tinged red. Histologically, myxomas are composed of loose connective tissue rich in mucopolysaccharides, capillaries, scattered fibroblasts, and smooth muscle cells (Fig. 5.23).

Malignant tumors of the heart are usually **metastases** from adjacent thoracic organs, such as the lungs, breast, and esophagus, or from distant sites (e.g., melanoma and lymphoma) (Fig. 5.24). Such tumors may involve any part of the heart. If located on the epicardium, these tumors are associated with pericardial effusion. Tumor cells can be found in aspirated pericardial fluid.

Tumors may originate from blood vessels. Such tumors may be benign (**hemangioma**) or malignant (**angiosarcoma**). **Angiofibroma** is a vascular tumor of the upper airways of young men (Fig. 5.25). Vascular tumors are commonly diagnosed in the skin, but may occur in any organ or tissue.

Diseases of the Aorta

The most important disease of the aorta is atherosclerosis, which was described previously (see Figs. 5.1 to 5.3). Atherosclerosis can involve all parts of the aorta. However, the abdominal aorta is most commonly affected by this process, which is typically complicated by calcifications and thrombosis and may lead to aneurysm formation (Diagram 5.8).

Among the degenerative diseases of clinical significance, one should mention cystic medial necrosis and the various congenital defects of connective tissue such as *Marfan syndrome*. Inflammatory diseases of the aorta may be infectious, such as syphilitic aortitis, or autoimmune, such as giant cell arteritis (*Takayasu disease*).

Cystic medial necrosis is a disease of unknown origin marked by degenerative changes in the media of the aorta. Slits and cystic spaces form between the layers of the aorta because of fragmentation of elastic fibers in the vessel wall (Fig. 5.26). The media is most often affected and shows accumulation of acid mucopolysaccharides between the fragmented and separated elastic fibers.

However, these changes are nonspecific and may occur in aorta affected by other diseases, including atherosclerosis and hypertension. *Marfan syndrome* is associated with similar changes.

Syphilis affects small nutrient blood vessels of the aorta (*vasa vasorum*). This obliterative microvasculitis causes multiple microscopic mural infarcts, which on gross examination cause the intima to resemble tree bark. This is most prominent in the ascending aorta and the arch of the aorta. Histologically, the small blood vessels of the tunica adventitia and media are surrounded by infiltrates of lymphocytes and plasma cells (Fig. 5.27). Additionally, they have narrowed or obliterated lumina (*obliterative vasculitis*). Weakening of the vessel wall predisposes to the formation of aneurysms,

which are usually saccular and affect the thoracic aorta.

Diseases of Peripheral Arteries and Veins

Small arteries and arterioles are especially susceptible to adverse effects of **hypertension**. Sustained chronic hypertension causes hyalinization of arterioles and initial fibrosis of arteries (Fig. 5.28). Sudden onset of hypertension (malignant hypertension) causes fibrinoid necrosis and hyperplastic arteriolitis (Fig. 5.29).

The most important disease of veins is thrombosis. It may begin as thrombosis of the veins (**phlebothrombosis**), or the clot formation may be secondary to the inflammation of the venous wall (**thrombophlebitis**). In a thrombosed vein that shows inflammation of its wall, it is impossible to tell which started first—thrombosis or inflammation. Venous thrombi are described in Chapter 3.

Vasculitis

Vasculitis includes immunologically mediated diseases and diseases of unknown etiology, all of which are characterized by a bacteriologically sterile inflammation of vessel walls. Vasculitis may involve the aorta and the major branches (*giant cell arteritis/Takayasu disease*); large elastic arteries; medium-sized and small arteries (*polyarteritis nodosa, Wegener granulomatosis, Kawasaki disease*); or venules, capillaries, and arterioles (*hypersensitivity vasculitis*). *Thromboangiitis obliterans* or *Buerger disease* involves medium-sized arteries and adjacent veins and nerves, usually in the lower extremities.

Giant cell arteritis most often affects the temporal artery, but it may involve other medium-sized vessels or the aorta (Takayasu disease). It is characterized by focal destruction of the elastic lamina by granulomatous inflammation in the vessel wall. The granulomas consist of macrophages, giant cells, and lymphocytes (Fig. 5.30).

Polyarteritis nodosa is caused by immune complexes formed between antibodies and antigen in the walls of the medium and small arteries. This reaction leads to the activation of complement. Consequent inflammation is mediated by inflammatory cells attracted to the site by chemotactic products of complement activation.

Histologically, the acute phase of the disease is characterized by focal fibrinoid necrosis and inflammation (Fig. 5.31). The inflammation heals but causes defects in the vessel wall, rupture of the lamina elastic interna or externa, and formation of microaneurysms.

Buerger disease, or *thromboangiitis obliterans*, is a disease of unknown origin that often affects certain ethnic groups (East European Jews, Indians). The disease is somehow related to tobacco products because it occurs almost exclusively in cigarette smokers. The disease affects the medium-sized and small arteries of the extremities and presents with thrombosis and inflammation of the vessel wall (Fig. 5.32). Microabscesses may also be seen in the vessel wall. The disease often extends to adjacent veins and may involve the major nerves as well.

Hypersensitivity (leukocytoclastic) vasculitis is an immune-mediated inflammation of small blood vessels, i.e., arterioles, venules, and capillaries. This systemic disease is typically associated with skin purpura and is often diagnosed by skin biopsy (Fig. 5.33).

PLATE 5.1. ATHEROSCLEROSIS

Figure 5.1. Early lesions of atherosclerosis. A. Accumulation of fat in intima. In paraffin-embedded tissue, the fat is wasted out, leaving behind empty space. Intima also contains fat-laden foamy macrophages. **B.** Intimal plaque composed of smooth muscle cells and fibroblasts.

Figure 5.2. Atheroma of aorta consists of amorphous material and "empty" spaces that previously contained lipid-rich material. Cholesterol clefts are recognized by their typical needle-shaped appearance.

Figure 5.3. Complicated atheroma. Calcification imparts a bluish tinge to the fibrosed vessel wall. A small thrombus (*T*) is seen in the lumen.

Diagram 5.2. Pathogenesis of atherosclerosis. A. Endothelial injury is accompanied by the attachment of monocytes, platelets, and thrombus formation. **B.** Macrophages in the intima phagocytize lipid and transform into foam cells. Macrophages also secrete growth factors that stimulate the proliferation of smooth muscle cells. **C.** Ruptured atheromas release thrombogenic material into the circulation, causing thrombus formation over the intimal ulceration.

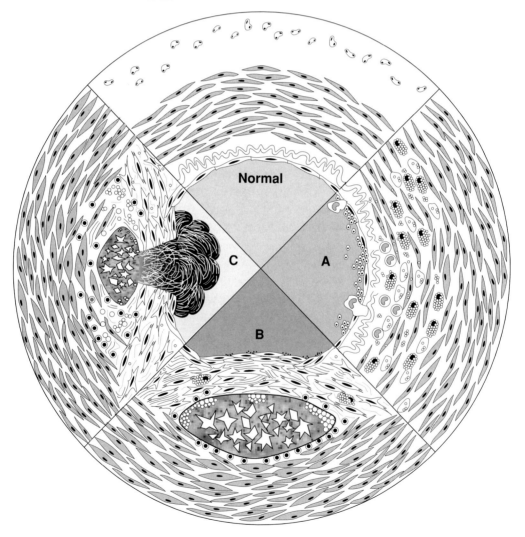

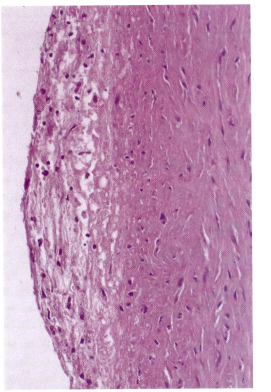

Figure 5.1A

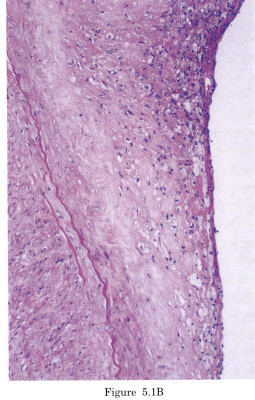

Figure 5.1B

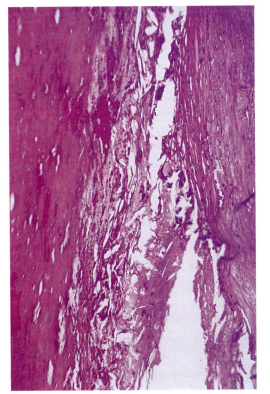

Figure 5.2

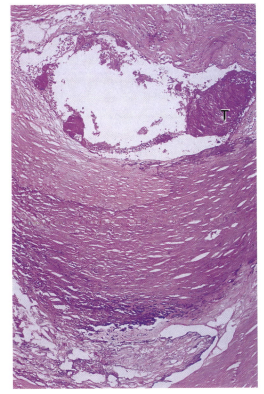

Figure 5.3

PLATE 5.2. CORONARY ATHEROSCLEROSIS AND MYOCARDIAL INFARCTS

Figure 5.4. Coronary thrombosis. The lumen of the vessel is occluded by a thrombus that developed over ruptured atheroma.

Figure 5.5. Myocardial infarct. A. Ten hours after occlusion of the coronary artery, the necrotic myocardial cells have lost their nuclei and appear eosinophilic in contrast to normal myocardial cells, which are seen to the right. **B.** Two-day-old myocardial infarct is infiltrated with neutrophils. **C.** Seven days after onset of anoxia, the necrotic myocardial cells have been removed and the field contains only macrophages, connective tissue, and blood vessels. **D.** Six weeks after onset of anoxia, a mature, acellular scar is formed, replacing the damaged myocardial cells.

Diagram 5.3. Myocardial infarct. Transmural infarcts are localized to defined anatomical sites corresponding to the supply areas of one of the three main coronary arteries. Hypotensive subendocardial infarcts are usually circumferential and do not correspond to an anatomical region supplied by a specific coronary artery. **A.** Occlusion of the descending branch of the left coronary artery. **B.** Occlusion of the circumflex branch of the left coronary artery. **C.** Occlusion of the right coronary artery. **D.** Hypotensive subendocardial infarct without any major artery occlusion.

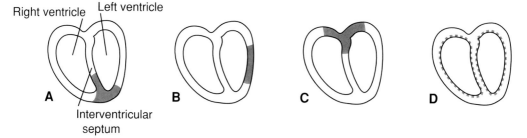

Diagram 5.4. Temporal sequence in the appearance of cells infiltrating a myocardial infarct.

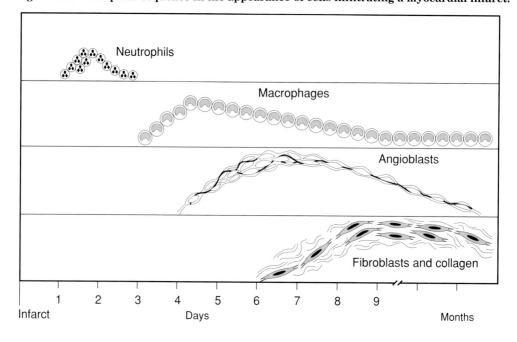

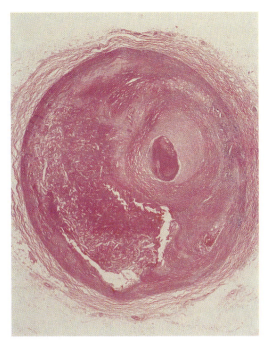

Figure 5.4

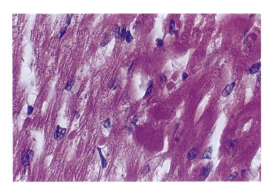

Figure 5.5A

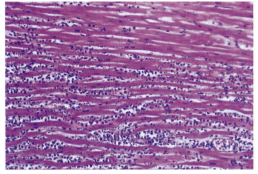

Figure 5.5B

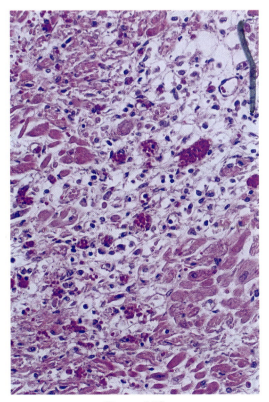

Figure 5.5C

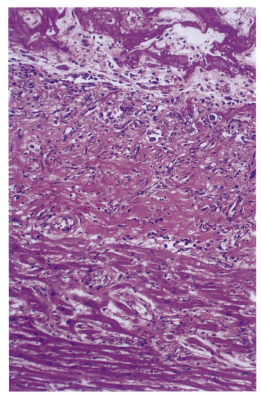

Figure 5.5D

PLATE 5.3. RHEUMATIC CARDITIS

Figure 5.6.   Rheumatic carditis. A. Acute endocarditis is characterized by thrombotic vegetations attached to the endocardial surface of the valve. The leaflet appears edematous, vascularized, and infiltrated with inflammatory cells. **B.** Aschoff body in the myocardium. It is composed of modified macrophages and a few scattered lymphocytes. **C.** Healing of rheumatic myocarditis leads to myocardial fibrosis and spindle-shaped scar formation. A few residual Aschoff bodies can be seen occasionally. **D.** Rheumatic pericarditis is characterized by exudation of fibrin. Granulation tissue grows into this exudate obliterating the pericardial cavity.

Diagram 5.5.   Rheumatic fever. Sensitization to streptococcal antigens during an upper respiratory tract infection elicits an untoward response characterized by the formation of antibodies to the body's own tissues and a cell-mediated immune reaction. Cardiac lesions include **endocarditis** (*verrucous valvulitis*), **myocarditis** with typical Aschoff bodies, and fibrinous **pericarditis.** Healing of inflammatory lesions results in fibrosis.

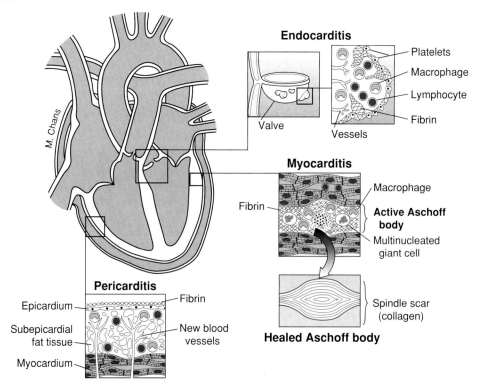

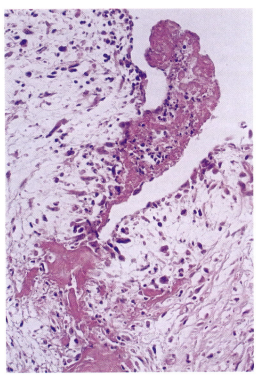

Figure 5.6A

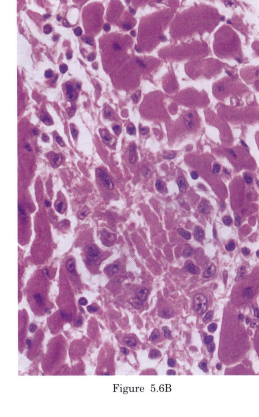

Figure 5.6B

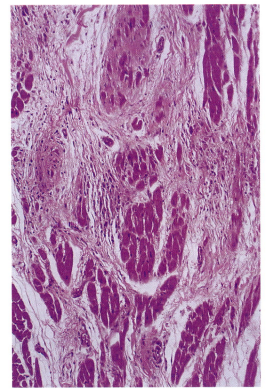

Figure 5.6C

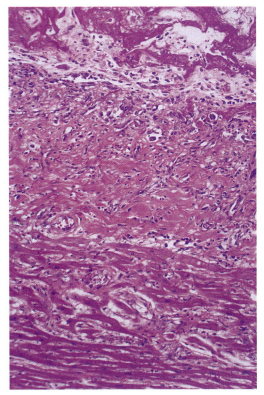

Figure 5.6D

PLATE 5.4. ENDOCARDITIS

Figure 5.7. Acute bacterial endocarditis. A. Acute inflammatory cells cover the endocardium. The surface of the exudate consists of fibrin and bacteria. **B.** Thrombotic vegetation contains numerous bacteria (blue).

Figure 5.8. Nonbacterial thrombotic endocarditis. An aggregate of fibrin covers the surface of the valve.

Figure 5.9. Carcinoid heart disease. The endocardium is marked by thickening due to fibrosis.

Diagram 5.6. Various forms of endocarditis. Bacterial endocarditis preferentially involves the aortic and mitral valves, except in drug addicts, who show a predilection to right-sided valvulitis. Mural endocarditis in most often a complication of congenital heart disease.

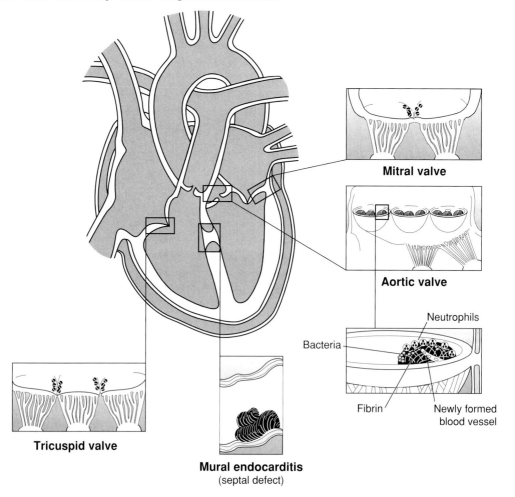

Mitral valve

Aortic valve

Neutrophils

Bacteria

Fibrin

Newly formed blood vessel

Tricuspid valve

Mural endocarditis
(septal defect)

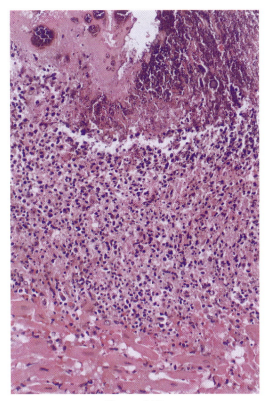

Figure 5.7A

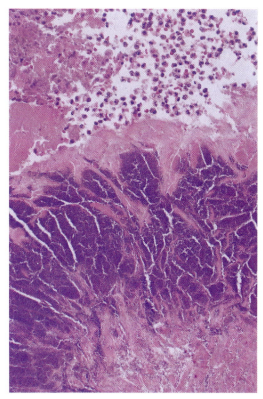

Figure 5.7B

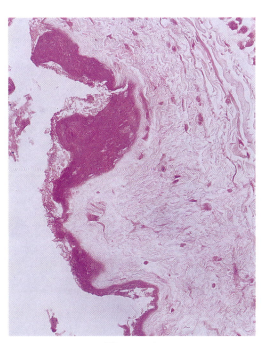

Figure 5.8

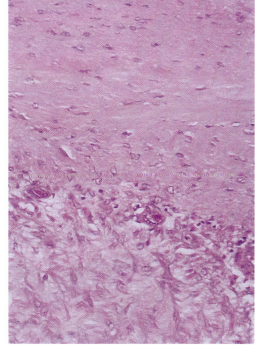

Figure 5.9

PLATE 5.5. MYOCARDITIS

Figure 5.10. Viral myocarditis. A. Infiltrates of mononuclear cells are scattered in the myocardium. **B.** The inflammatory cells and interstitial edema separate myocardial cells, some of which are undergoing necrosis.

Figure 5.11. Chagas disease. Myocardial cells contain the protozoon *Trypanosoma cruzi.*

Figure 5.12. Bacterial abscess in the myocardium in AIDS.

Figure 5.13. Cardiac transplant rejection. The myocardium is focally infiltrated with lymphocytes and macrophages.

Figure 5.14. Giant cell myocarditis. The infiltrate replacing myocardial cells consists of lymphocytes, macrophages, and multinucleated giant cells.

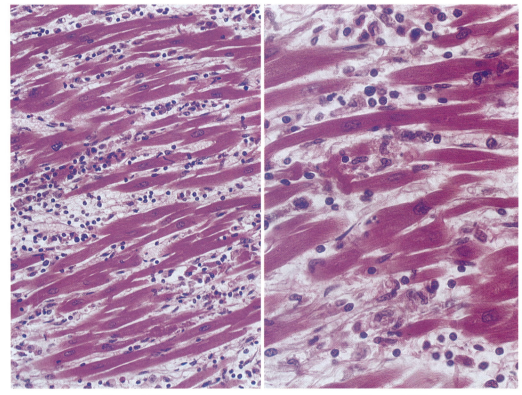

Figure 5.10A   Figure 5.10B

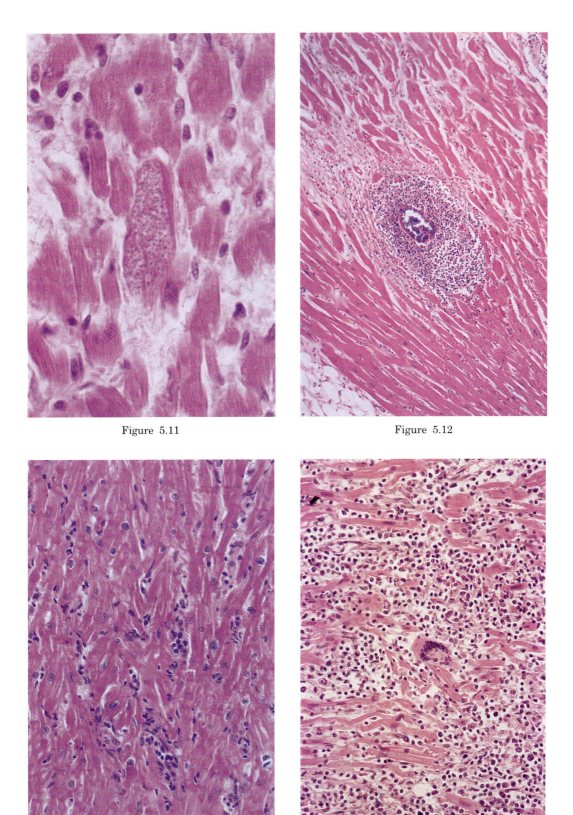

Figure 5.11

Figure 5.12

Figure 5.13

Figure 5.14

PLATE 5.6. CARDIOMYOPATHY

Figure 5.15.   Congestive dilated cardiomyopathy. Endocardial fibrosis extends into the myocardium.

Figure 5.17.   Pompe disease. This genetic disorder of metabolism is characterized by accumulation of glycogen in the myocardium. The myocardial cells appear pale.

Figure 5.19.   Cardiac amyloidosis. A. Amyloid deposits appear like homogeneous eosinophilic material. **B.** This slide, stained with Congo red and photographed under polarizing light, shows birefringent greenish material in the interstitial spaces and in the wall of the vessels. The collagen is also birefringent but it appears as white fluorescing fibers.

Figure 5.16.   Autosomal dominant hereditary cardiomyopathy. The myocardial cells are hypertropic and are in disarray, rather than regular bundles.

Figure 5.18.   Hemosiderosis. The specimen in this slide was stained with the Prussian blue reaction. The myocardial cell contains the prominent blue granules of hemosiderin in their cytoplasm.

Diagram 5.7.   Cardiomyopathy. A. Normal heart. **B.** Congestive (dilated) cardiomyopathy. **C.** Hypertrophic cardiomyopathy. **D.** Restrictive cardiomyopathy.

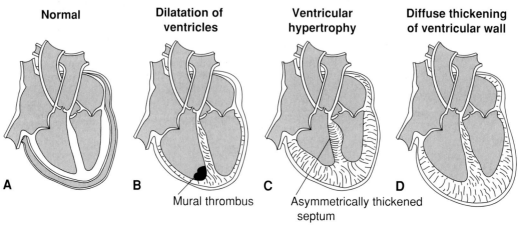

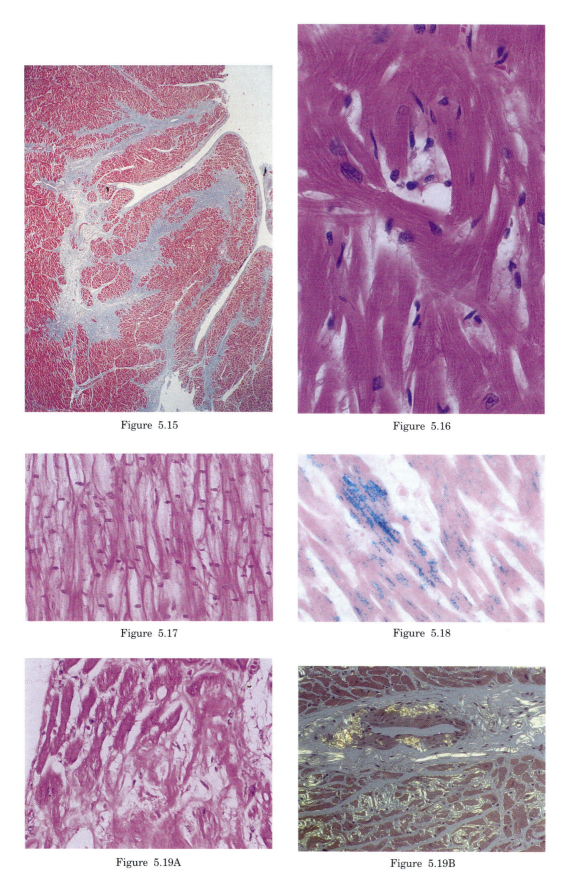

Figure 5.15

Figure 5.16

Figure 5.17

Figure 5.18

Figure 5.19A

Figure 5.19B

PLATE 5.7. PERICARDITIS

Figure 5.20.   Fibrinous pericarditis. A. The inflamed pericardium is covered with fibrin. **B.** Organizing fibrinous pericarditis is characterized by granulation tissue that invades the fibrin and obliterates the pericardial cavity.

Figure 5.21.   Epicardial fibrosis. The epicardium shows fibrovascular scarring.

Figure 5.22.   Tuberculous pericarditis. There is extensive caseous necrosis surrounded by granuloma. The surface of epicardium is covered with fibrin (top).

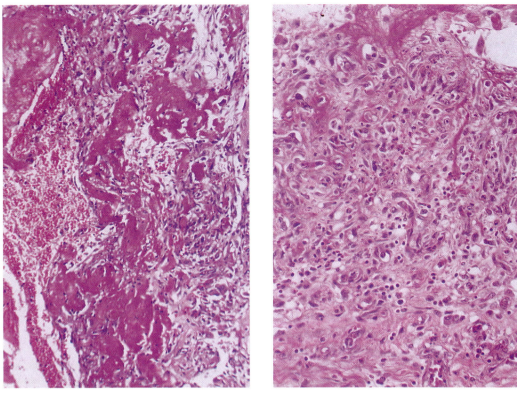

Figure 5.20A Figure 5.20B

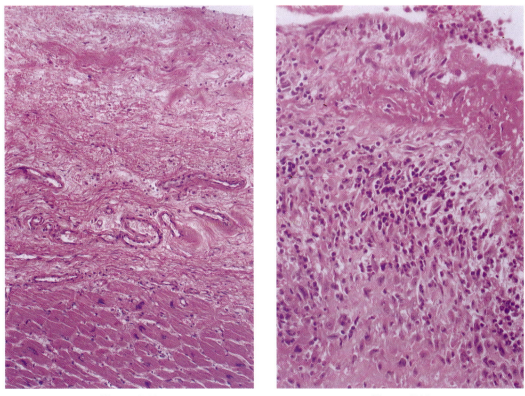

Figure 5.21 Figure 5.22

PLATE 5.8. NEOPLASMS OF THE CARDIOVASCULAR SYSTEM

Figure 5.23. Myxoma of the heart. This benign tumor is composed of loosely arranged elongated and stellate mesenchymal cells, macrophages, and blood vessels embedded in a loose stroma.

Figure 5.24. Metastatic carcinoma in the heart.

Figure 5.25. Tumors of blood vessels. A. Angiofibroma is a nasopharyngeal tumor composed of dilated blood vessels, surrounded by fibroblasts. **B.** Angiosarcoma composed of malignant spindle cells forming irregular vascular spaces.

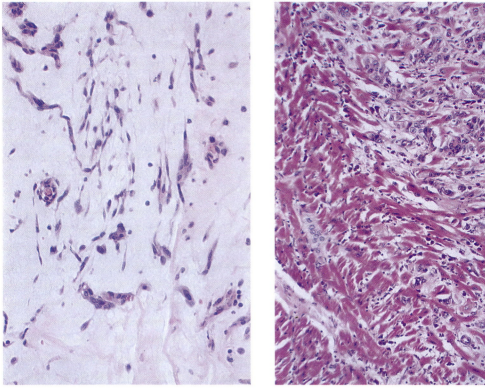

Figure 5.23

Figure 5.24

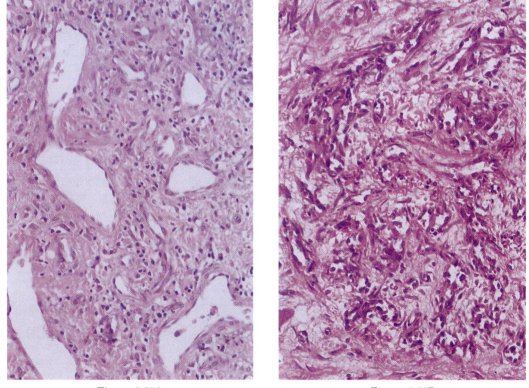

Figure 5.25A

Figure 5.25B

PLATE 5.9. DISEASES OF THE AORTA AND ITS MAJOR BRANCHES

Figure 5.26.   Cystic medial necrosis of the aorta. A. The elastic fibers of the media are separated from one another by loose amorphous material. **B.** Dissecting aneurysm develops because of blood entering between the layers of the aortic wall. **C.** Elastic stain better shows the fraying and separation of layers of the vessel wall.

Figure 5.27.   Syphilitic aortitis. A. The *vasa vasorum* are surrounded by lymphocytes and plasma cells. **B.** Elastic stain shows foci of destruction and loss of elastic fibers in the media.

Diagram 5.8.   Diseases involving the aorta. A. Atherosclerosis is most prominent in the abdominal aorta, where it may produce aneurysms. **B.** Cystic medial necrosis and Marfan syndrome are marked by dissecting aneurysms. Dissecting aneurysms also develop as a complication of atherosclerosis and hypertension. **C.** Syphilis causes aneurysms of the thoracic aorta. **D.** Giant cell aortitis involves the aortic arch and major branches originating from it.

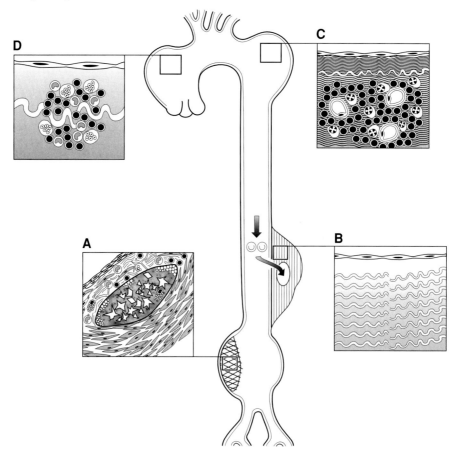

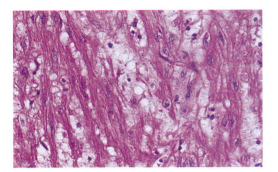

Figure 5.26A

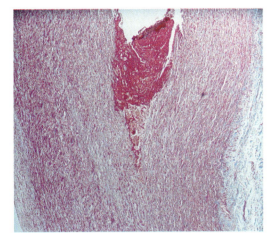

Figure 5.26B

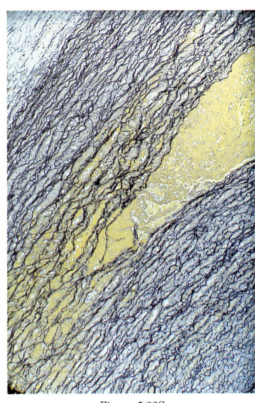

Figure 5.26C

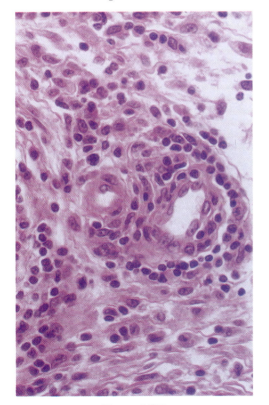

Figure 5.27A

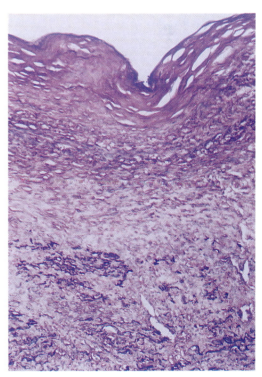

Figure 5.27B

PLATE 5.10. VASCULAR CHANGES CAUSED BY HYPERTENSION

Figure 5.28.   Benign hypertension. The arteriole shows hyalinosis of its wall and narrowing of the lumen.

Figure 5.29.   Malignant hypertension. A. Concentric layering of smooth muscle cells in small renal arteries and arterioles. **B.** Fibrinoid necrosis of afferent arteriole of the glomerulus. **C.** A parallel slide stained with fluorescein-treated antibodies to fibrin shows that the wall of the vessel is impregnated with fibrin (yellow).

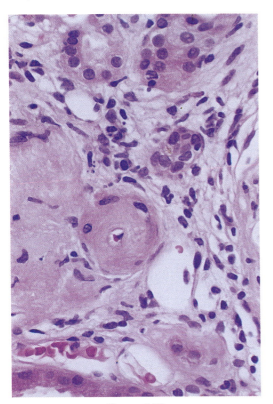

Figure 5.28

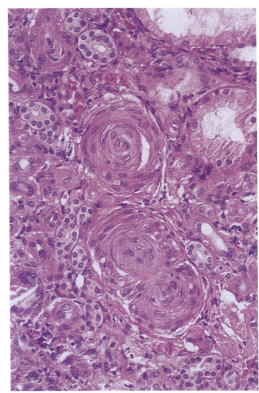

Figure 5.29A

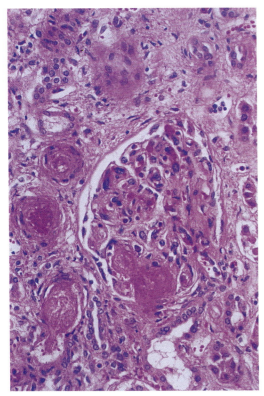

Figure 5.29B

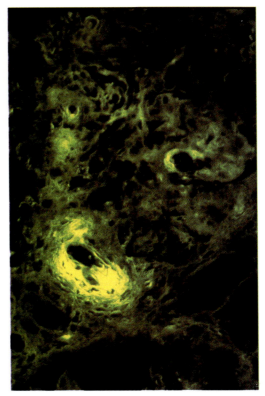

Figure 5.29C

PLATE 5.11. VASCULITIS

Figure 5.30. **Giant cell arteritis. A.** The wall of the aorta is infiltrated with macrophages, giant cells, and lymphocytes. **B.** Higher-magnification view of the granuloma shows numerous multinucleated giant cells.

Figure 5.31. **Polyarteritis nodosa. A.** The acute phase of the disease is characterized by fibrinoid necrosis and inflammation. **B.** In the chronic phase, the vessel shows focal destruction of the elastic laminae.

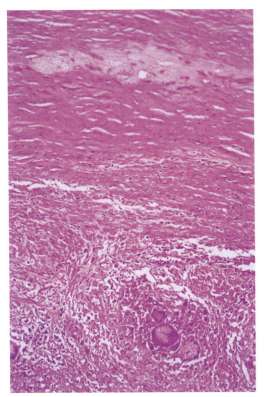

Figure 5.30A

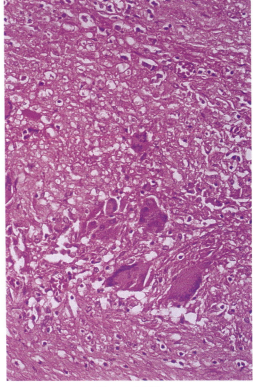

Figure 5.30B

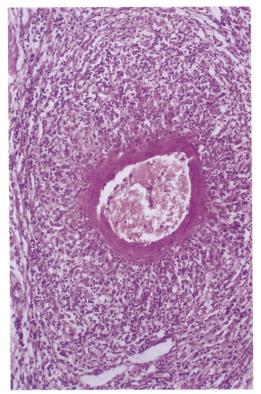

Figure 5.31A

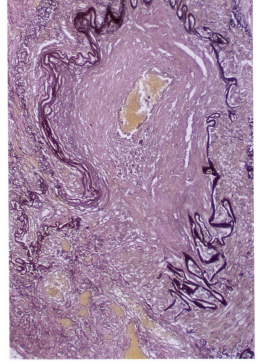

Figure 5.31B

PLATE 5.12. VASCULITIS

Figure 5.32.   Buerger disease. A. The artery is obliterated and the vein has a thickened fibrosed wall. The vessels are surrounded by fibrous tissue also encasing the nerve. **B.** The lumen of this previously thrombosed artery has been recanalized with newly formed blood vessels. **C.** The site of attachment of the thrombus to the vessel wall contains a microabscess. The inflammation extends through the vessel wall into the surrounding tissue (bottom portion of the photograph).

Figure 5.33.   Hypersensitivity vasculitis. The wall of the dermal small vessels is infiltrated with neutrophils ("leukocytoclastic reaction"). Extravasation of red blood cells causes purpura.

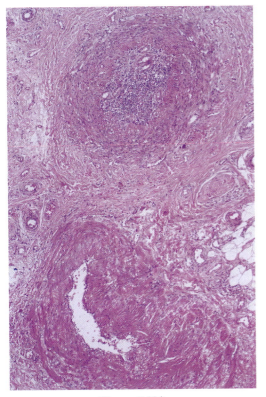

Figure 5.32A

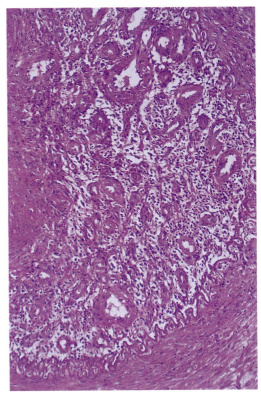

Figure 5.32B

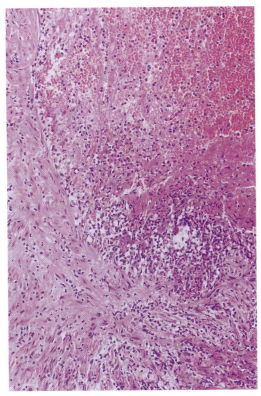

Figure 5.32C

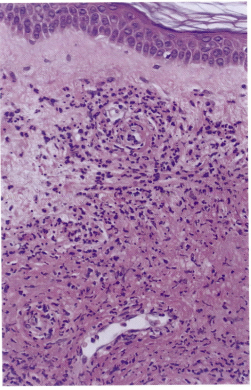

Figure 5.33

NOTES

CHAPTER 6

Pulmonary System

NORMAL HISTOLOGY

The respiratory system includes the nose, the pharynx, and the larynx, called the *upper respiratory tract*; and the trachea and the major bronchi and the lungs, called the *lower respiratory tract* (Diagram 6.1).

The nasal mucosa is lined by stratified squamous epithelium in the vestibule and by pseudostratified ciliated columnar epithelium in the respiratory and the olfactory regions. The pharynx, which is common to both the respiratory and the digestive systems, is lined by pseudostratified ciliated epithelium in the upper part (nasopharynx) and squamous epithelium in the lower part. The upper part of the larynx is lined by squamous epithelium and the lower part with pseudostratified ciliated columnar epithelium. Pseudostratified ciliated columnar epithelium also lines the trachea and the major bronchi. The bronchioles are lined by simple columnar cuboidal epithelium, which extends all the way to the terminal bronchioles and parts of the respiratory bronchioles. The alveoli are lined by simple flattened cells (pneumocytes type I, which allow passage of gasses from the inhaled air into the circulation and vice versa) and by cuboidal cells (pneumocytes type II, which secrete pulmonary surfactant). Approximately 90% of the alveolar surface is lined by pneumocytes type I. The lung is encased in pleura, which consists of mesothelium and underlying connective tissue.

The respiratory mucosa is in most parts enclosed by submucosa and support structures. In the upper respiratory tract, the external layers contain striated muscle and, in many places, cartilage. Cartilage is found in the nose and larynx. The trachea, major bronchi, and their intrapulmonary branches also contain cartilage. Bronchioli and the air passages distal to them do not contain cartilage in their walls. The alveolar wells are thin and consist of epithelial cells on both sides of centrally located capillaries with no intervening connective tissue stroma.

OVERVIEW OF PATHOLOGY

The most important diseases of the respiratory system are:

- Diseases that damage alveoli and impede air exchange in alveoli, such as neonatal and adult respiratory distress syndrome
- Infections, such as pneumonia
- Immunological diseases, such as asthma, extrinsic allergic alveolitis, and sarcoidosis
- Diseases related to inhalation of pollutants from air and smoking, such as pneumoconioses and chronic obstructive pulmonary disease
- Neoplasms

Neonatal Lung Diseases

During fetal life, the lungs mature gradually. By the end of pregnancy, the lungs have usually reached a level at which they can maintain respiration if exposed to air. The fetal lungs are filled with amniotic fluid, which is expectorated upon delivery. If the respiratory movements of the neonate are weak, the amniotic fluid will remain in the alveoli (Fig. 6.1). This is incorrectly called **amniotic fluid aspiration**, although it actually represents inadequate clearance of amniotic fluid from the neonatal lungs.

Neonatal respiratory distress syndrome, also known as *hyaline membrane disease,* develops in prematurely born infants as a consequence of pulmonary immaturity (Diagram 6.2). Because of inadequate production of pulmonary surfactant by the pneumocytes type II, the alveoli of the newborn infant do not open to maintain respiration and remain collapsed. Owing to the atelectasis of alveoli, gas exchange occurs through the epithelium of alveolar ducts and respiratory bronchioli, which is injured in this process and undergoes necrosis. Necrotic cells are sloughed off and the defects are covered with fibrin, which forms the so-called *hyaline membranes* (Fig. 6.2). Hyaline membranes may show brownish tinge from meconium. Such brown hyaline membranes are found in infants born after

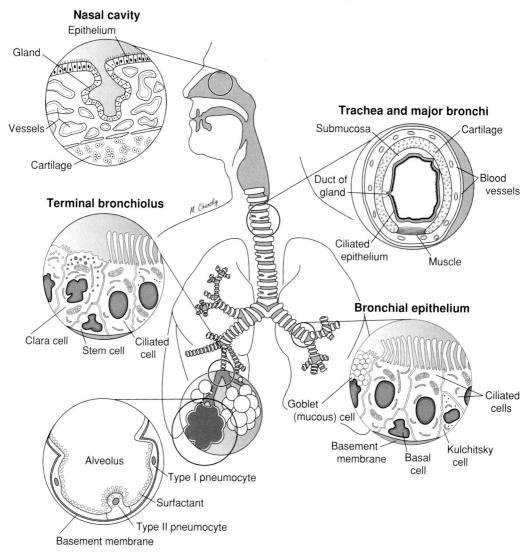

Diagram 6.1. Normal respiratory system.

Nasal cavity
Epithelium
Gland
Vessels
Cartilage

Trachea and major bronchi
Submucosa
Cartilage
Duct of gland
Blood vessels
Ciliated epithelium
Muscle

Terminal bronchiolus
M. Chansky

Clara cell
Stem cell
Ciliated cell

Bronchial epithelium

Goblet (mucous) cell
Ciliated cells
Basement membrane
Basal cell
Kulchitsky cell

Alveolus
Type I pneumocyte
Surfactant
Type II pneumocyte
Basement membrane

prolonged labor and intrauterine anoxia accompanied by a discharge of meconium into the amniotic fluid.

Adult Respiratory Syndrome

Adult respiratory distress syndrome (ARDS), also known as *diffuse alveolar damage (DAD)*, results from acute injury of the alveoli and the breakdown of the alveolar air-blood barrier. The injury can be initiated by inhalants that damage the alveolar lining cells or by endogenous mediators of inflammation that damage the endothelial cells in the alveolar capillaries (Diagram 6.2). Cell injury allows transudation of the fluid into the alveoli and formation of pulmonary edema, which is rich in fibrin. Fibrin contributes to the formation of hyaline membranes that cover the damaged alveolar epithelium or the defects that have developed because of alveolar cell necrosis (Fig. 6.3). Despite the high mortality of ARDS, some patients survive and show signs of repair of the alveolar damage. The hyaline membranes are organized by the ingrowing granulation tissue, which, however, obliterates the respiratory spaces. Such lung injury is permanent since the normal alveolar structure has not been restored. Dyspnea persists for life because of a loss injury of alveolar respiratory surfaces.

Pneumonia

Pneumonia is an infection of the lungs that may occur in several forms and can be classified according to several criteria:

- Duration—acute or chronic
- Etiology—bacterial, viral, fungal, or protozoal
- Location of lesions—alveolar or interstitial
- Extent of lesions—lobular or lobar

In general terms, bacterial and fungal infections are characterized by intra-alveolar exudates, whereas viruses and *Mycoplasma pneumoniae* cause pneumonia that is predominantly interstitial.

Bacterial pneumonia usually begins in the bronchi and adjacent alveoli of a single lobule (Diagram 6.3). Such localized lobular pneumonia is also called **bronchopneumonia** (Fig. 6.4) to indicate that bronchi are also involved and filled with inflammatory exudate. The bronchial exudate is expectorated and accounts for the purulent sputum typically found in such patients.

In debilitated, immunocompromised patients or those whose natural defenses are weakened, such as alcoholics, the infection of the lungs tends to spread through the entire lobe, resulting in **lobar pneumonia** (Fig. 6.5). Virulent organisms may also cause massive destruction of the pulmonary parenchyma, resulting in necrotizing pneumonia. Pathogens such as *Staphylococcus aureus* tend to produce pulmonary **abscesses** (Fig. 6.6).

Viral pneumonia is characterized by alveolar cell injury (Diagram 6.4), which usually elicits a predominantly interstitial inflammatory infiltrate (Fig. 6.7). The damaged alveolar septa are leaky, and this results in the formation of intra-alveolar edema. The loss of damaged alveolar cells causes defects that are covered with fibrin. Fibrin exudation contributes to the formation of hyaline membranes. Viruses are not seen in routine histology sections except for cytomegalovirus, which forms intranuclear and intracytoplasmic inclusions and enlargement of the infected cells.

***Pneumocystis carinii* pneumonia** is a common complication of AIDS, but it occurs in many other conditions characterized by immunosuppression and extreme debilitation. This parasite has low invasiveness and remains inside the alveoli, causing a protein-rich exudate, which typically has a bubbly appearance (Fig. 6.8). The cysts and sporozoites of *Pneumocystis carinii* can be recognized in this exudate by special stains (e.g., silver impregnation) or immunohistochemically. The inflammatory response to the infection includes lymphocytes, plasma cells, and macrophages, which are confined to the alveolar septa. In terminally ill, immunosuppressed AIDS patients, this inflammatory response may be very weak or nonexistent.

Pulmonary tuberculosis is the most common human form of infection with *Mycobacterium tuberculosis* (Diagram 6.5). The infection begins as a localized pulmonary inflammation extending to bronchial lymph nodes (*Ghon complex*). It is characterized by the formation of necrotizing granulomas (Fig. 6.9) called *caseous granulomas* because of their cheese-like appearance. Such granulomas contain *M. tuberculosis*, demonstrable by special stains. These granulomas may heal and transform into fibrotic scars. Granulomas also tend to become confluent, destroying the parenchyma and giving rise to large cavities (*cavernous tuberculosis*). The wall of these cavities is composed of fibrous tissue and contains active and healing granulomas. Healing granulomas often calcify.

Widespread dissemination of *M. tuberculosis* through the lymphatic or blood circulation or through the airways results in the formation of numerous small nodules the size of millet seeds, which are therefore called *miliary tubercles*. These have the same histological appearance as the primary granulomas in the Ghon complex and may show extensive necrosis with a scant inflammatory response.

Fungal pneumonia is also found in immunocompromised and debilitated persons, but in some forms (e.g., histoplasmosis), it may occur in persons with no known risk factors. The most important pathogens are *Candida albicans, Aspergillus fumigatus,*

Histoplasma capsulatum, and *Coccidioides immitis.* The infection may produce several forms of inflammatory reaction, which depend on the type of fungus and the host response. *Candida* and *Aspergillus* tend to grow in the bronchi but may also extend into the alveoli, causing a mixed inflammatory response. *Histoplasma* and *Coccidioides* tend to produce granulomas that may be indistinguishable from tuberculosis. Fungi can be demonstrated in the infected lungs by special stains (Fig. 6.10).

Chronic pneumonia results from incompletely resolved acute lung injuries such as bacterial and viral pneumonia, ARDS, toxic injury, or lung diseases of unknown etiology (Diagram 6.6). Granulation tissue invading the alveoli is most prominent in bacterial pneumonias and is characterized by massive exudation of fibrin. This fibrin cannot be easily reabsorbed and serves as a template for the ingrowing granulation tissue formed from angioblasts and fibroblasts (Fig. 6.11). The massive pulmonary tissue destruction by virulent pathogens cannot be repaired, and the granulation tissue that grows into the damaged area completely obliterates the normal architecture, to the extent that few normal tissue components are retained (Fig. 6.12).

Bronchiolitis obliterans-organizing pneumonia (BOOP) is a form of focal chronic pneumonia involving the bronchioli and adjacent alveoli. It represents a nonspecific reaction to injury caused by a variety of pathogens, most of which are usually not identified clinically. BOOP is characterized by an obstruction of bronchioli with granulation tissues (Fig. 6.13). Obstruction of the airways impedes the discharge of pulmonary surfactant, other secretions, and cellular detritus, which are taken up by macrophages. This results in *endogenous lipid pneumonia.*

Immunological Lung Diseases

The respiratory system may be affected by all four types of immune-mediated hypersensitivity reactions (Diagram 6.7). **Type I reaction** is mediated by immunoglobulin E (IgE) and mast cells. Principal chemical mediators of inflammation are biogenic amines such as histamine and serotonin and arachidonic acid derivatives such as leukotrienes or slow-reacting substances of anaphylaxis (SRS-A). This reaction is the basis for asthma and hay fever. **Type II reaction,** mediated by cytotoxic antibodies, is the basis for Goodpasture syndrome. **Type III reaction,** mediated by immune complexes, is the basis for extrinsic allergic pneumonitis caused by inhaled allergens, as in pigeon breeders' lung disease and farmers' lung. **Type IV reaction,** which is cell-mediated, is characterized by the formation of granulomas and is the basis of sarcoidosis or berylliosis.

Asthma is a chronic allergic disease affecting the bronchi and bronchioli (Fig. 6.14). Histologically, it is characterized by hypersecretion of mucus from hyperplastic mucous cells in the bronchial mucosa and bronchial glands, hypertrophy and hyperplasia of bronchial smooth muscle cells, and chronic inflammation of the bronchial wall. The inflammatory infiltrates in the bronchial wall consist of neutrophils, lymphocytes, macrophages, basophils, and numerous eosinophils.

Extrinsic allergic pneumonitis is an immunological response to inhaled allergens. It is rarely diagnosed in the early stages of the disease, which rapidly evolve into a chronic interstitial pneumonitis. The histological features of allergic pneumonitis are nonspecific, irrespective of its etiology. Occasionally, in response to particulate allergens, the chronic interstitial inflammatory infiltrates will contain not only lymphocytes, plasma cells, and macrophages but also foreign body giant cells (Fig. 6.15).

Sarcoidosis is a disease of unknown etiology characterized by noncaseating granulomas (Fig. 6.16). These granulomas are prototypical of type IV immune reaction, which has prompted the hypothesis that sarcoidosis represents a delayed cell-mediated immune reaction to some unidentified pathogens.

Wegener granulomatosis is an immune disease that involves the lungs, upper respiratory tract, and kidneys. However, the pathogenesis of this disease is not known, and it cannot be classified into one of the above categories of hypersensitivity. In the lungs, Wegener granulomatosis causes a granulomatous angiitis that leads to widespread infarcts and necrosis (Fig. 6.17).

Interstitial Pneumonia and Pneumoconioses

Chronic interstitial pneumonia may develop without obvious reasons, but may also be caused by inhaled minerals. In the former case it is considered idiopathic, and in the latter it is classified as pneumoconiosis.

Idiopathic chronic interstitial pneumonia occurs in several forms, the most important of which are the *usual interstitial pneumonia* (UIP), *desquamative interstitial pneumonia* (DIP), and *lymphocytic interstitial pneumonia* (LIP) (Diagram 6.6).

UIP is the most common of these diseases. It is characterized by patches of alveolar fibrosis and chronic inflammation, adjacent to more or less normal lung parenchyma (Fig. 6.18). This fibrosis distorts the terminal respiratory bronchioli, which are often dilated cystically and conflated with alveolar duct ("honeycomb lung").

DIP is characterized by accumulation of macrophages in the alveoli (Fig. 6.19). Alveolar septa are normal or only slightly inflamed.

Pneumoconioses include a variety of lung diseases that are caused by minerals inhaled in contaminated air, such as silicosis or asbestosis (Diagram 6.8).

Asbestosis is caused by inhaled asbestos fibers that lodge in the terminal airways and cause fibrosis of the lungs (Fig. 6.20). The fibrotic lung parenchyma contains typical asbestos bodies, which appear as brown, beaded rods. Asbestos exposure also results in pleural plaques and predisposes to the formation of lung carcinoma (especially in smokers) and mesothelioma.

Silicosis is a chronic fibrosing lung disease caused by inhaled silicon dioxide crystals (better known as quartz). The disease most often presents with multiple small fibrotic nodules that contain silica and coal particles, **anthracosilicosis**. Such nodules are composed of collagen, fibroblasts, and scattered lymphocytes (Fig. 6.21). Quartz crystals are retained between the fibers and are not evident by routine microscopy but can be seen under polarized light.

Chronic Obstructive Pulmonary Disease

Chronic obstructive pulmonary disease (COPD) includes two closely related entities that often occur together in the same patient: chronic bronchitis and emphysema. Both of these diseases are most often caused by smoking, but many other chronic irritants and chronic infections can produce similar pathological changes. Emphysema also may be caused by a congenital deficiency of alpha-1-antitrypsin.

Chronic bronchitis is characterized by a thickening of the bronchial wall, hyperplasia and hypertrophy of bronchial glands, and chronic inflammation of the bronchial mucosa and submucosa (Diagram 6.9 and Fig. 6.22). The inflammation extends into the bronchioli as well as into the trachea. The surface epithelium may also be thickened and contain prominent goblet cells or it may undergo squamous metaplasia.

Emphysema is a loss of lung parenchyma distal to the terminal bronchioles. Histologically, there are several types of emphysema, the most important of which are the centrolobular emphysema and panacinar emphysema (Diagram 6.10). In histological sections, it is difficult to precisely diagnose the various forms of emphysema. The diagnosis is best made on wholemount preparations of the entire lung or with specially prepared lung tissue examined with a dissecting microscope (Fig. 6.23). Emphysema and chronic bronchitis may be associated with pneumoconioses, as typically seen in coal miners (Fig. 6.24).

Neoplasms

Lung carcinomas account for the vast majority of primary lung tumors. Most of the tumors originate from the bronchial or bronchiolar epithelium and mimic, with some exceptions, the cells normally found in the epithelium (Diagram 6.11).

Several histological types of lung cancer are recognized: squamous cell carcinoma, adenocarcinoma, bronchioloalveolar carcinoma, large cell undifferentiated carcinoma, and small cell carcinoma (oat cell carcinoma). Carcinoid tumors are considered separately because of their low-grade malignant potential. Mesotheliomas originate from the pleura.

Squamous cell carcinoma originates from the bronchial epithelium. Normal bronchi do not contain squamous cells. However, chronic exposure to tobacco smoke leads to squamous metaplasia, which may gradually evolve into carcinoma in situ and invasive squamous cell carcinoma. Such tumors may be moderately well differentiated or poorly differentiated (Fig. 6.25). Histologically, the lung tumors do not differ from squamous cell carcinomas in other sites.

Adenocarcinoma may originate from bronchial epithelium, from bronchiolar cells in the periphery of the lungs, or from mucosal glands of major bronchi. The peripheral subpleural tumors often originate in scars that contain entrapped bronchial epithelium (Fig. 6.26). Histologically, the primary lung tumors do not differ from adenocarcinomas in other organs. Accordingly, primary adenocarcinomas of the lung cannot be distinguished with certainty from metastatic adenocarcinoma.

Bronchioloalveolar carcinoma is a tumor originating from stem cells of the terminal bronchioli. Tumor cells spread into the alveoli, replacing the alveolar lining cells (Fig. 6.27). The tumor cells resemble those normally derived from stem cells in terminal bronchioli: mucus-secreting cells, Clara cells, or pneumocytes type II. Bronchioloalveolar carcinoma could be considered a variant of adenocarcinoma characterized by a peculiar intra-alveolar growth pattern. Some metastatic carcinomas may also assume this growth pattern.

Large cell undifferentiated carcinoma is composed of poorly differentiated, large anaplastic cells (Fig. 6.28). Some tumor cells show ultrastructural or immunohistochemical features suggestive of squamous, adenocarcinomatous, and even neuroendocrine differentiation.

Small cell carcinoma, also known as *oat cell carcinoma*, is a tumor composed of poorly differentiated neuroendocrine cells (Fig. 6.29). Light microscopy reveals that these cells have small hyperchromatic oval or round nuclei and very little cytoplasm. Electron microscopy shows that these tumor cells may contain neuroendocrine granules. Immunohistochemistry uncovers typical neuroendocrine markers such as neuroendocrine matrix proteins (e.g., synaptophysin), various polypeptide hormones (e.g., adrenocorticotropic hormone), and neuropeptides (e.g., endorphin) can be demonstrated in these tumors by immunohistochemistry.

Carcinoid tumors are locally invasive tumors of low malignant potential. Histologically, these tumors are composed of monomorphic cells that have round to slightly oval nuclei of uniform appearance and a moderate amount of cytoplasm (Fig. 6.30). These tumor cells, which appear cytologically benign, are arranged into nests, columns, and tubules. Carcinoids tend to invade the surrounding tissues and even metastasize to local lymph nodes. Ultrastructurally, they contain neuroendocrine granules; immunohistochemically, they show evidence of neuroendocrine differentiation.

Mesothelioma is a malignant tumor of the pleura. Similar tumors can originate from the peritoneum or the pericardium, although less commonly. The tumor may occur in three histological forms: as an epithelial malignancy resembling carcinoma, as a mesenchymal malignancy resembling sarcoma, and as a biphasic tumor composed of both carcinomatous and sarcomatous components (Fig. 6.31).

NOTES

PLATE 6.1.   ALVEOLAR DAMAGE AND ATELECTASIS

Figure 6.1.   Amniotic fluid aspiration. The neonatal lungs are filled with amniotic fluid, which contains squames of fetal skin.

Figure 6.2.   Neonatal respiratory distress syndrome. Hyaline membranes line the alveolar ducts, and the alveoli are collapsed.

Figure 6.3.   Adult respiratory distress syndrome (ARDS). A. The alveoli appear dilated, evidence that the space was filled with edema fluid that was washed out during processing. Hyaline membranes line the alveoli, which are partially necrotic. **B.** Alveolar fibrosis develops in patients who have survived ARDS.

Diagram 6.2.   Respiratory distress syndrome. A. Normal alveolus. **B.** Neonatal respiratory distress syndrome is caused by immaturity of pneumocytes II unable to secrete surfactant. Alveoli collapse (atelectasis). Hyaline membranes cover the focally damaged epithelium of respiratory bronchioli. **C.** Adult respiratory distress syndrome is caused by the injury of the alveolar-capillary unit. This lesion may reflect an injury of pneumocyte (e.g., fumes) or endothelial capillary cells (e.g., endotoxin). The alveoli contain edema fluid due to leakiness of the alveolocapillary barrier and necrotic cells, and scavenger macrophages. Epithelial defects are covered with hyaline membranes.

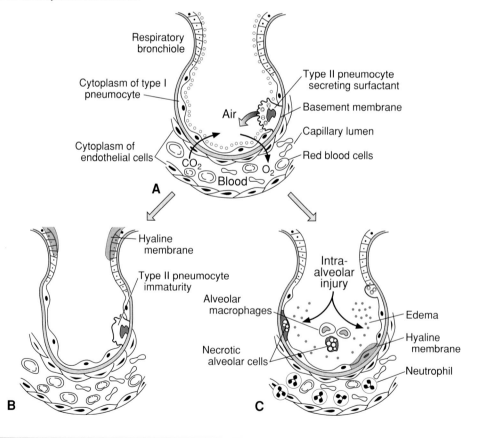

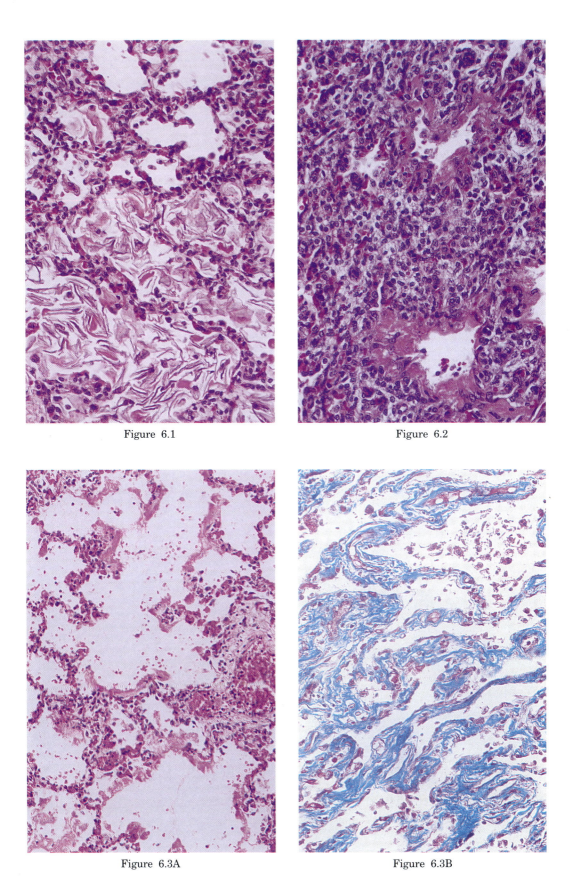

Figure 6.1

Figure 6.2

Figure 6.3A

Figure 6.3B

PLATE 6.2. BACTERIAL PNEUMONIA

Figure 6.4. A. Bronchopneumonia. The bronchus and the surrounding alveoli are filled with polymorphonuclear leukocytes. **B.** The alveoli contain numerous polymorphonuclear leukocytes.

Figure 6.5. Lobar pneumonia. All the alveoli are filled with polymorphonuclear leukocytes and fibrin.

Figure 6.6. Pulmonary abscess. The center of the cavity filled with necrotic amorphous material (upper part) and neutrophils.

Diagram 6.3. Bacterial pneumonia has several phases and may present as localized bronchopneumonia (lobular pneumonia) or diffuse lobar pneumonia. Initially, the alveoli contain bacteria, edema fluid, and scattered neutrophils. Massive exudation of neutrophils causes consolidation (gray hepatization). In the resolution phase, the exudate is taken up by scavenger macrophages and expectorated or reabsorbed.

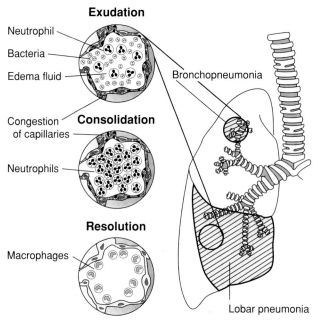

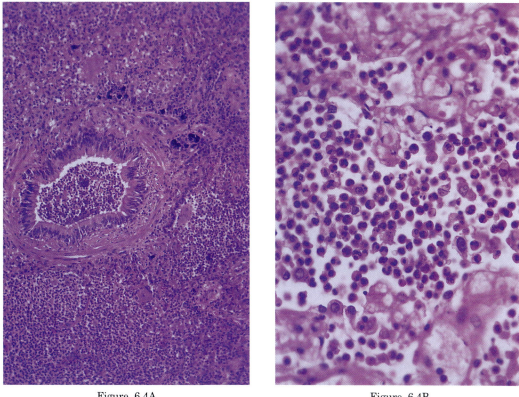

Figure 6.4A

Figure 6.4B

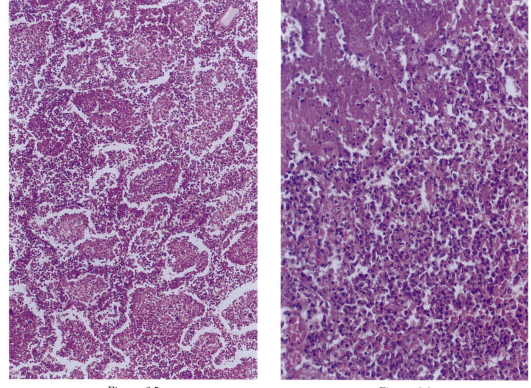

Figure 6.5

Figure 6.6

PLATE 6.3. VIRAL AND PARASITIC PNEUMONIA

Figure 6.7.   Viral pneumonia. A. The infiltrate is predominantly interstitial. The alveoli contain proteinaceous edema fluid and hyaline membranes. **B.** Higher-magnification view of the alveolar septa, which are widened and infiltrated with lymphocytes and macrophages. The edema fluid stains with eosin because it contains proteins in high concentration. **C.** Cytomegalovirus in desquamated alveolar cells that are surrounded with blood.

Figure 6.8.   *Pneumocystis carinii* pneumonia. A. The alveoli are filled with a bubbly, protein-rich exudate. **B.** The cysts of *Pneumocystis carinii* in the exudate are impregnated with silver and appear black.

Diagram 6.4.   Viral pneumonia. The damage of alveolar cells represents the primary lesion to which all other changes are related. The infiltrate of mononuclear inflammatory cells is limited to alveolar septa. Alveoli contain desquamated damaged epithelial cells and scattered scavenger cells (macrophages). There is also intra-alveolar edema. Hyaline membranes are formed focally. CMV, cytomegalovirus.

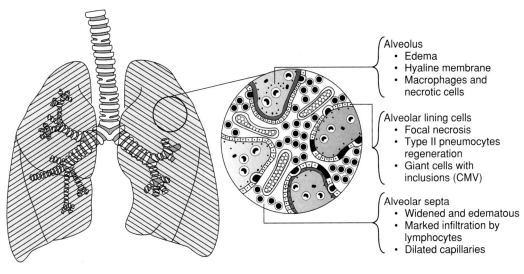

Alveolus
- Edema
- Hyaline membrane
- Macrophages and necrotic cells

Alveolar lining cells
- Focal necrosis
- Type II pneumocytes regeneration
- Giant cells with inclusions (CMV)

Alveolar septa
- Widened and edematous
- Marked infiltration by lymphocytes
- Dilated capillaries

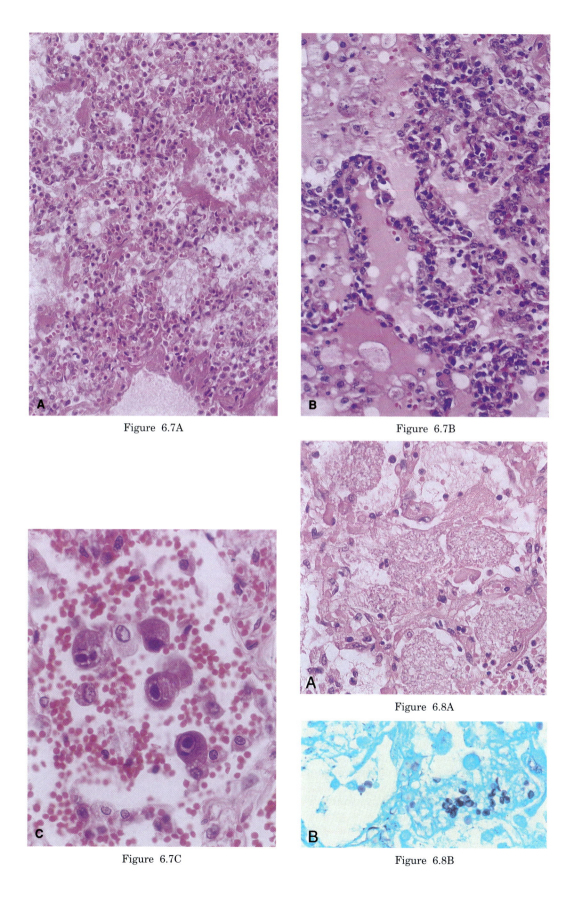

Figure 6.7A

Figure 6.7B

Figure 6.7C

Figure 6.8A

Figure 6.8B

PLATE 6.4. TUBERCULOSIS AND FUNGAL PNEUMONIA

Figure 6.9.   Pulmonary tuberculosis. A. Granulomas of early tuberculosis show extensive necrosis. **B.** Ziehl-Neelsen stain shows *M. tuberculosis* as red rods. **C.** Fibrotic scar in the wall of a tuberculous cavity consists of fibroblasts, collagen, and scattered Langerhans giant cells. **D.** The wall of tuberculous cavity contains foci of calcification replacing the caseating granulomas.

Figure 6.10.   Aspergillosis. Fungal hyphae are impregnated with silver and appear as branching strands.

Diagram 6.5.   Pulmonary tuberculosis. Primary tuberculosis consists of Ghon focus. Secondary tuberculosis may present in several forms.

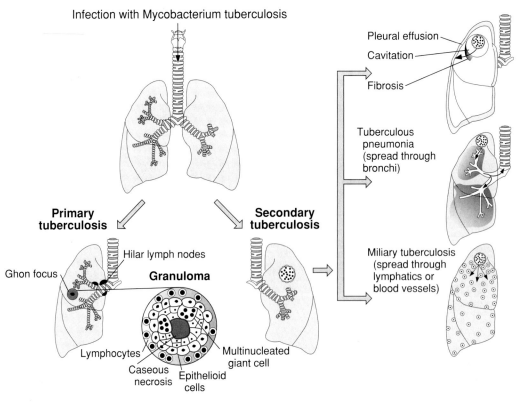

Infection with Mycobacterium tuberculosis

Pleural effusion
Cavitation
Fibrosis

Tuberculous pneumonia (spread through bronchi)

Miliary tuberculosis (spread through lymphatics or blood vessels)

Primary tuberculosis

Secondary tuberculosis

Ghon focus

Hilar lymph nodes

Granuloma

Lymphocytes

Caseous necrosis

Epithelioid cells

Multinucleated giant cell

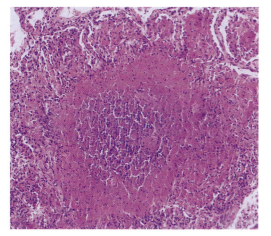

Figure 6.9A

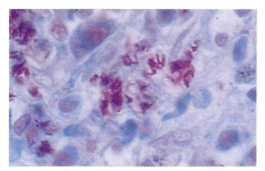

Figure 6.9B

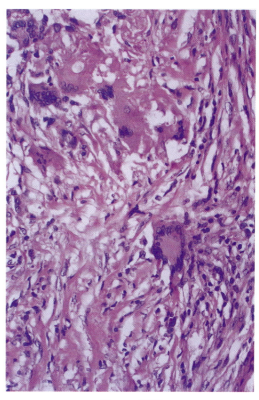

Figure 6.9C

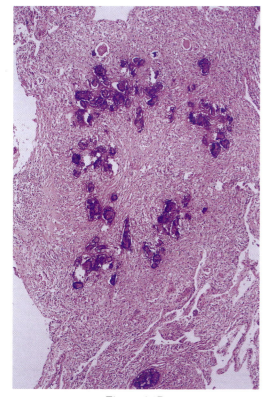

Figure 6.9D

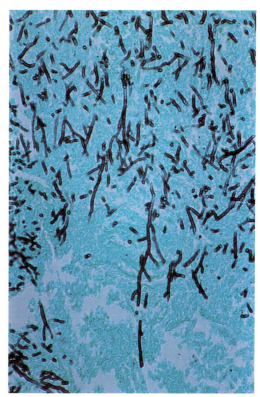

Figure 6.10

PLATE 6.5. CHRONIC PNEUMONIA

Figure 6.11. Organizing pneumonia. The alveoli contain fibrin and granulation tissue.

Figure 6.12. Chronic pulmonary fibrosis. Normal lung architecture has been lost. The alveolar walls have been distorted by fibrous tissue.

Figure 6.13. Bronchiolitis obliterans-organizing pneumonia (BOOP). A. The bronchiole is partially obliterated by granulation tissue. **B.** Bronchioli and adjacent alveoli contain whorls of fibroblasts, collagen, and chronic inflammatory cells.

Diagram 6.6. Chronic pneumonia. A. Normal lung. **B.** Usual interstitial pneumonia. There are numerous fibroblasts and interstitial fibrosis infiltrated with lymphocytes and macrophages. The alveoli are lined by an increased number of pneumocytes type II. **C.** Desquamative pneumonia. The alveoli contain numerous macrophages. **D.** Lymphocytic interstitial pneumonia. The interstitial septa are infiltrated with lymphocytes.

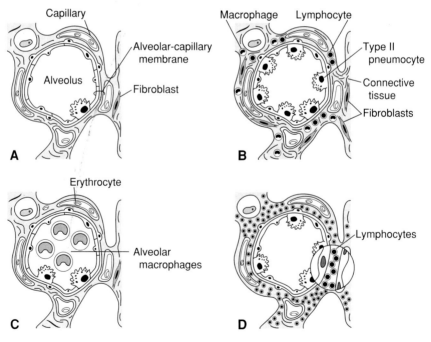

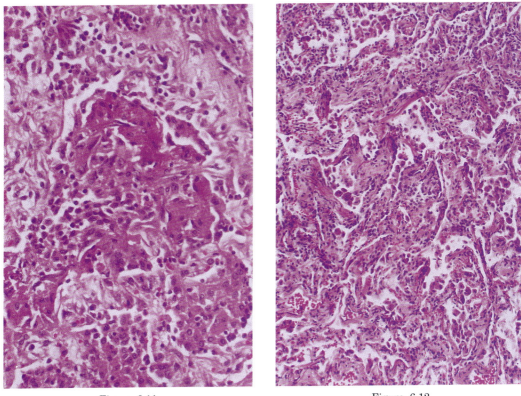

Figure 6.11

Figure 6.12

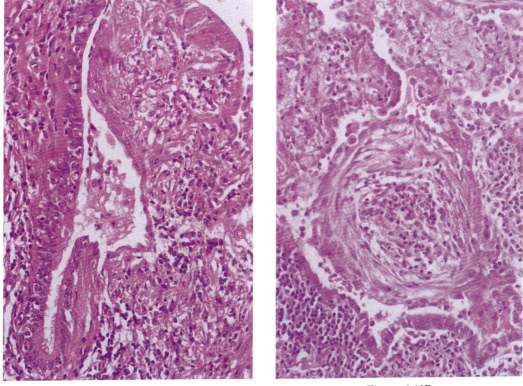

Figure 6.13A

Figure 6.13B

PLATE 6.6. IMMUNE–MEDIATED LUNG DISEASES

Figure 6.14. **Asthma.** The bronchial wall contains prominent smooth muscle cells. The bronchial epithelium forms invaginations and is lined with enlarged mucous cells.

Figure 6.16. **Sarcoidosis.** The tissue contains granulomas composed of epithelioid macrophages and only a few lymphocytes and giant cells. There is no central necrosis.

Figure 6.15. **Extrinsic allergic pneumonitis.** The lung shows interstitial inflammation.

Figure 6.17. **Wegener granulomatosis.** The consolidated lung parenchyma has a "geographical appearance" due to irregular areas of inflammation, necrosis, and hemorrhage.

Diagram 6.7. **Immunological lung injury.** Lungs may be affected by all four types of hypersensitivity reaction: Type I—asthma; Type II—Goodpasture syndrome; Type III—allergic pneumonitis; Type IV—sarcoidosis.

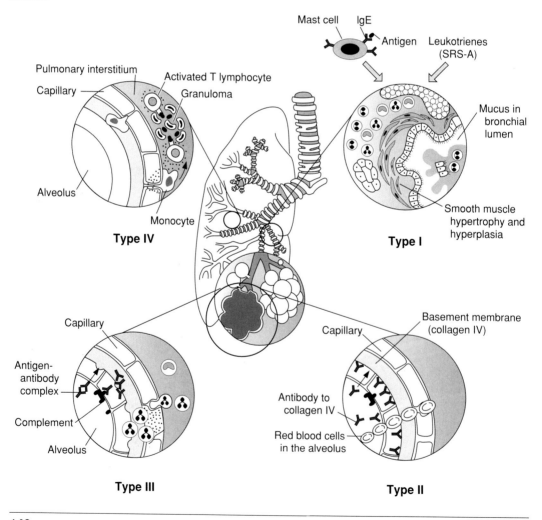

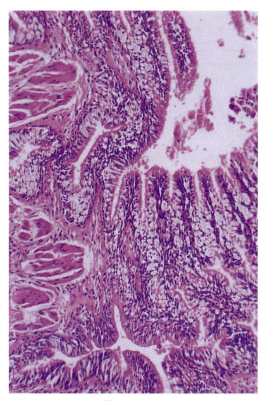

Figure 6.14

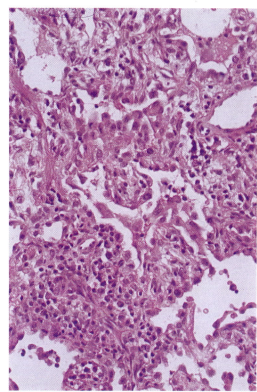

Figure 6.15

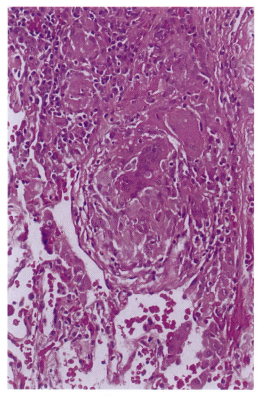

Figure 6.16

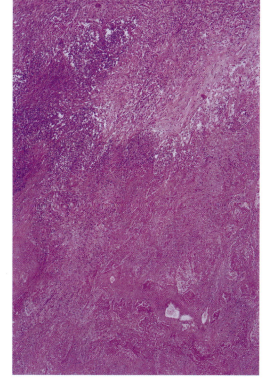

Figure 6.17

PLATE 6.7. CHRONIC INTERSTITIAL PNEUMONIA

Figure 6.18. Usual interstitial pneumonia (UIP). The normal lung architecture has been lost and is replaced with strands of fibrosis and chronic inflammatory infiltrates.

Figure 6.20. Asbestosis. A. Asbestosis-induced pulmonary fibrosis. Fibrous tissue appears blue in this trichrome-stained slide. **B. Inset** shows an asbestos body. These bodies appear as brown, beaded, dumbbell-shaped rods.

Figure 6.19. Desquamative interstitial pneumonia. The alveoli contain numerous macrophages.

Figure 6.21. Anthracosilicosis. A. The disease is characterized by fibrotic nodules. The black pigment represents coal particles. **B. Inset** shows silica particles photographed under polarized light. These particles appear as birefringent crystals.

Diagram 6.8. Pneumoconioses. Silicosis is caused by chronic inhalation of quartz crystals. These crystals act on the alveolar macrophage to produce fibroblast stimulating cytokines, which results in the formation of fibrotic nodules. **Asbestosis** is caused by asbestos fibers that enter the alveoli and are taken up by macrophages. Interaction of macrophages and asbestos leads to the formation of asbestos bodies and fibrosis of the lung and pleura. Pleural fibrosis may result in formation of fibrotic plaques.

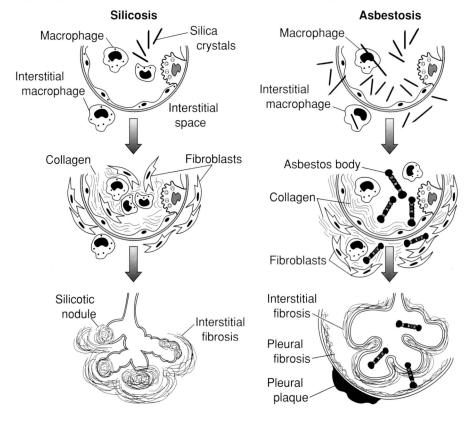

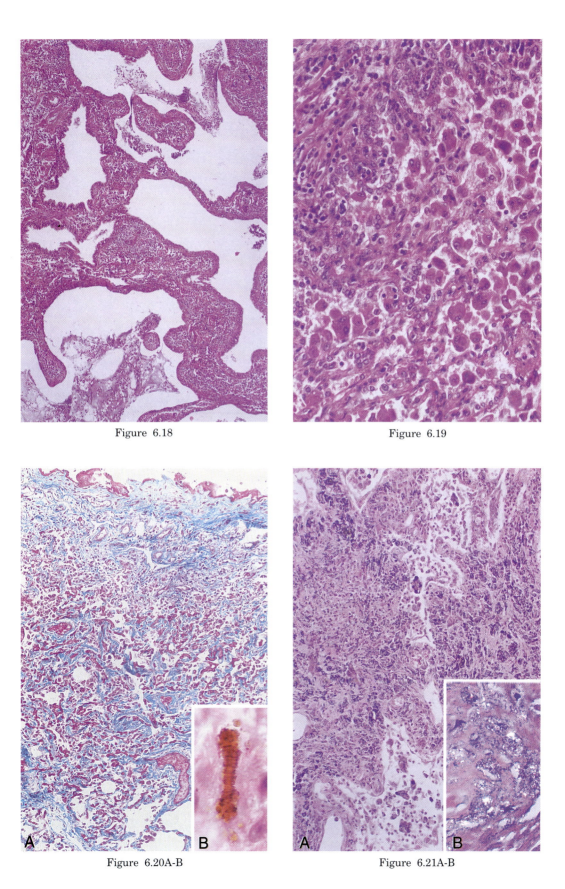

Figure 6.18

Figure 6.19

Figure 6.20A-B

Figure 6.21A-B

PLATE 6.8. CHRONIC OBSTRUCTIVE PULMONARY DISEASE

Figure 6.22. Chronic bronchitis. A. The thickened bronchial wall is infiltrated with inflammatory cells and contains enlarged glands. **B.** The submucosa of a dilated bronchiolus is densely infiltrated with inflammatory cells, and the lumen contains an inflammatory exudate.

Figure 6.23. Emphysema. Centrolobular emphysema is characterized by a loss of septa lining the respiratory bronchioles distal to the terminal bronchiole. The wall of the terminal bronchiole usually contains anthracotic pigment and chronic inflammatory cells.

Figure 6.24. Coal workers' lung disease. The lung shows confluent nodules of anthracosilicosis and focal loss of alveolar septa typical of emphysema (Courtesy of Dr. W. M. Thurlbeck, Vancouver).

Diagram 6.9. Chronic bronchitis shows inflammatory changes and thickening of the bronchial wall.

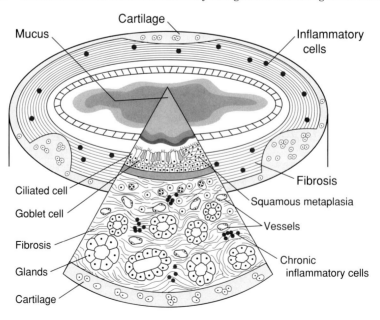

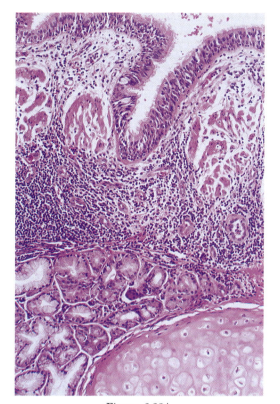

Figure 6.22A

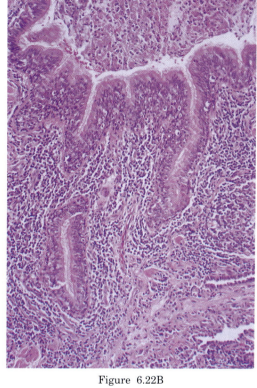

Figure 6.22B

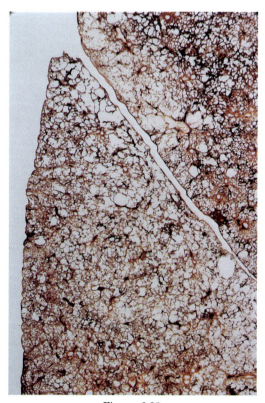

Figure 6.23

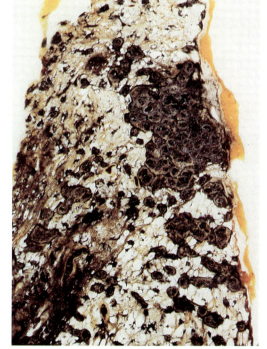

Figure 6.24

PLATE 6.9. NEOPLASMS OF THE LUNG

Figure 6.25. Squamous cell carcinoma of the bronchus. Carcinoma (bottom) arises from the metaplastic bronchial epithelium.

Figure 6.27. Bronchioloalveolar carcinoma. The neoplastic tumor cells are lining the alveoli, which contain proteinaceous fluid.

Figure 6.26. Adenocarcinoma. This peripheral lung tumor arose in a subpleural scar. Hence, the neoplastic glandular structures are encased in connective tissue stroma.

Figure 6.28. Large cell undifferentiated carcinoma. The tumor is composed of large cells that are arranged without any specific pattern.

Diagram 6.10. Emphysema occurs in two major forms, both of which show widening of airspaces distal to the terminal bronchiole. **A.** Normal lung. **B.** *Centrolobular emphysema*, which primarily affects the airspaces surrounding the respiratory bronchioli. **C.** *Panacinar emphysema*, which affects the respiratory bronchioli. alveolar ducts, and acini.

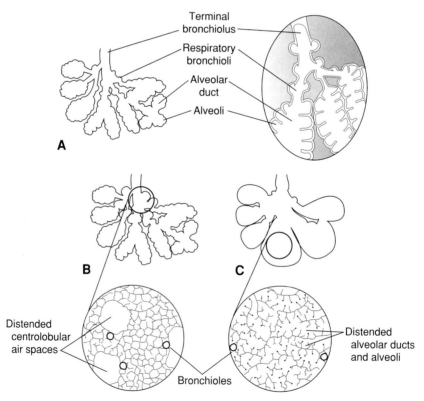

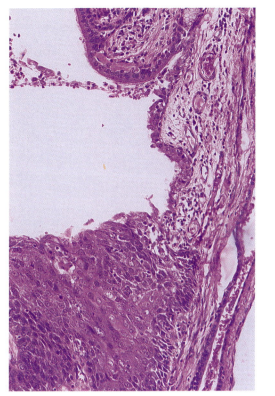

Figure 6.25

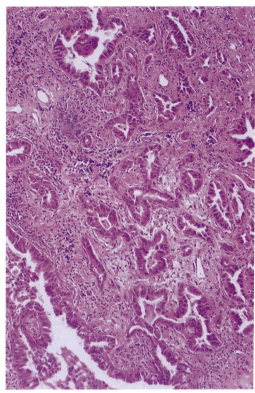

Figure 6.26

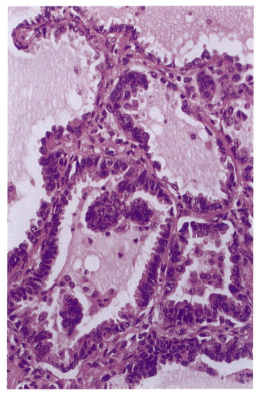

Figure 6.27

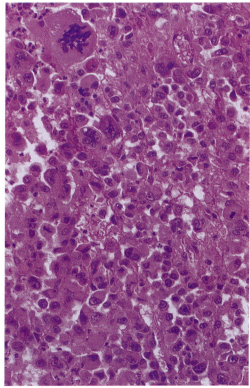

Figure 6.28

PLATE 6.10. NEOPLASMS OF THE LUNG AND PLEURA

Figure 6.29. Small cell carcinoma ("oat cell carcinoma"). The tumor is composed of small cells that have elongated nuclei. These nuclei appear round on cross-sectioning. The tumor cells have very little cytoplasm. Foci of necrosis are common (left upper corner).

Figure 6.30. Carcinoid. The tumor is composed of uniform cells that have round nuclei and are arranged into well delineated nests surrounded with scant stroma.

Figure 6.31. Mesothelioma. Epithelial mesothelioma consists of columnar cells lining tissue spaces and forming papillary protrusions. **B.** Biphasic mesothelioma consists of spindle shaped cells and flattened epithelial cells lining tissue clefts.

Diagram 6.11. Lung cancer. Most tumors are bronchogenic and are composed of cells found in the normal or pathologically altered bronchial epithelium. *Squamous cell carcinoma* corresponds to foci of squamous metaplasia in chronic bronchitis. *Adenocarcinoma* is composed of cells that may resemble the ciliated or mucous cells of bronchial mucosa and cells forming the bronchial glands. *Small cell (oat cell) carcinoma* and *carcinoid tumors* correspond to neuroendocrine cells. *Large cell carcinoma* has no equivalent benign cell and is probably equivalent to altered bronchial stem cells that could differentiate into glandular squamous or neuroendocrine cells. *Bronchioloalveolar carcinoma* probably originates from cells in the bronchioli. The neoplastic cells grow into the alveoli and line the terminal air spaces. *Mesothelioma* is a biphasic tumor composed of fibroblastic subpleural cells and cells that resemble epithelial-like surface mesothelial cells of the pleura.

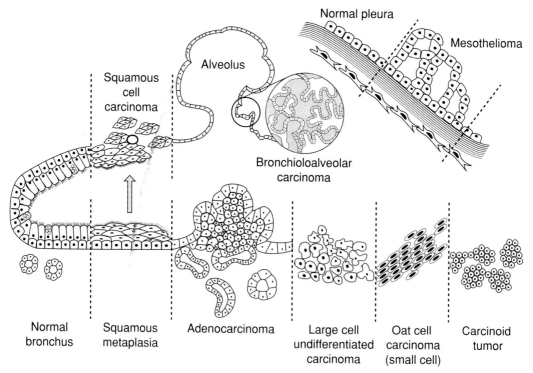

Normal pleura

Mesothelioma

Alveolus

Squamous
cell
carcinoma

Bronchioloalveolar
carcinoma

| Normal bronchus | Squamous metaplasia | Adenocarcinoma | Large cell undifferentiated carcinoma | Oat cell carcinoma (small cell) | Carcinoid tumor |

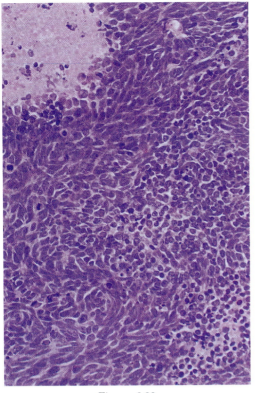

Figure 6.29

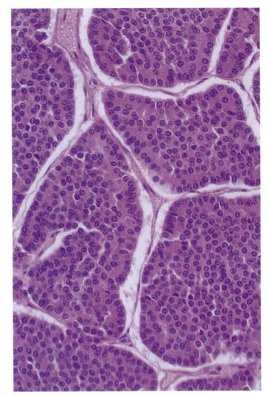

Figure 6.30

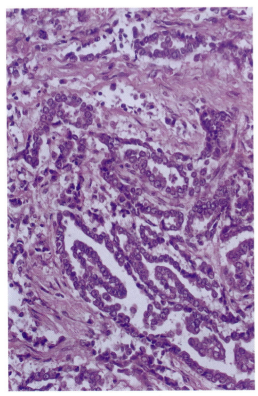

Figure 6.31A

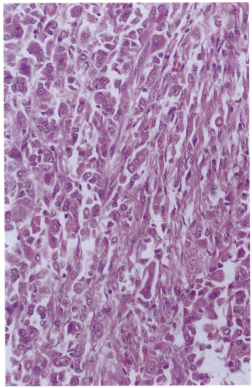

Figure 6.31B

N O T E S

CHAPTER 7

Hematopoietic System

NORMAL HISTOLOGY

Circulating blood cells, erythrocytes, or red blood cells; leukocytes or white blood cells; and thrombocytes or platelets (Diagram 7.1) are formed in the bone marrow, which is the primary hematopoietic organ. In a broader sense, the hematopoietic system also includes the lymph nodes and organ-related lymphoid tissue, the spleen, the thymus, and even the liver, which all partake in hematopoiesis during fetal life and even in adults have hematopoietic potential. The lymph nodes, organ-related lymphoid tissue, spleen, and thymus are composed of lymphoid cells and are important for lymphocytopoiesis and trafficking of lymphocytes. The spleen and the liver are the primary site for the removal of aged red blood cells (Diagram 7.2).

OVERVIEW OF PATHOLOGY

The most important diseases of the hematopoietic system include:

- Anemia
- Myeloproliferative syndromes and leukemia
- Lymphoma and related disorders such as Hodgkin disease and plasma cell neoplasms

Anemia

Anemia is a deficiency of red blood cells (RBCs). The diagnosis of anemia is made by counting the RBCs in peripheral blood, measuring the concentration of hemoglobin, and examining the morphology of RBCs in peripheral smears. Additional tests that are sometimes needed include, among numerous others: bone marrow biopsy, electrophoretic studies of hemoglobin, and molecular biological studies of genes controlling heme and globin synthesis.

Morphologically, anemias can be classified on the basis of the size and shape of RBCs in peripheral smears (Table 7.1) and their content of hemoglobin (Diagrams 7.3 and 7.4).

In **microcytic hypochromic anemia**, most often secondary to iron deficiency, the RBCs have a low hemoglobin content and appear small with a wide central pale area (Fig. 7.1). The RBCs also show poikilocytosis, i.e., vary in size and shape. The deficiency of iron can be confirmed best by bone marrow biopsy. Typically, the bone marrow contains no hemosiderin, as one would normally expect, since hemosiderin is the principal storage form of iron in the bone marrow.

In **macrocytic anemia**, caused by vitamin B_{12} or folate deficiency, the RBCs are larger than normal (Fig. 7.2). The deficiency of these essential nutrients affects DNA synthesis and impedes the maturation of all hematopoietic cells. In the peripheral blood smears, this is reflected in macrocytosis, anisocytosis, and poikilocytosis of erythrocytes, and in hypersegmentation of polymorphonuclear leukocytes. The bone marrow is hypercellular (*compensatory erythroid hyperplasia*) and contains numerous *megaloblasts* replacing the normal erythroid precursors (normoblasts). Megaloblasts have large nuclei and very little cytoplasm because of asynchrony in the maturation of nuclei and the cytoplasm of erythroid precursors. The precursors of leukocytes are also enlarged, and the inhibition of thrombocytopoiesis results in hypersegmentation of megakaryocytes.

Spherocytosis is a feature of hereditary spherocytosis, a chronic congenital hemolytic anemia caused by RBC abnormality. Instead of the normal biconcave shape of normal RBC, the spherocytes are round. In the peripheral blood smears, the spherocytes lack the central pale area and appear homogeneously red (Fig. 7.3).

Sickle cells are typical of sickle cell anemia, a defect in the synthesis of beta globin that leads to the formation of S-hemoglobin. This abnormal hemoglobin polymerizes in deoxygenated blood, thus causing RBC deformities (Fig. 7.4). **Acanthocytosis**, characterized by spur-like surface projections,

Diagram 7.1. Normal blood cells in circulation.

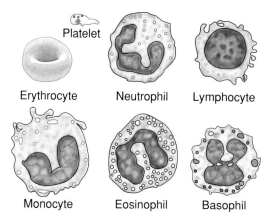

Platelet

Erythrocyte   Neutrophil   Lymphocyte

Monocyte   Eosinophil   Basophil

Table 7.1
Morphological Classification of Anemias

Classification	Examples
1. Normocytic-normochromic	Aplastic anemia Posthemorrhagic anemia Hemolytic anemia Anemia of chronic disease
2. Microcytic-hypochromic anemia	Iron-deficiency anemia Sideroblastic anemia Thalassemia
3. Macrocytic-normochromic anemia	Pernicious anemia (lack of vitamin B_{12}) Folate deficiency

Diagram 7.2. Hematopoietic and lymphoid organs—thymus, lymph node, spleen, bone marrow.
FC, fat cells; MEG, megalocytes; RBC, red blood cell; WBP, white blood cell precursor; WBC, white blood cell.

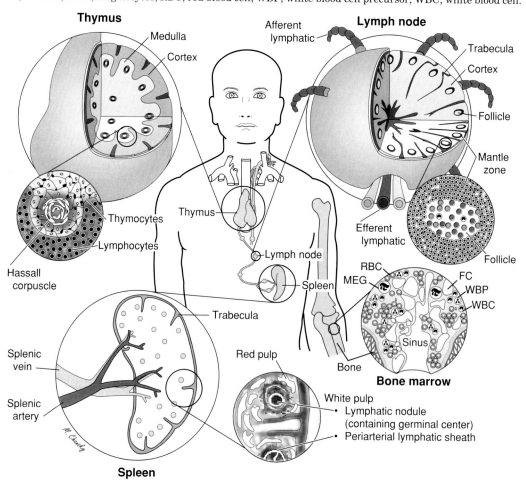

are found in abetalipoproteinemia and chronic liver diseases (Fig. 7.5). The abnormal cell shape is caused by derangements of lipoprotein metabolism in the cell membrane of RBCs.

Morphology of RBC can be changed by external factors as well. Acquired deformities of RBC are rather common. These deformities take many forms and are described by such names as *burr cells*, *schistocytes*, and *helmet* cells. Distorted RBCs and RBC fragments are found in **microangiopathic anemia,** typical of disseminated intravascular coagulation, or in patients with intravascular hemolysis due to mechanical RBC injury, such as those with mechanical heart valves (Fig. 7.6).

Abnormal hemoglobins that may present inside the RBCs appear as cytoplasmic inclusions, or densities. In **thalassemia**, a congenital microcytic hypochromic anemia caused by a defect of the globin alpha or beta gene, the abnormal hemoglobin accumulation results in the formation of *target cells* (Fig. 7.7).

Anemia is usually associated with morphological changes in the bone marrow, which vary depending on whether the bone marrow pathology is the cause of anemia or a compensatory reaction to RBC deficiency (Diagram 7.5).

Aplastic anemia is characterized by a depletion of all hematopoietic cells (Fig. 7.8). The term is used as a synonym for bone marrow failure because it involves not only the precursors of RBCs, but the white blood cells and platelets as well. **Myelofibrosis** is characterized by an overgrowth of the bone marrow with fibroblasts (Fig. 7.9). **Myelophthisic anemia** is caused by tumors infiltrating the bone marrow and replacing the normal hematopoietic cells (Fig. 7.10).

Hemolytic anemia or any **chronic blood loss** leads to erythroid cell hyperplasia in the bone marrow. The ratio of myeloid to erythroid cells is reduced from a normal 4:1 to 2:1 and even lower (Fig. 7.11). The release of immature RBCs, which are exported from bone marrow at an increased rate to compensate for the anemia, results in the appearance of immature RBCs called reticulocytes. Reticulocytes can be recognized in special stains because of basophilic stippling of their cytoplasm that contains precipitated RNA and proteins. The normal peripheral blood contains less than 0.1% reticulocytes; an increased number of these cells is a good sign that the bone marrow is responding to increased demands for RBC production.

The lesions caused by anemia may be seen in many organs, although such changes usually are nonspecific and inconspicuous in routinely prepared histological sections. Tissue hypoxia, the most important consequence of anemia, usually produces only minor morphological changes, such as fatty change of the heart and kidneys. More prominent are changes caused by complications of specific forms of anemia and treatment used to correct the specific defect.

Extramedullary hematopoiesis is a complication of myelofibrosis and myelophthisic anemia. Because the bone marrow is replaced by fibrosis or tumor cells, compensatory hematopoiesis occurs in the spleen and liver, and less often in other sites (Fig. 7.12).

Sickle cell anemia is often associated with formation of thrombi in small blood vessels and **microinfarcts**. These infarcts mostly lead to scarring prominent in the spleen (Fig. 7.13), which may lead to splenic atrophy and shrinkage ("autosplenectomy"). Ischemic microinfarcts occur in other organs as well, causing many clinical complications, the most important of which pertain to cerebral ischemia.

Hemolytic anemia is associated with hepatosplenomegaly. In hereditary spherocytosis, the splenic sinusoids contain an increased number of RBCs (Fig. 7.14). The fragments of hemolyzed RBCs are taken up by tissue macrophages. The sinusoidal cells of the spleen and the Kupffer cells contain increased amounts of hemosiderin, which appears as brown pigment that becomes blue following the Prussian blue staining reaction.

Intravascular hemolysis differs from the hemolytic anemias caused by corpuscular defects of RBCs or antibodies, in that it generates large amounts of free hemoglobin in circulation. Since this free hemoglobin cannot be taken up fast enough by the phagocytic cells of the liver and spleen, it is excreted through the glomeruli, causing *hemoglobinuria*. Hemoglobin in the primary glomerular filtrate is partially taken up by the proximal tubular cells and transformed into the hemosiderin inside the lysosome, causing renal hemosiderosis (Fig. 7.15).

Acute Leukemia

Acute leukemias comprise two main categories: *acute myeloblastic leukemia* (AML) and *acute lymphoblastic leukemia* (ALL). According to the French-American-British (FAB) classification, each of these categories comprises several subtypes that are defined on the basis of their cell morphology and differentiation (Diagram 7.6).

Acute myeloblastic leukemia is subdivided according to the FAB criteria into seven subtypes labeled M1 to M7 (Fig. 7.16). M1 is composed of least differentiated cells, which show no evidence of differentiation. M2 to M7 variants contain blasts that show some form of differentiation from promyelocytes, monocytes, erythroblasts, or megakaryocytes.

Acute lymphoblastic leukemia differs from AML in that its cells do not show any signs of differentiation (Fig. 7.17). According to FAB classification, ALL is divided into three subcategories: L1, L2, or L3. ALL characterized by small blasts is classified as L1. In L2, the blast cells vary in size of the nuclei and the amount of cytoplasm and usually have prominent nucleoli. This category also includes adult T-cell leukemias. In the L3 variant, the nuclei vary in size but are always surrounded by well developed cytoplasm that typically contains vacuoles similar to those in Burkitt lymphoma. Acute lymphoblastic leukemia is positive for terminal deoxynucleotidyl transferase, which can be demonstrated by enzyme histochemistry in the cytoplasm of neoplastic cells.

Chronic Leukemia

Chronic leukemia comprises *chronic myelogenous leukemia* and *chronic lymphocytic leukemia* (CLL), which includes several variants such as *hairy cell leukemia* and *Sézary syndrome.*

In **chronic myelogenous leukemia**, the peripheral blood smears show an increased number of granulocytes in excess of 50,000 per microliter in all stages of maturation (Fig. 7.18). In addition to segmented neutrophils, the peripheral blood smears contain myeloblasts, promyelocytes, myelocytes, metamyelocytes, and band forms, but also basophils. In about two-thirds of cases, the disease ends in a blast crisis and death.

Chronic lymphocytic leukemia is characterized by an increased number of lymphocytes in the circulating blood and lymph nodes, spleen, and liver. Neoplastic cells resemble mature lymphocytes and express surface immunoglobulins such as normal B cells, from which they differ only slightly (Fig. 7.19). In addition to lymphocytosis, the peripheral blood films often show "smear cells," an artifact typical of CLL, probably reflecting the increased fragility of leukemia cells.

Hairy cell leukemia is a B-cell leukemia that can be recognized morphologically and that presents with a clinically distinct picture. The neoplastic cells contain round nuclei and well developed cytoplasm that has a ruffled surface extending into short villi ("hairs") (Fig. 7.20).

Chronic T-cell leukemia, also called *Sézary syndrome,* is characterized by the appearance of relatively mature T cells in the circulating blood. Such cells have deeply indented or lobulated nuclei and scant cytoplasm (Fig. 7.21).

The bone marrow of patients with myelogenous leukemia appears hypercellular and is infiltrated with neoplastic cells (Fig. 7.22). Leukemic cells may infiltrate other tissues, most prominently the spleen and the liver, and form tumors of soft tissues called *chloromas.* Lymphoblastic leukemia infiltrates hematopoietic organs and is usually associated with an enlargement of the spleen and lymph nodes. CLL (Fig. 7.23) also infiltrates lymph nodes and the white pulp of the spleen, but it may involve the bone marrow and the liver as well. Hairy cell leukemia typically infiltrates the spleen, diffusely obliterating its normal architecture (Fig. 7.24). T-cell leukemia tends to infiltrate the skin, which is known as *mycosis-fungoides* (Fig. 7.25).

Lymphoma

The term malignant lymphoma includes a variety of neoplastic disorders of lymphoid cells, which are subdivided into two groups: non-Hodgkin lymphoma and Hodgkin lymphoma. All these disorders represent clonal proliferation of T or B lymphocytes and their common or distinctly specific precursors. Malignant lymphomas can be immunohistochemically classified as B- or T-cell derived and several other classifications, of which the most widely used is the National Cancer Institute Working Formulation.

Non-Hodgkin Lymphoma. According to the National Cancer Institute Working Formulation, this group of malignant tumors is divided into three main categories: low-grade malignancy, intermediate-grade malignancy, and high-grade malignancy (Table 7.2). These categories include morphologically recognizable entities distinguished from one another by the cellular composition and the histological patterns displayed by the affected lymph node.

Cytologically, lymphoma cells can be classified as small or large. Their nuclei can be small or large, round or vesicular, and they may be further subclassified according to whether the nuclei are cleaved or noncleaved, whether the chromatin is condensed or finely granular, whether the nucleolus is prominent or not, and whether the cytoplasm is well developed or scant (Diagram 7.7).

Histologically, lymphomas are classified as follicular or diffuse. Figures 7.26 to 7.29 show typical examples of malignant lymphomas.

Lymphoma of low-grade malignancy may be follicular or diffuse. These neo-plasms are composed of well differentiated lymphocytes resembling those normally found in lymph nodes.

Lymphomas of intermediate-grade malignancy may be follicular, composed of large cells, or more often diffuse and composed of small cleaved cells, mixed small and large cells, or only large cells.

Lymphoma of high-grade malignancy is typically composed of highly anaplastic cells, which may show immunoblastic (plasmacytoid) differentiation or no differentiation at all, as in Burkitt lymphoma.

Lymphoma typically involves the lymph nodes. However, the infiltrates often spread into other organs, such as bone marrow, spleen, and soft tissues.

Hodgkin Disease. Hodgkin disease is a form of lymphoma that occurs in four histological types, listed in Table 7.3 and illustrated in Figure 7.30. All four subtypes of Hodgkin disease (Diagram 7.8) contain the diagnostic Reed-Sternberg cells, which are typically bilobed and have prominent nucleoli surrounded by a clear halo.

Plasma Cell Neoplasia

Neoplastic monoclonal proliferation of plasma cells and preneoplastic plasma cell

---

Table 7.2
National Cancer Institute Working Formulation

Low-Grade Lymphoma
Malignant lymphoma small lymphocytic (consistent with chronic lymphocytic leukemia or plasmacytoid)
Malignant lymphoma, follicular, predominantly small cleaved cell
Malignant lymphoma, folicular, mixed, small cleaved and large cell

Intermediate-Grade Lymphoma
Malignant lymphoma, follicular predominantly large cell
Malignant lymphoma, diffuse small cleaved cell
Malignant lymphoma, diffuse mixed, small and large cell
Malignant lymphoma, diffuse large cell, cleaved cell, non-cleaved cell

High-Grade Lymphoma
Malignant lymphoma, large cell, immunoblastic
  • Plasmacytoid
  • Polymorphous
Malignant lymphoma, lymphoblastic
Malignant lymphoma, small noncleaved cell
  • Burkitt lymphoma

Table 7.3
Histological Classification of Hodgkin's Disease

Type	Histological Features
Lymphocyte-predominant	Lymphocytes predominant Few Reed-Sternberg cells Tumor infiltrates surrounded by collagen extending from nodule capsule Mixed cell infiltrate Characteristic "lacunar" cells
Mixed cellularity	Numerous Reed-Sternberg cells Intermediate number of lymphocytes Mixed cell infiltrate, composed of lymphocytes plasma cells, eosinophils
Lymphocyte-depleted	Few lymphocytes: "Reticular pattern" with predominant Reed-Sternberg cells Diffuse fibrosis with disordered connective tissue and infrequent Reed-Sternberg cells

---

Table 7.4
Plasma Cell Disorders

Monoclonal gammopathy of unknown significance (MGUS)
Solitary plasmacytoma
Multiple myeloma
Waldenström macroglobulinemia

dyscrasias can occur in several forms (Table 7.4). Clinically and pathologically, these entities are related. For example, monoclonal gammopathy of unknown significance may evolve into multiple myeloma.

Plasma cell neoplasia develops because of malignant transformation and subsequent expansion of a single clone of plasma cells. Infiltrates of these neoplasmic cells are found most often in the bone marrow (Fig. 7.31). Cells found in monoclonal gammopathy of unknown significance (MGUS), solitary plasmacytoma, and most multiple myelomas resemble plasma cells. In addition to well differentiated plasma cells, the bone marrow may contain atypical and even multinucleated plasmacytoid cells. These neoplastic clones secrete immunoglobulin G (IgG), IgA, IgM, IgD, or IgE. Since the IgG-secreting cells predominate under normal conditions, MGUS and multiple myeloma composed of IgG-secreting cells are the most common plasma cell disorders.

All plasma cellular neoplasms cause monoclonal gammopathy, which can be recognized by electrophoresis of serum proteins. The immunoglobulins produced by neoplastic plasma cells are filtered through the glomeruli and accumulate as intratubular protein casts. These casts damage the tubular cells and cause tubular obstruction. The light chain of immunoglobulin may also be deposited in the kidney tissue as AL amyloid, which is morphologically indistinguishable from other forms of amyloid. Amyloid deposits are most prominent in the glomeruli and renal blood vessels.

Waldenström macroglobulinemia is a malignancy of IgM-secreting plasmacytoid cells that appear less differentiated than those of other plasma cell neoplasms. Waldenström macroglobulinemia cells have features intermediate between lymphoma and plasma cells (Fig. 7.32).

NOTES

PLATE 7.1. ANEMIA

Figure 7.1. **Microcytic hypochromic anemia. A.** Peripheral smear contains small RBCs with a wide central pale area. The cigar-shaped and tear-shaped poikilocytes are also seen. **B.** The bone marrow aspirate is devoid of stainable iron as shown in this Prussian blue–stained slide. (For comparison see **C.**) **C.** Normal iron stores in the bone marrow. Iron is stored as hemosiderin, which appears as blue dots in this Prussian blue–stained slide.

Figure 7.2. **Macrocytic-megaloblastic anemia. A.** Peripheral blood smear shows macrocytosis, anisocytosis, and poikilocytosis of erythrocytes. **B.** Neutrophils have hypersegmented nuclei. **C.** Aspiration of bone marrow. Megaloblasts are large erythroid cells not normally found in the bone marrow. Normal maturation of erythroid cells is recognized by the pink cytoplasm (hemoglobin) and clumping of the nuclei, which ultimately results in the expulsion of the nucleus before the erythrocyte leaves the bone marrow. In megaloblasts, such maturation does not occur and the nucleus remains disproportionately large and "lacy," which indicates its immaturity.

Diagram 7.3. **Morphology of RBCs in various forms of anemia.**

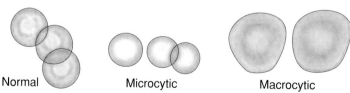

Normal   Microcytic   Macrocytic

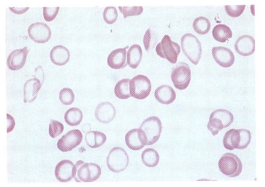

Figure 7.1A

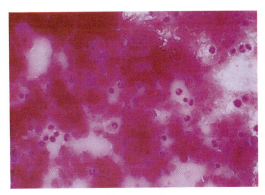

Figure 7.1B

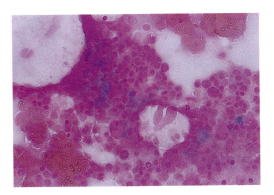

Figure 7.1C

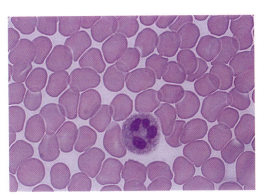

Figure 7.2A

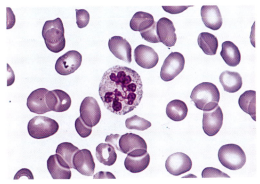

Figure 7.2B

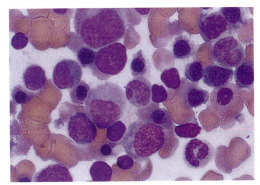

Figure 7.2C

PLATE 7.2. ANEMIA

Figure 7.3.   Spherocytosis. The spherocytes are smaller than normal RBCs. The abnormal cells appear round and homogeneously red. Spherocytes do not have a central pale area.

Figure 7.5.   Acanthocytosis of liver disease. The smear contains typical "spur-cells" with numerous spikes on their surface.

Figure 7.7.   Thalassemia. The peripheral blood smear contains microcytic hypochromic erythrocytes, some of which appear as target cells.

Figure 7.4.   Sickle cell anemia. A. The abnormal red cells are semilunar or form sickles. **B.** Sickle cells seen by electron microscopy. **C.** At higher magnification, one may see cytoplasmic filaments ("tactoids") formed from polymerized hemoglobin S.

Figure 7.6.   Microangiopathic anemia. The smear contains numerous helmet-shaped acanthocytes and other deformed RBCs and RBC fragments.

Diagram 7.4.   Morphology of RBCs in various forms of anemia.

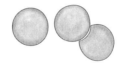

Spherocytosis

Target cells
(thalassemia)

Elliptocytosis

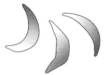

Sickle cell

Microangiopathic

Tear drop cells
(myelofibrosis)

Lead toxicity

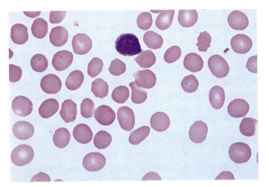

Figure 7.3

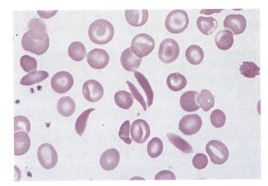

Figure 7.4A

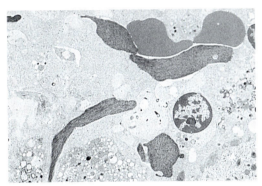

Figure 7.4B

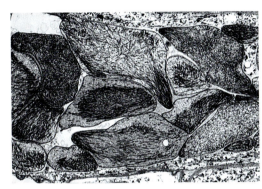

Figure 7.4C

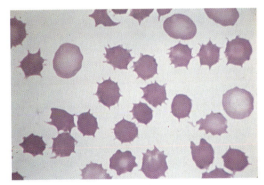

Figure 7.5

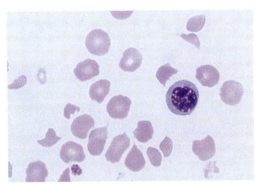

Figure 7.6

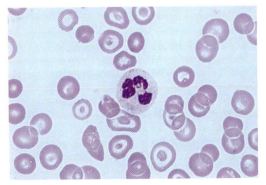

Figure 7.7

PLATE 7.3. BONE MARROW CHANGES IN ANEMIA

Figure 7.8. Aplastic anemia. The bone marrow is depleted of hematopoietic cells. Only stromal cells, fat cells, and sinusoids filled with blood remain.

Figure 7.9. Myelofibrosis. The bone marrow is infiltrated with fibroblasts and contains few hematopoietic cells.

Figure 7.10. Myelophthisic anemia. Tumor cells and fibrous tissue surrounding them replace the normal hematopoietic marrow.

Figure 7.11. Erythroid hyperplasia. A. The bone marrow contains an excess of erythroid cells. The erythroid cells are recognized by their dark round nuclei and bluish cytoplasm. The cytoplasm of the most mature cells, normoblast, has a red tinge due to nascent hemoglobin. **B.** The peripheral blood smear contains an increased number of reticulocytes. Reticulocytes show stippling of their cytoplasm, which can be seen only by special staining.

Diagram 7.5. Bone marrow in anemia.

COLOR ATLAS OF HISTOPATHOLOGY

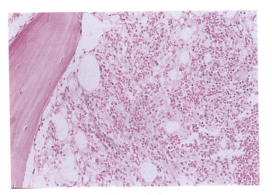

Figure 7.8

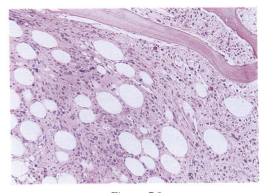

Figure 7.9

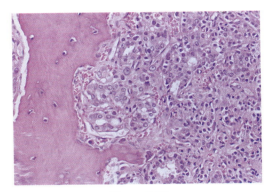

Figure 7.10

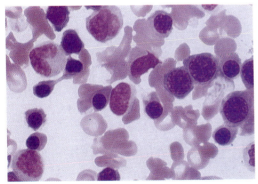

Figure 7.11A

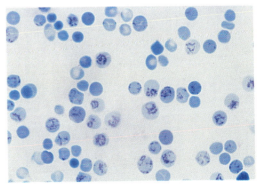

Figure 7.11B

PLATE 7.4. CONSEQUENCES AND COMPLICATIONS OF ANEMIA

Figure 7.12. Extramedullary hematopoiesis. Liver sinusoids contain foci of hematopoietic cells. The large cells are megakaryocytes. Erythroid precursors have dark round nuclei. The white blood cell precursors have bean-shaped nuclei with finely dispersed chromatin.

Figure 7.13. Sickle cell anemia. The spleen shows marked pooling of blood in the sinusoids and foci of fibrosis. The fibrous scar tissue is impregnated with iron and calcium and appears black.

Figure 7.14. Hemolytic anemia. A. Splenomegaly of hereditary spherocytosis typically shows marked congestion of splenic sinusoids. **B.** Hemolysis is accompanied by hemosiderin accumulation in the splenic and hepatic macrophages.

Figure 7.15. Hemoglobinuria of intravascular hemolysis. The excess free hemoglobin is filtered through glomeruli, resulting in hemoglobinuria and hemosiderosis of proximal tubular cells. Hemosiderin appears as blue granules stained with the Prussian blue reaction.

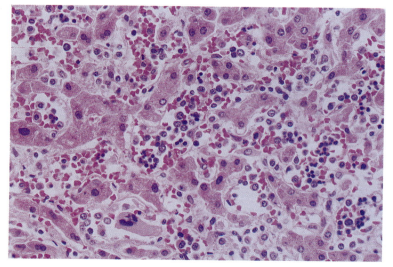

Figure 7.12

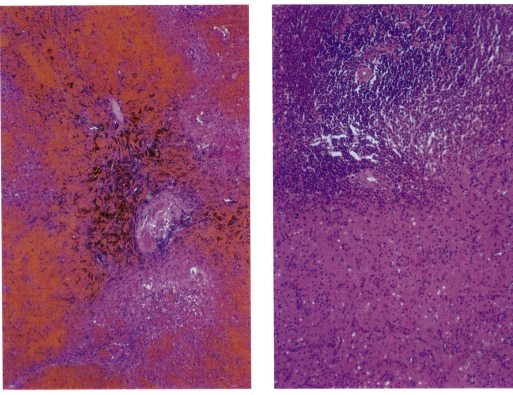

Figure 7.13

Figure 7.14A

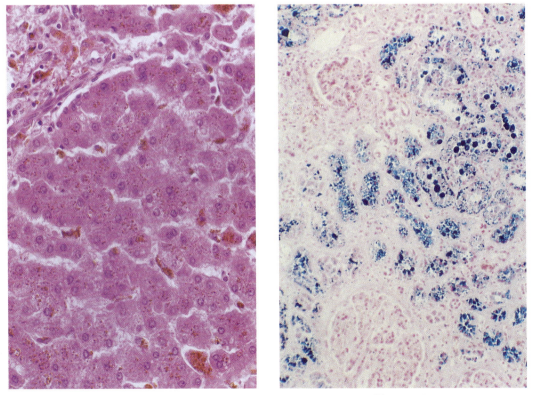

Figure 7.14B

Figure 7.15

PLATE 7.5. ACUTE LEUKEMIAS

Figure 7.16. **Acute myeloblastic leukemia.** The peripheral smear and the bone marrow contain immature myeloid cells. No segmented neutrophils are seen. **A.** Myeloblastic cells with no evidence of maturation (M1). **B.** Myeloblastic cells with maturation (M2). **C.** Promyelocyte with Auer bodies in cytoplasm (M3). **D.** Monocyte-like cells (M5).

Figure 7.17. **Acute lymphoblastic leukemia. A.** The peripheral blood smear contains small blasts (L1). **B.** The nuclei of tumor cells have loosely structured chromatin, vary in size, and have prominent nucleoli (L2). **C.** The tumor cell nuclei vary in size. The cytoplasm contains vacuoles. **D.** The cells express terminal deoxynucleotidyl transferase, which was demonstrated by enzyme histochemistry as pink cytoplasmic granules.

Diagram 7.6. **FAB classification of acute leukemias.**

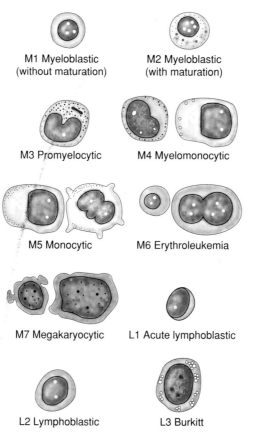

M1 Myeloblastic
(without maturation)

M2 Myeloblastic
(with maturation)

M3 Promyelocytic

M4 Myelomonocytic

M5 Monocytic

M6 Erythroleukemia

M7 Megakaryocytic

L1 Acute lymphoblastic

L2 Lymphoblastic

L3 Burkitt

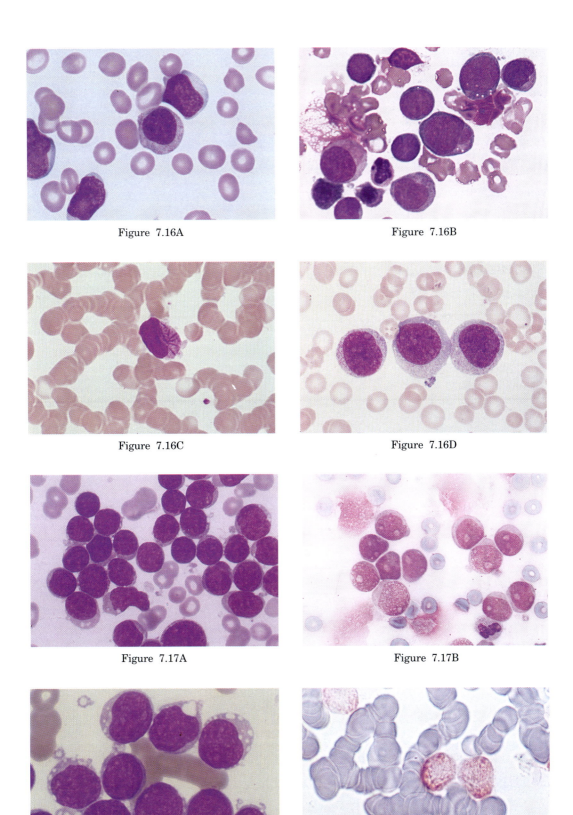

Figure 7.16A

Figure 7.16B

Figure 7.16C

Figure 7.16D

Figure 7.17A

Figure 7.17B

Figure 7.17C

Figure 7.17D

PLATE 7.6. CHRONIC LEUKEMIAS

Figure 7.18. **Chronic myelogenous leukemia. A.** The peripheral blood smear shows an increased number of myeloid precursors in all stages of maturation. **B.** Advanced stages of myeloid maturation. Some cells have segmented nuclei.

Figure 7.19. **Chronic lymphocytic leukemia. A.** Lymphocytosis, as evidenced by an increased number of lymphocytes in the peripheral blood. **B.** Leukemic cells have small round or slightly irregular nuclei with a small rim of cytoplasm. The chromatin is condensed, and the nucleoli are not prominent

Figure 7.20. **Hairy cell leukemia. A.** Peripheral smear shows cells with surface projections of their cytoplasm. The cell to the left is a normal lymphocyte. **B.** Electron microscopy shows microvilli of the cell membrane.

Figure 7.21. **T-cell leukemia (*Sézary* syndrome). A.** In the peripheral blood smear, the lobes of the lymphocyte nucleus seem to overlap. **B.** Electron microscopy shows that the nucleus is deeply indented ("cerebriform," i.e., like gyri of the brain).

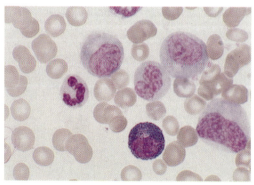

Figure 7.18A

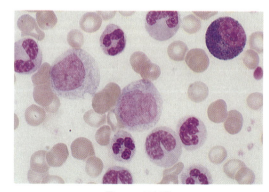

Figure 7.18B

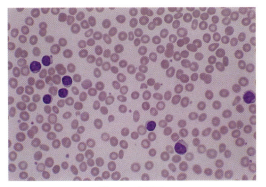

Figure 7.19A

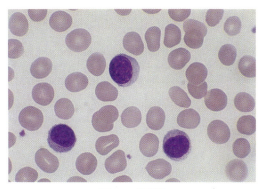

Figure 7.19B

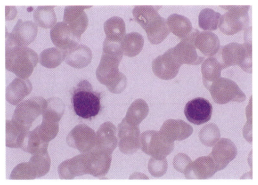

Figure 7.20A

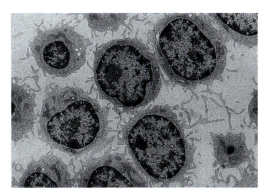

Figure 7.20B

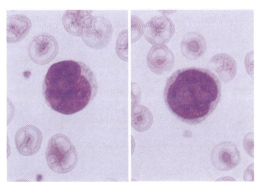

Figure 7.21A

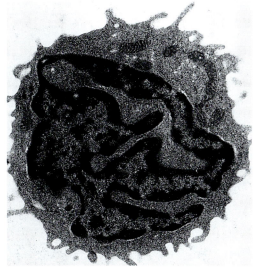

Figure 7.21B

PLATE 7.7. TISSUE INFILTRATES IN LEUKEMIA

Figure 7.22.   Myelogenous leukemia. A. The bone marrow of chronic myelogenous leukemia appears hypercellular. **B.** Neoplastic myeloid cells have vesicular nuclei. **C.** Acute myelogenous leukemia infiltrating the spleen. The neoplastic cells have bean-shaped vesicular nuclei.

Figure 7.23.   Chronic lymphocytic leukemia.
The hepatic infiltrate of neoplastic lymphoid cells is limited to the portal tract.

Figure 7.24.   Spleen in hairy cell leukemia.
The white and the red pulp are diffusely infiltrated.

Figure 7.25.   Mycosis fungoides. A. The skin is infiltrated with malignant lymphoid cells. **B.** Intraepidermal tumor cells form a so-called Pautrier abscess.

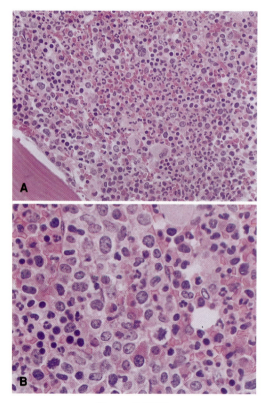

Figure 7.22AB

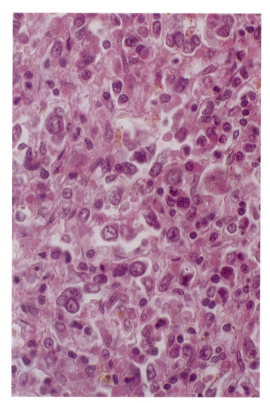

Figure 7.22C

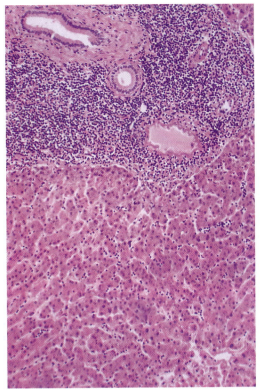

Figure 7.23

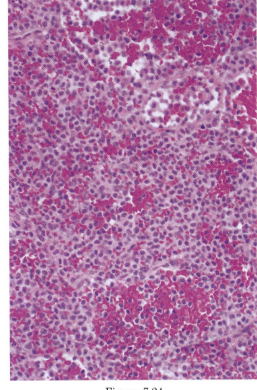

Figure 7.24

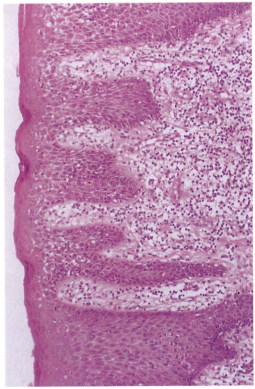

Figure 7.25A

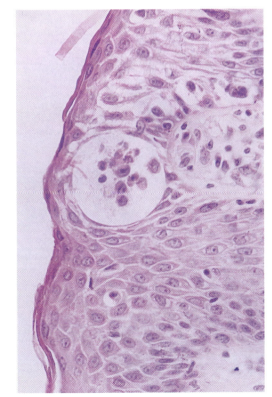

Figure 7.25B

PLATE 7.8. MALIGNANT LYMPHOMA

Figure 7.26. Follicular lymphoma. The neoplastic cells are arranged into large lymphoid follicles but also infiltrate the perifollicular spaces.

Figure 7.27. Diffuse well differentiated cell lymphoma. The small lymphoid cells infiltrate the lymph node, obliterating its normal architecture.

Figure 7.28. Diffuse lymphoma of intermediate malignancy. The tumor is composed of small cleaved cells.

Figure 7.29. Lymphoma of high-grade malignancy. Burkitt lymphoma composed of small noncleaved cells. The infiltrate also contains scattered macrophages, which accounts for the typical "starry-sky" pattern.

Diagram 7.7. Cells of malignant lymphomas.

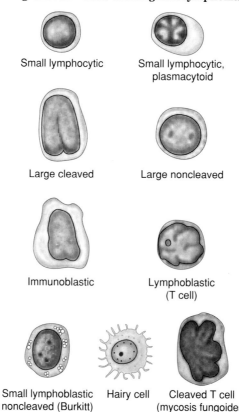

Small lymphocytic

Small lymphocytic, plasmacytoid

Large cleaved

Large noncleaved

Immunoblastic

Lymphoblastic (T cell)

Small lymphoblastic noncleaved (Burkitt)

Hairy cell

Cleaved T cell (mycosis fungoides)

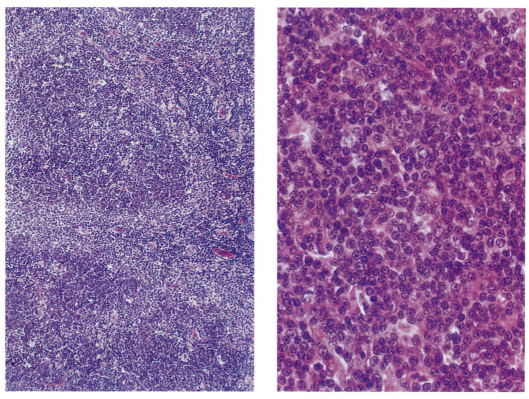

Figure 7.26

Figure 7.27

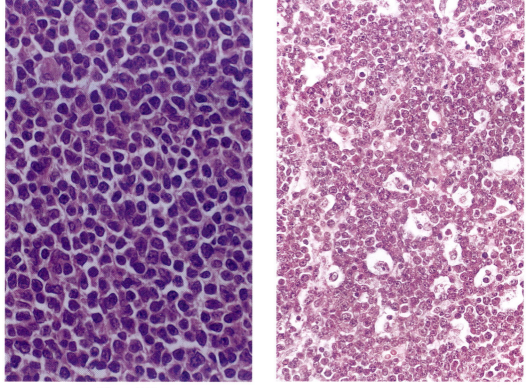

Figure 7.28

Figure 7.29

PLATE 7.9. HODGKIN DISEASE (HD)

Figure 7.30. **A.** Lymphocyte predominance HD. The lymph node is densely infiltrated with lymphocytes and contains a few scattered Reed-Sternberg cells. **B. Inset.** Reed-Sternberg cells have two or multilobed nuclei and prominent nucleoli. **C.** Nodular sclerosis HD. The lymph node infiltrates are subdivided by broad strands of fibrous tissue. **D. Inset.** Higher magnification shows pale "lacunar cells" typical of this variant. The infiltrate is mixed. **E.** Mixed cellularity HD. The infiltrate contains numerous Reed-Sternberg cells. Note eosinophils, plasma cells, and lymphocytes. **F.** Lymphocyte-depleted HD. Stromal fibrosis overshadows the cellular infiltrate, which consists of a few Reed-Sternberg cells and eosinophils.

Diagram 7.8.   Histopathology of Hodgkin disease.

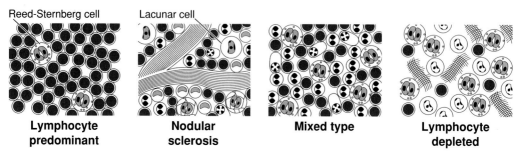

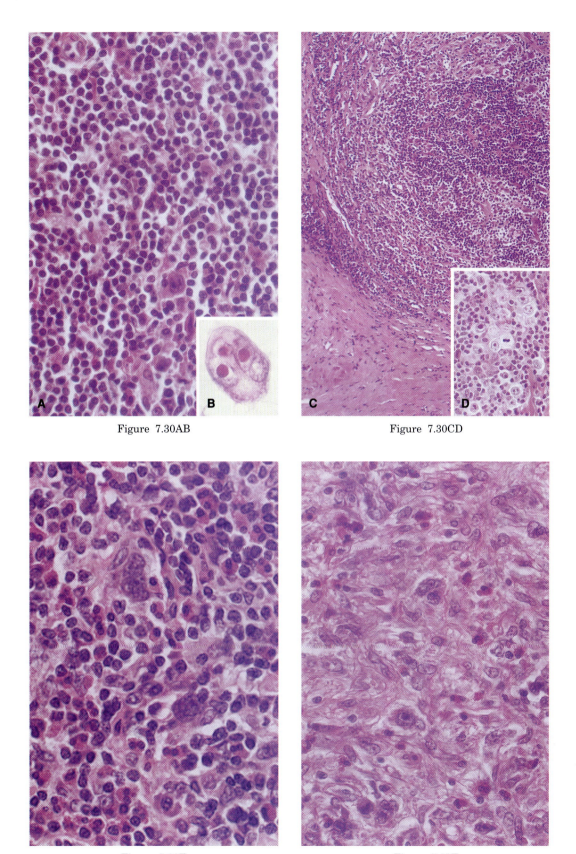

Figure 7.30AB

Figure 7.30CD

Figure 7.30E

Figure 7.30F

PLATE 7.10. PLASMA CELL NEOPLASIA

Figure 7.31. Multiple myeloma. A. Bone marrow is infiltrated with atypical plasma cells. **B. Inset.** Bone marrow aspirate shows atypical plasma cells that vary in size and shape. **C.** Myeloma kidney disease. The tubules contain protein casts and appear disrupted. Multinucleated cells represent a response to tubular casts. **D.** Amyloidosis leads to obliteration of normal glomerular architecture. **E.** Amyloid deposits stain brick red with Congo red. **F.** Congo red–positive amyloid has a greenish color under polarized light.

Figure 7.32. Waldenström macroglobulinemia. A. The bone marrow aspirate contains plasmacytoid cells intermediate between lymphocytes and plasma cells, and small immature blasts. **B.** Neoplastic lymphoid cells in peripheral blood are surrounded by erythrocytes that form rouleaux due to hyperviscosity of the plasma.

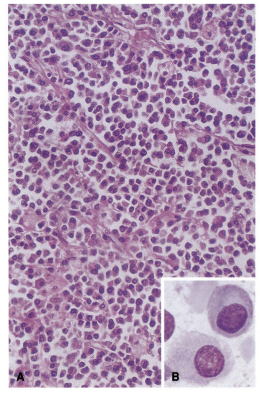

Figure 7.31AB

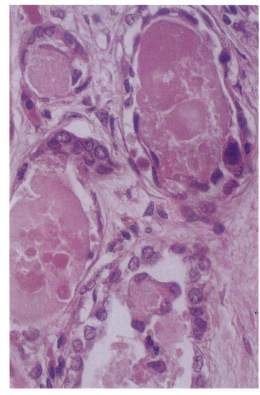

Figure 7.31C

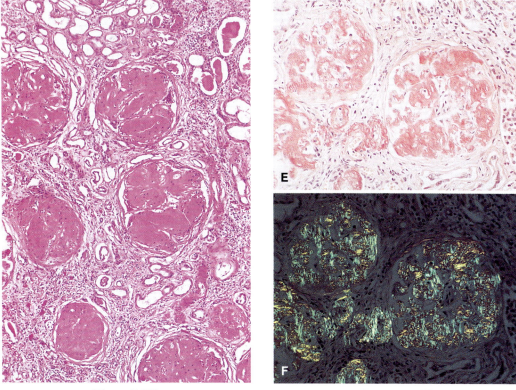

Figure 7.31D

Figure 7.31EF

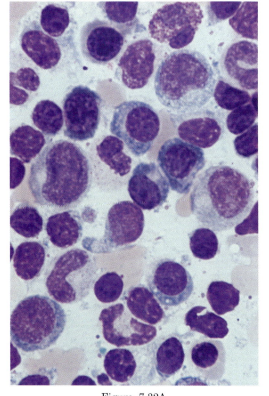

Figure 7.32A

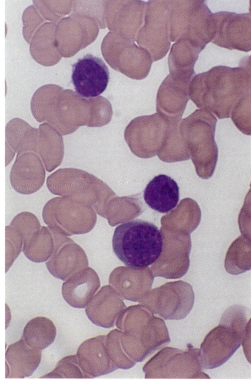

Figure 7.32B

NOTES

CHAPTER 8

Digestive System

NORMAL HISTOLOGY

The digestive, or alimentary, system includes the mouth, pharynx, esophagus, stomach, duodenum, small intestine, large intestine, and anus. The liver, the biliary tract, and the pancreas also belong to the digestive system but are described separately in Chapters 9 (liver and biliary tract) and 10 (pancreas).

The digestive system is a hollow tube that has a stereotypical structure. The tube consists of a mucosa, a variably developed submucosa, a muscularis, and an outer layer known as adventitia or serosa (Diagram 8.1). In the mouth, pharynx, and esophagus, the mucosa is lined by squamous epithelium. The stomach and intestines are lined by glandular cuboidal epithelium that shows special site-specific features reflecting the unique secretory or absorptive functions of these parts.

Despite these anatomical and functional variations, the response of various parts of the gastrointestinal system are rather predictable and nonspecific. For example, infectious lesions of the mouth and esophagus resemble similar lesions in other squamous epithelia, and the squamous cell carcinoma originating in these sites has the same features as squamous cell carcinoma in other organs, such as skin or uterine cervix. To avoid repetition, this chapter presents only the most typical and the most unique lesions.

OVERVIEW OF PATHOLOGY

Important diseases of the digestive system include:

- Inflammatory conditions
- Conditions that change the lumen or wall of the digestive system
- Circulatory disturbances
- Neoplasms

MOUTH, SALIVARY GLANDS, AND ESOPHAGUS

Inflammation of the Upper Digestive System

The most common causes of inflammation of the upper digestive system are presented in Diagram 8.2.

Stomatitis or inflammation of the oral mucosa presents as a mucosal ulcer or leukoplakia (white plaque). Histologically, such leukoplakia consists of a focus of thickened squamous epithelium and underlying chronic inflammation (Fig. 8.1).

Periodontitis is an inflammation of the gums and the tissue forming the tooth socket. This inflammation may progress to purulent gingivitis and periodontal abscess formation. Apical dental abscess may be a complication of tooth decay caused by caries. The infection is usually caused by saprophytic bacteria residing in the mouth. Histologically, such abscesses consist of a pus-filled cavity surrounded by granulation tissue that separates it from the surrounding jaw bone (Fig. 8.2). Only occasionally do such lesions show diagnostic features. For example, the periodontal abscess caused by *Actinomyces israelii* contains diagnostic "sulfur granules" composed of strands of bacteria.

Sialadenitis, i.e., inflammation of the salivary glands, can be caused by infections reaching the gland through the excretory ducts from the mouth, or hematogenously as in mumps. Chronic sialadenitis may also be caused by autoimmune mechanisms, as in Sjögren syndrome.

Esophagitis is an inflammation of the esophagus. Squamous epithelium of the esophagus is resistant to infections. Nevertheless, superficial or ulcerating esophagitis caused by fungi and viruses may occur in debilitated patients and those suffering from cancer or AIDS (Fig. 8.3).

Diagram 8.1.   Normal digestive system.

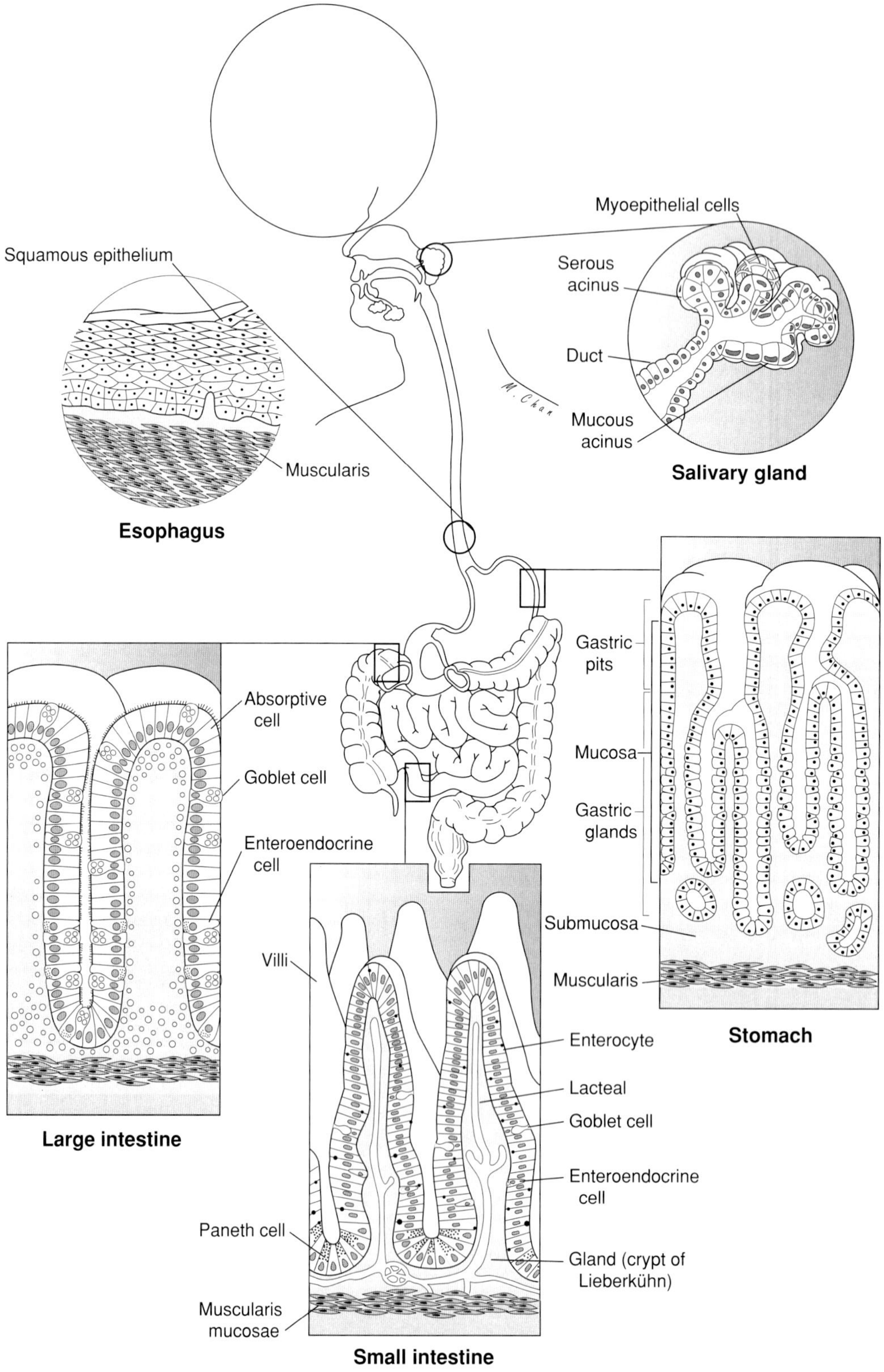

Squamous epithelium

Muscularis

Esophagus

Myoepithelial cells

Serous
acinus

Duct

Mucous
acinus

Salivary gland

M. Chan

Absorptive
cell

Goblet cell

Enteroendocrine
cell

Large intestine

Villi

Paneth cell

Muscularis
mucosae

Small intestine

Enterocyte

Lacteal

Goblet cell

Enteroendocrine
cell

Gland (crypt of
Lieberkühn)

Gastric
pits

Mucosa

Gastric
glands

Submucosa

Muscularis

Stomach

Neoplasms

Squamous cell carcinoma is the most important and most common malignant tumor of the upper alimentary system (Fig. 8.4). All squamous cell carcinomas appear alike whether they originate from the lips, tongue, or esophagus.

Ameloblastoma is a benign but locally invasive oral tumor derived from remnants of the fetal odontogenic epithelium (Fig. 8.5). Histologically, the tumor is composed of epithelial nests or cords embedded into loose connective tissue ("stellate reticulum"). These features are reminiscent of the fetal enamel organ in the tooth primordium.

Carcinoma of the nasopharynx, also called *lymphoepithelial carcinoma*, is a poorly differentiated squamous carcinoma. It consists of epithelial cells that are typically intermixed with reactive lymphoid cells (Fig. 8.6). This lymphoid stroma sometimes obscures the epithelial islands, and such tumors may be misdiagnosed as lymphoma.

Salivary gland tumors occur in several histological forms: pleomorphic adenoma, monomorphic adenoma, Warthin tumor (cystadenoma lymphomatosum), acinic cell carcinoma, mucoepidermoid carcinoma, and adenocarcinoma of excretory ducts (Fig. 8.7). The most common is **pleomorphic adenoma**, which accounts for two-thirds of all salivary gland tumors. Pleomorphic adenomas are benign but locally invasive tumors. These tumors may evolve into a frank malignancy ("carcinoma ex pleomorphic adenoma"). Histologically, pleomorphic adenomas are composed of islands, strands, and cords of epithelial and myoepithelial cells surrounded by a variety of stromal cells. The stromal cells may be arranged loosely and appear myxomatous or densely grouped into cartilage-like structures. **Warthin tumor** is composed of cuboidal cells lining cystic spaces surrounded by stroma densely infiltrated with lymphocytes. **Acinic cell carcinoma** is composed of well-differentiated cuboidal cells arranged into acini reminiscent of normal serous glands. Warthin tumor is benign. Acinic cell carcinoma is a low-grade malignancy.

STOMACH AND DUODENUM

Gastritis and Peptic Ulcer

Gastritis may be classified as erosive gastritis and nonerosive gastritis (Diagram 8.3).

Erosive gastritis is usually acute and characterized by superficial mucosal defects (*erosions*) (Fig. 8.8). These defects are caused by chemicals and drugs such as aspirin, circulatory disturbances (e.g., shock), or bacteria such as *Helicobacter pylori* (Fig. 8.9).

Nonerosive gastritis is a chronic disease that may be present in two forms: *atrophic*, the more common form, or *hypertropic*, which is extremely rare.

Two types of **atrophic** gastritis are recognized: antral and fundic. **Antral gastritis** involves the pyloric antrum and is typically associated with achlorhydria. **Fundic gastritis** is associated with a reduced number of parietal cells in the body of the stomach and pernicious anemia. Histologically, these two forms of gastritis have similar features. The mucosa contains fewer glands and is therefore thinner than normal. The mucosa also shows intestinal metaplasia, whereby the gastric epithelium is replaced by intestinal glands. These glands resemble those of the small intestine and contain goblet and Paneth cells (Fig. 8.10). The mucosa also shows signs of chronic inflammation and contains infiltrates of lymphocytes and plasma cells.

Peptic ulcer is a multifactorial disease characterized by a deep defect of the mucosa extending into the submucosa, and even into the muscularis of the stomach or duodenum (Fig. 8.11). The mucosal defect contains inflammatory cells and granulation tissue (Diagram 8.4). Ulcers may heal by scarring and re-epithelialization of the overlying mucosal defect. Erosion of blood vessels at the bottom of the ulcer may lead to bleeding.

Extension of ulcer through the serosa leads to perforation and subsequent peritonitis.

Gastric Neoplasms

Gastric tumors are classified as:

- *Epithelial tumors.* These include benign adenomatous polyps and carcinomas.

- *Stromal tumors.* The most important among the benign tumors are leiomyomas and leiomyoblastomas, and among the malignant ones, leiomyosarcomas.
- *Lymphomas.* These can be primary gastrointestinal lymphomas or secondary gastrointestinal lymphomas due to extension into the gut of systemic lymphoma.

The neoplasms of the stomach are presented in Diagram 8.5. **Epithelial neoplasms** account for the vast majority of all gastric tumors.

Adenomatous polyp is composed of irregular but nevertheless benign glands arranged into a polypoid, usually broadly based exophytic mass (Fig. 8.12).

Adenocarcinoma of the stomach is composed of atypical and pleomorphic cells that form neoplastic glands (Fig. 8.13). The tumor usually begins as a strictly mucosal lesion (*superficial carcinoma*). The tumor cell growth may be exophytic or endophytic, resulting in either polypoid or invasive lesions. The tumors usually are both exophytic and endophytic and appear as crater-like ulcers with indurated margins. Tumors that diffusely permeate the entire wall of the stomach are called *linitis plastica*.

Carcinoma of the stomach may be composed of nondescript cuboidal or cylindrical cells, or cells resembling various specialized gastrointestinal cells. Mucus-secreting cells are often prominent. Since these tumor cells have a semilunar nucleus displaced to the peripherally by the cytoplasmic mucus, they are called *signet ring carcinoma cells*.

SMALL INTESTINE

Inflammation of the small intestine is rarely seen in pathology samples, even though enteritis is a common disease. First of all, biopsy is rarely used to confirm the clinical diagnosis of enteritis. Second, in postmortem material, intestinal mucosa rapidly undergoes autolysis and thus cannot be properly evaluated at autopsy. Finally, many toxigenic bacteria that cause diarrhea, such as cholera, affect the function of intestinal cells but do not produce morphological signs of mucosal inflammation. Nevertheless, many intestinal inflammatory processes have characteristic morphological features that can be documented by biopsy.

For example, pathogens such as *Giardia lamblia* can be identified in intestinal biopsy (Fig. 8.14).

Malabsorption

Malabsorption is the most important consequence of small intestinal diseases. Small intestinal causes of malabsorption that can be diagnosed by intestinal biopsy are outlined in Diagram 8.6.

Whipple disease is systemic bacterial inflammatory disease that produces typical intestinal changes and is usually accompanied by malabsorption. Bacteria are phagocytosed by intestinal macrophages, which can be seen as mucosal aggregates of cells with granular cytoplasm (Fig. 8.15). These bacteria are best seen by electron microscopy.

Celiac disease is characterized by malabsorption that develops because of hypersensitivity to gluten. In contrast to the normal small intestinal mucosa, which has prominent villi, the mucosa affected by celiac disease shows villous atrophy (Fig. 8.16). The atrophy of villi and the chronic mucosal inflammation can be cured by placing the patient on a gluten-free diet. Under this treatment, the mucosal architecture will revert to normal. Patients with celiac disease are, nevertheless, at an increased risk for intestinal lymphoma.

Intestinal lymphoma is the most common malignancy associated with malabsorption. The intestinal mucosa or the entire wall may be infiltrated with neoplastic lymphocytes, which destroy the normal epithelium.

LARGE INTESTINE

Inflammatory Bowel Disease

This term includes two diseases of unknown etiology: *ulcerative colitis* and *Crohn's disease*. The most important histological features of these two diseases are listed in Table 8.1.

Ulcerative colitis is a disease of the large intestine that may also produce pathological changes in the appendix and distal ileum ("backwash ileitis"). The early changes are confined to intestinal crypts that are invaded by polymorphonuclear leukocytes (Fig. 8.17). These lesions are

Table 8.1
Histological Features of Ulcerative Colitis and Crohn Disease

	Ulcerative Colitis	Crohn Disease
Mucosal inflammation	+ +	+ +
Ulceration	+ +	+ +
Crypt abscess	+ +	+
Granulomas	–	+ +
Inflammation of the muscularis	–	+ +
Serosal inflammation	–	+ +
Epithelial atypia	+ +	+/–

called *crypt abscesses*. The inflammation spreading over the mucosal surface leads to the formation of broad confluent ulcers that surround remnants of inflamed mucosa. The regeneration of mucosal epithelial islands leads to the formation of *inflammatory pseudopolyps* that protrude into the lumen of the intestine. Prolonged regeneration predisposes to *epithelial dysplasia*. The dysplastic glands may progress into invasive adenocarcinoma.

Crohn's disease involves either the terminal ileum, the colon, or both. Initial mucosal changes may be indistinguishable from those of ulcerative colitis. However, in the fully established disease, the inflammation is *transmural* and extends to the serosal surface (Fig. 8.18), in contrast to ulcerative colitis, which is limited to the mucosa. The lesions contain *granulomas* in 50% of cases. Fistulas are a common complication. Adenocarcinoma is also a late complication but it occurs less often than in ulcerative colitis.

Circulatory Disturbances

Intestinal ischemia may be acute or chronic. **Acute ischemia** results from the occlusion of major arteries or veins, which is typically caused by thrombi or emboli. Such occlusion leads to **transmural infarction** of the intestine (Fig. 8.19), which is usually hemorrhagic (Diagram 8.7). Acute hypotension due to heart failure or shock causes hypoperfusion of the intestine and results in **multifocal necrosis** of the superficial mucosa.

Chronic ischemia caused by smaller branches of the intestinal arteries or chronic hypoperfusion in heart failure leads to multifocal patchy necrosis of the mucosa (Fig. 8.20). Ischemic mucosa sloughs off and ulcerates.

Diverticulosis

Diverticulosis is a focal dilatation of the intestine in which the mucosa protrudes through a defect in a muscle layer (Fig. 8.21). Such outpouchings of the mucosa are prone to inflammation, which is then called *diverticulitis*.

Intestinal Infections

Infections of the intestine may be caused by viruses, bacteria, or parasites. Diffuse infections are called enterocolitis, while localized infections bear site specific names, e.g., ileitis, proctitis (infection of the rectum), appendicitis.

Appendicitis is one of the most common bacterial infection of the intestines (Diagram 8.8). The infection is initially limited to the luminal surface and is typically caused by bacteria retained in the lumen of an obstructed appendix (Fig. 8.22). The obstruction may be caused by hardened feces (*fecalith*), hyperplastic lymphoid tissue (particularly in children), or worms. The inflammation permeates the entire thickness of the wall leading to gangrene and perforation. The perforation is associated with localized peritonitis involving the serosa of the appendix and adjacent organs, but it may progress into a *perityphlitic abscess* or **diffuse peritonitis** (Fig. 8.23). Similar bacterial peritonitis can obviously develop following rupture of any other part of the gastrointestinal tract.

Amebic colitis is caused by *Entamoeba histolytica*. Trophozoites released from the ingested amebic cysts invade the mucosa and form "flask-shaped" ulcers extending into the submucosa. Such ulcers contain an inflammatory exudate rich in neutrophils and scattered amebas (Fig. 8.24).

Polyps and Neoplasms

The most important non-neoplastic and neoplastic polyps and neoplasms of the colon are listed in Table 8.2 and presented in Diagrams 8.9 and 8.10.

Non-neoplastic polyps comprise congenital and inflammatory lesions that produce polypoid lesions of distinct histological appearance.

Table 8.2
Polyps of the Large Intestine

Non-neoplastic polyps
  Hyperplastic polyp
  Juvenile polyp
  Peutz-Jeghers polyp
  Lymphoid polyp
  Inflammatory pseudopolyp (Ulcerative colitis)
Neoplastic polyps
  Tubular adenoma
  Villous adenoma
  Tubulovillous adenoma

Hyperplastic polyps are the most common non-neoplastic polyps. These polyps appear as small, slightly elevated nodules of the mucosa usually measuring 1–5 mm in diameter. Histologically, these polyps consist of hyperplastic, slightly disorganized glands (Fig. 8.25) lined by normal colonic epithelium, which appears serrated because of cellular overcrowding.

Juvenile polyps are composed of dilated, often obstructed glands that are enclosed in inflamed connective tissue (Fig. 8.26). These polyps are hamartomas or developmental abnormalities of the intestinal mucosa.

The polyps of **Peutz-Jeghers syndrome** are also congenital and related to focal abnormal development of the intestinal wall. Such polyps are composed of irregularly shaped glands enclosed by connective tissue and strands of smooth muscle cells (Fig. 8.27). The glands often contain an increased number of mucous cells.

Lymphoid polyps are composed of mucosal lymphoid follicles that are enlarged to the point where they elevate the overlying mucosa, causing a small polypoid protrusion (Fig. 8.28).

Neoplastic Polyps

Neoplastic polyps are principally of two types: *tubular adenomas* and *villous adenomas* (Diagram 8.10). These two patterns of growth may be intermixed, resulting in *mixed tubulovillous adenomas*.

Tubular adenomas are typically pedunculated, i.e., attached to the mucosa with a stalk. The head of the polyp is composed of abnormally shaped glands lined with columnar or cuboidal cells that differ from normal colonic cells in that they do not contain mucus. The nuclei appear hyper-chromatic, crowded, and stratified (Fig. 8.29). Benign tubular adenomas have a small but definite chance of malignant transformation. Malignant change, recognized in 1–3% of tubular adenomas, is characterized by the appearance of highly irregular glands lined with hyperchromatic cells that typically invade the stalk and/or extend into the wall of the intestine.

Villous adenoma is a sessile, broad-based lesion composed of finger-like elongated villi (Fig. 8.30). These villi are lined by cylindrical cells that have hyperchromatic stratified nuclei and often show signs of mucin production. Villous adenomas have a high propensity for malignant transformation, which is recognized in early stages by the irregularity of glands that invade the muscularis.

Carcinoma of the Colon

Adenocarcinomas account for 95% of all malignant neoplasms of the colon. Histologically, these tumors resemble adenocarcinomas in other sites (Fig. 8.31) and are classified as well, moderately, or poorly differentiated. The tumor cells produce carcinoembryonic antigen (CEA), which is also released into the blood and may serve as a diagnostic tumor marker. CEA can be demonstrated immunohistochemically on cell membranes and in the lumen of neoplastic glands.

Carcinoid Tumors

Carcinoids are tumors of neuroendocrine cells (Fig. 8.32). These tumors can arise in any part of the intestine but are most often found in the appendix. Histologically, carcinoids are composed of well differentiated neuroendocrine cells that typically have round nuclei. The cells appear uniform and benign. Nevertheless, all carcinoids are locally invasive, and those larger than 2 cm tend also to metastasize most often to the local lymph nodes and the liver. Carcinoids may also secrete serotonin, histamine, and various polypeptide hormones (e.g., glucagon, adrenocorticotropic hormone, vasoactive intestinal polypeptide). These polypeptide hormones can be demonstrated immunohistochemically in the tumor cells. Electron microscopy reveals that carcinoids contain neuroendocrine granules.

NOTES

PLATE 8.1. INFLAMMATION OF THE UPPER DIGESTIVE SYSTEM

Figure 8.1. Stomatitis. An area of chronic inflammation is seen in the connective tissue underneath the thickened surface epithelium. Such epithelial thickening appears clinically as leukoplakia.

Figure 8.2. Periodontitis. A. The wall of the periodontal abscess consists of granulation tissue. **B.** Abscess caused by *Actinomyces israelii* contains diagnostic sulfur granules composed of strands of bacteria.

Figure 8.3. Esophagitis. Ulceration of esophageal mucosa.

Diagram 8.2. The most common infections of the upper digestive tract.

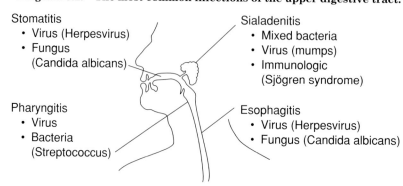

Stomatitis
- Virus (Herpesvirus)
- Fungus
  (Candida albicans)

Pharyngitis
- Virus
- Bacteria
  (Streptococcus)

Sialadenitis
- Mixed bacteria
- Virus (mumps)
- Immunologic
  (Sjögren syndrome)

Esophagitis
- Virus (Herpesvirus)
- Fungus (Candida albicans)

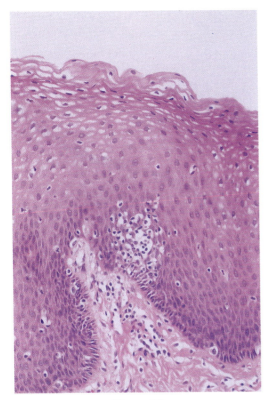

Figure 8.1

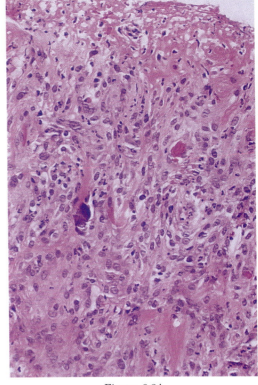

Figure 8.2A

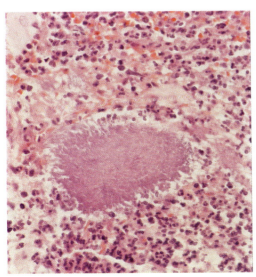

Figure 8.2B

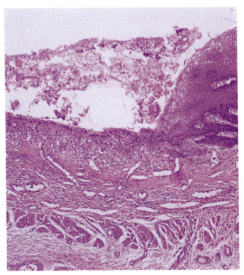

Figure 8.3

PLATE 8.2. NEOPLASMS OF THE UPPER DIGESTIVE SYSTEM

Figure 8.4. Squamous cell carcinoma of the tongue. Similar squamous cell carcinomas occur on the lips, mouth, and esophagus.

Figure 8.6. Lymphoepithelial carcinoma of the pharynx. Large tumor cells are intermixed with lymphocytes.

Figure 8.5. Ameloblastoma. The tumor is composed of nests of stellate and spindle-shaped cells.

Figure 8.7. Salivary gland tumors. A. Pleomorphic adenoma is composed of epithelial and myoepithelial cells and loose myxomatous stroma. **B.** Warthin tumor is composed of acidophilic epithelial cells and stroma that contain lymphocytes. **C.** Acinic cell carcinoma is composed of cuboidal glandular cells.

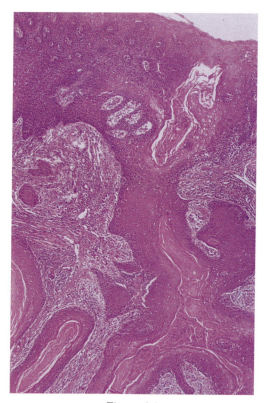

Figure 8.4

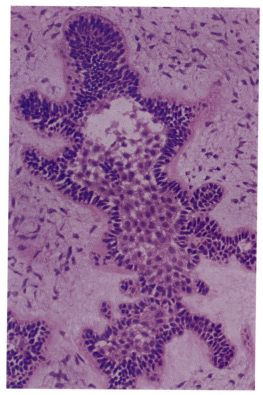

Figure 8.5

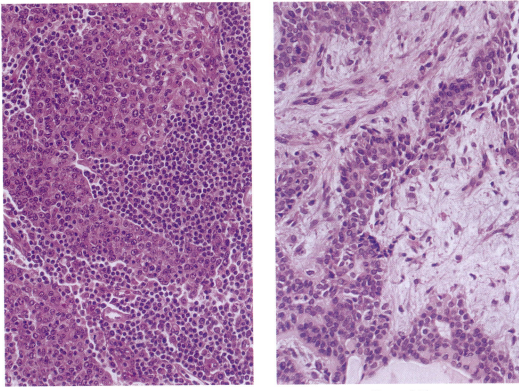

Figure 8.6

Figure 8.7A

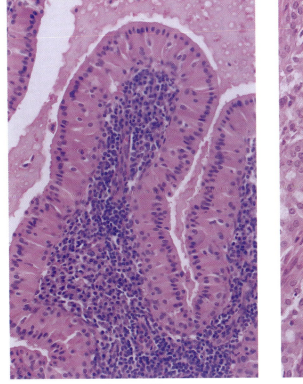

Figure 8.7B

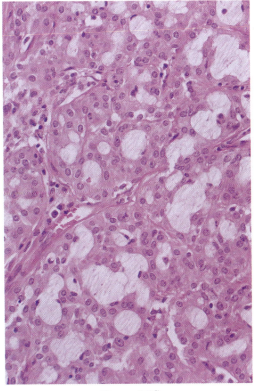

Figure 8.7C

PLATE 8.3. GASTRITIS

Figure 8.8. Erosive gastritis. Superficial loss of normal mucosa is accompanied by congestion and hemorrhage.

Figure 8.9. Gastritis caused by *Helicobacter pylori.* The bacilli are attached to the apical surface of gastric cells. (Courtesy Dr. R. Genta, Houston, Texas.)

Figure 8.10. Antral atrophic gastritis. A. The mucosa contains fewer glands than normal and the stroma is infiltrated with chronic inflammatory cells. **B.** The glands show intestinal metaplasia characterized by goblet cells (G) and Paneth cells (P).

Diagram 8.3. Gastritis and peptic ulcer. A. Normal gastric mucosa. **B.** Erosive gastritis. **C.** Atrophic gastritis. **D.** Hyperplastic gastritis. **E.** Peptic ulcer.

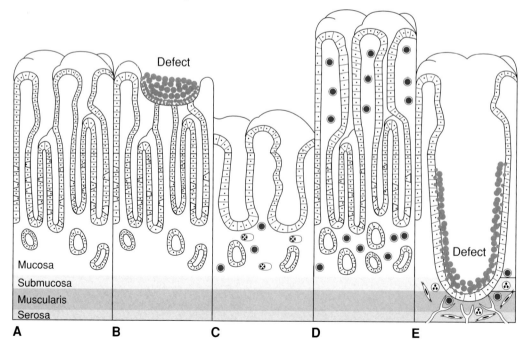

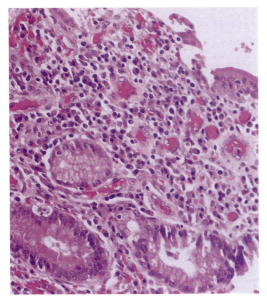

Figure 8.8

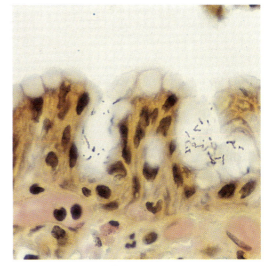

Figure 8.9

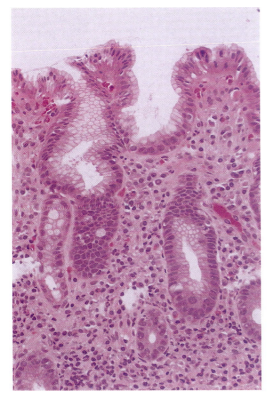

Figure 8.10A

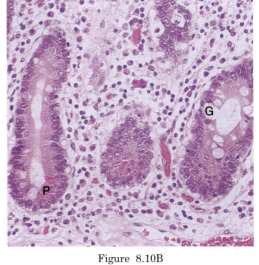

Figure 8.10B

PLATE 8.4. PEPTIC ULCER

Figure 8.11.   Peptic ulcer. A. The defect of mucosa extending into the muscularis contains granulation tissue. (From Grundmann E, Geller SA. Histopathology. Munich: Urban & Schwarzenberg, 1989.) **B.** Higher-magnification view of the superficial layers of an ulcer. The surface layer consists of necrotic tissue; underneath it is a layer rich in blood vessels and chronic inflammatory cells. **C.** The bottom of chronic peptic ulcer contains an artery, the wall of which has been eroded. The overlying granulation tissue has sloughed off, exposing the artery to the action of peptic juices. The artery has probably bled, but its lumen is now occluded with a fibrin thrombus.

Diagram 8.4.   Peptic ulcer. The bottom of the mucosal defect consists of several layers: necrotic material, acute inflammatory exudate, vascular granulation tissue, and fibrous scarring. The inflammation may erode arteries and cause profuse bleeding.

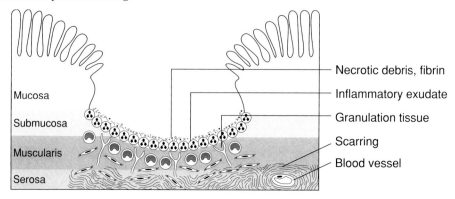

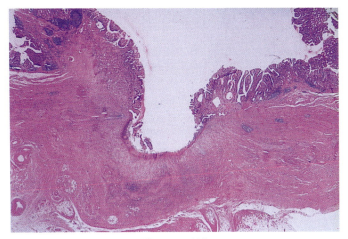

Figure 8.11A

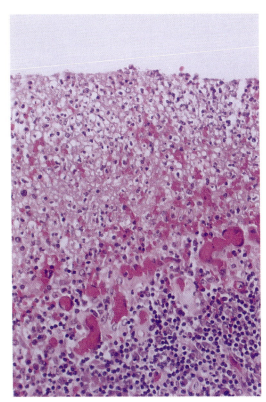

Figure 8.11B

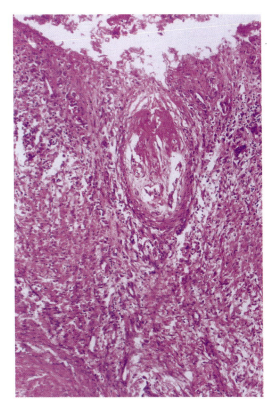

Figure 8.11C

PLATE 8.5. TUMORS OF THE STOMACH

Figure 8.12.   Adenomatous polyp of the stomach. This benign tumor is composed of irregular, dilated glands.

Figure 8.13.   Adenocarcinoma of the stomach. A. Well differentiated adenocarcinoma limited to the surface epithelium. **B.** Linitis plastica. The tumor cells infiltrate between the smooth muscle cells of the muscle layer of the stomach. **C.** Signet ring cell carcinoma. The tumor cells are filled with mucus, which displaces the nucleus and imparts to it a semilunar shape.

Diagram 8.5.   Gastric neoplasms. A. Adenoma grows like an exophytic polyp. **B.** Superficial adenocarcinoma. **C.** Invasive, ulcerated (crater-like) adenocarcinoma. **D.** Diffusely infiltrating carcinoma (linitis plastica) composed of signet ring cells. **E.** Primary lymphoma involving the mucosa and submucosa. **F.** Leiomyomas (leiomyoblastomas) and leiomyosarcomas originate from the smooth muscle cells of the muscularis.

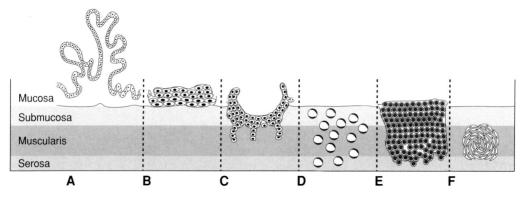

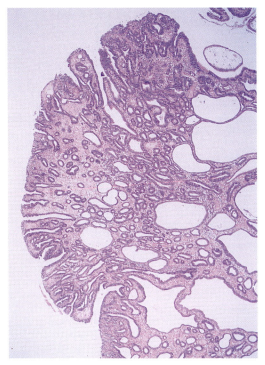

Figure 8.12

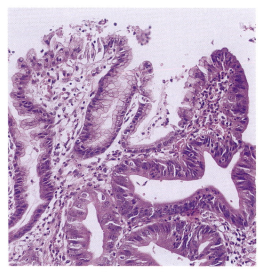

Figure 8.13A

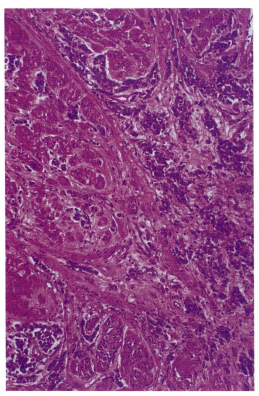

Figure 8.13B

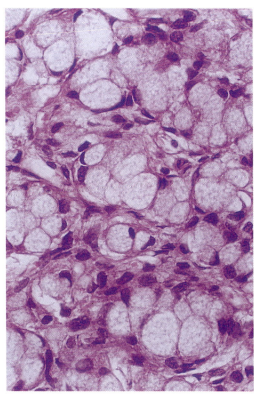

Figure 8.13C

PLATE 8.6. SMALL INTESTINAL LESIONS ASSOCIATED WITH MALABSORPTION

Figure 8.14.   Giardiasis of small intestine. The protozoa *(Lamblia giardia)* can be seen in the lumen and attached to the mucosal cells.

Figure 8.15.   Whipple disease. A. The mucosa contains prominent macrophages with granular cytoplasm. The lymphatics are dilated. **B. Inset** shows the electron microscopic appearance of the bacilli in the cytoplasm of mucosal histiocytes. (Courtesy of Dr. N. Ectors, Leuven, Belgium.)

Figure 8.16.   Celiac disease. A. Loss of villi is accompanied by chronic mucosal inflammation. **B.** Almost normal intestinal mucosa is seen following treatment, which included removal of gluten from the diet.

Diagram 8.6.   Small intestinal lesions associated with malabsorption. A. Normal mucosa shows long villi lined by typical intestinal epithelium. **B.** Abetalipoproteinemia is marked by clear, lipid-laden epithelial lining cells. **C.** Celiac disease shows atrophy of villi and chronic inflammation. **D.** Lymphoma is characterized by mucosal infiltrates of malignant lymphocytes. **E.** Whipple diseases is characterized by mucosal infiltrates of macrophages. **F.** *Giardia lamblia* is a superficial mucosal parasite. **G.** Scleroderma or amyloidosis cause stromal changes.

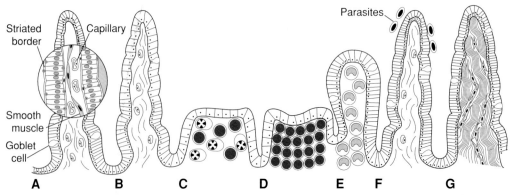

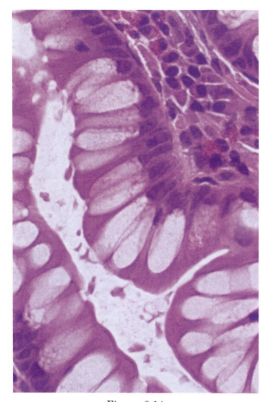

Figure 8.14

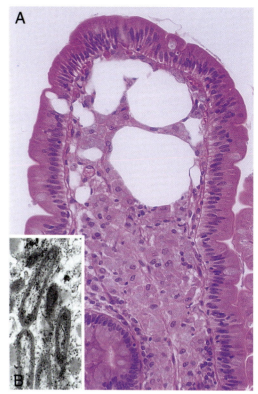

Figure 8.15A,B

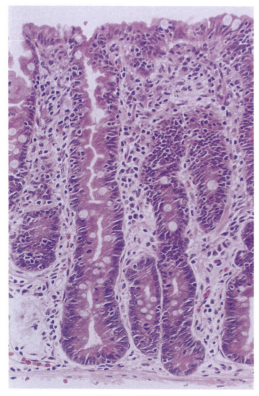

Figure 8.16A

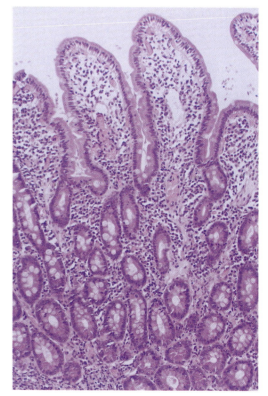

Figure 8.16B

PLATE 8.7. INFLAMMATORY BOWEL DISEASE

Figure 8.17. **Ulcerative colitis. A.** Crypt abscess. **B.** Ulceration of the mucosa. **C.** Inflammatory pseudopolyps consist of inflamed mucosa protruding above ulcerated mucosa. **D.** Epithelial dysplasia. The cells form irregular glands. The size and shape of nuclei vary mildly.

Figure 8.18. **Crohn's disease. A.** Transmural inflammation. **B.** Granulomas.

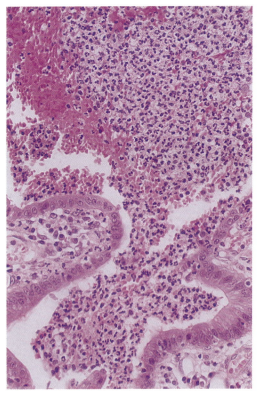

Figure 8.17A

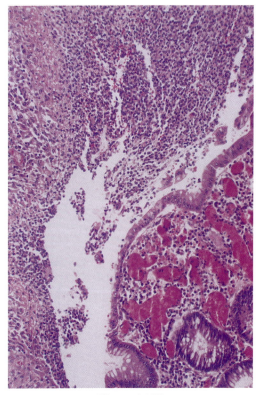

Figure 8.17B

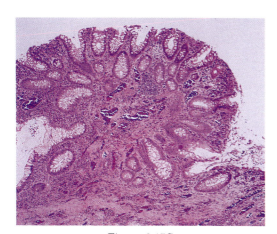

Figure 8.17C

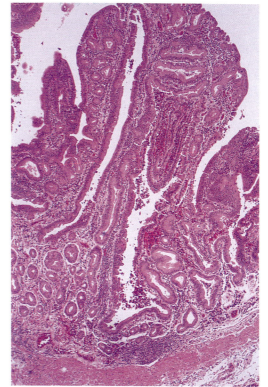

Figure 8.17D

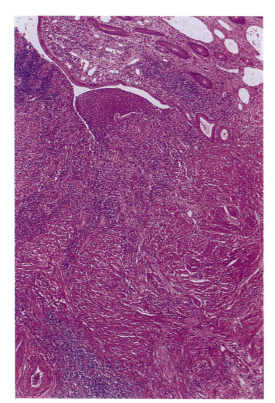

Figure 8.18A

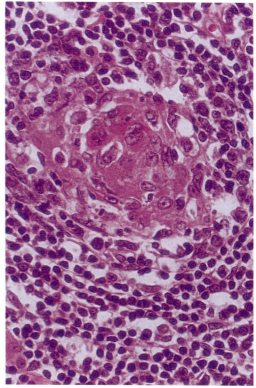

Figure 8.18B

PLATE 8.8. CIRCULATORY DISORDERS AND DIVERTICULOSIS

Figure 8.19.   Infarction of the intestine. A. The entire intestine is necrotic, and part of it is permeated with blood. **B.** Focal ischemia of the mucosal surface.

Figure 8.20.   Ischemic colitis. Ulceration is a late consequence of an infarct that has destroyed a segment of intestinal mucosa.

Figure 8.21.   Diverticulosis. The mucosa protrudes through the muscle layer.

Diagram 8.7.   Circulatory disturbances of the intestine. A. Arterial occlusion leads to infarction of the entire intestine. **B.** Occlusion of veins also causes an infarction of the entire intestine. **C.** Hypertension caused by heart failure or circulatory collapse in shock leads to necrosis of superficial mucosa.

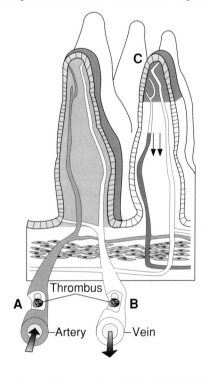

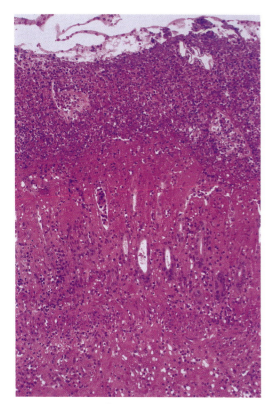

Figure 8.19A

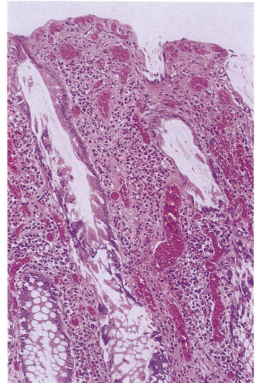

Figure 8.19B

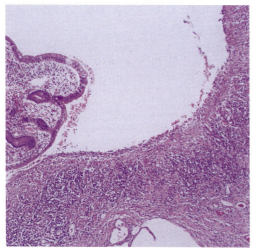

Figure 8.20

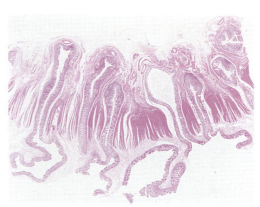

Figure 8.21

PLATE 8.9. INTESTINAL INFECTIONS

Figure 8.22. Appendicitis. Transmural inflammation extending into the mesoappendix.

Figure 8.23. Peritonitis. Gangrene of the appendix is associated with a serosal exudate of acute inflammatory cells and fibrin.

Figure 8.24. Amebic colitis. A. The ulcer is referred to as "flask-shaped," because it undermines the mucosa. **B.** The ulcer contains amebas. These trophozoites typically ingest erythrocytes, which can be recognized in their cytoplasm.

Diagram 8.8. Appendicitis. The disease evolves through several stages. **A.** Obstruction of the lumen and retention of bacteria leads to mucosal inflammation. **B.** Ulceration develops. **C.** The transmural spread of infection ultimately leads to rupture of the appendix. **D.** Peritonitis develops as a complication of appendiceal rupture or massive transmural inflammation.

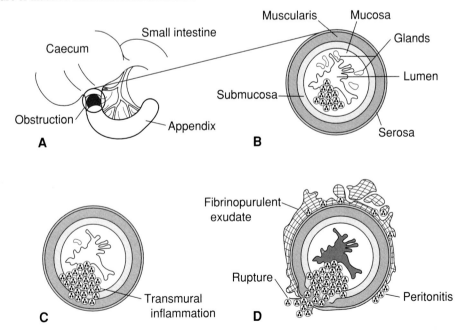

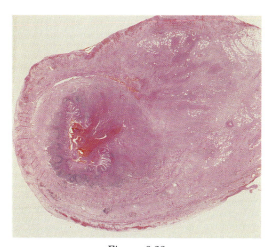

Figure 8.22

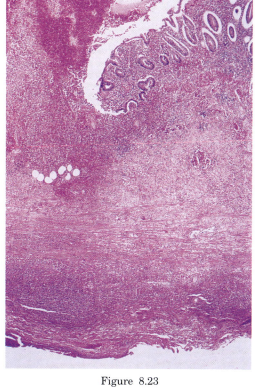

Figure 8.23

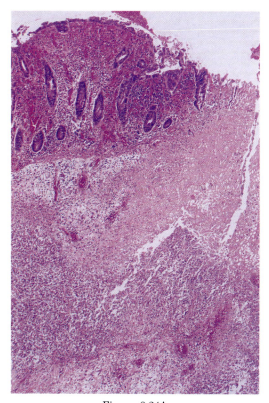

Figure 8.24A

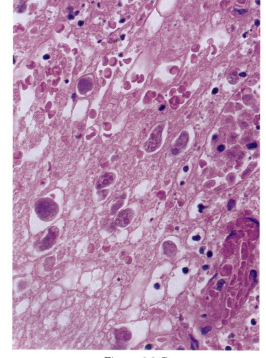

Figure 8.24B

PLATE 8.10. NON–NEOPLASTIC POLYPS

Figure 8.25. Hyperplastic polyp. The epithelium is composed of normal cells, which are crowded and impart to the lumen a serrated appearance ("corkscrew-like"). Goblet cells are prominent.

Figure 8.26. Juvenile polyp. The surface of this polyp is ulcerated and covered with granulation tissue. The stroma of the polyp also contains inflammatory cells, blood vessels, and dilated glands lined by normal colonic epithelium.

Figure 8.27. Peutz-Jeghers polyp. The glands embedded between strands of smooth muscle cells are lined by normal epithelium rich in goblet cells.

Figure 8.28. Lymphoid polyp. Lymphocytes form a follicle in the mucosa.

Diagram 8.9. Non-neoplastic intestinal polyps. A. Normal mucosa. **B.** Hyperplastic polyp. **C.** Peutz-Jeghers polyp. **D.** Juvenile polyp. **E.** Lymphoid polyp.

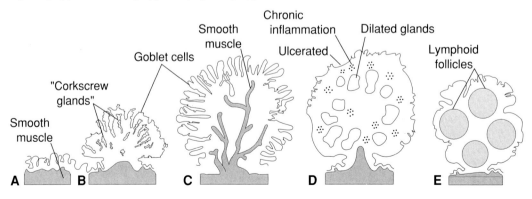

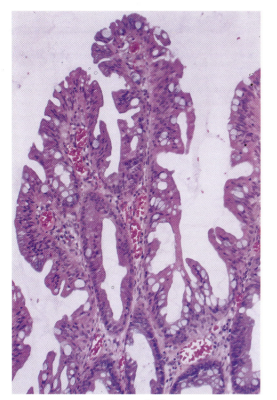

Figure 8.25

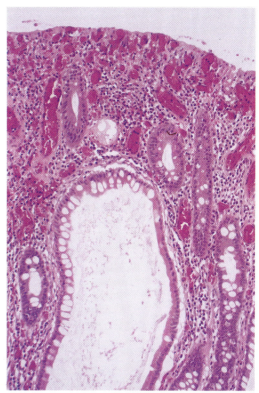

Figure 8.26

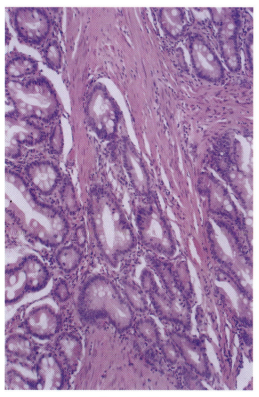

Figure 8.27

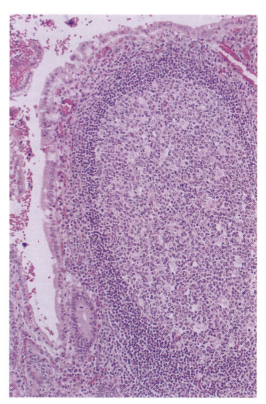

Figure 8.28.

PLATE 8.11. NEOPLASTIC POLYPS

Figure 8.29. Tubular adenoma. A. The tumor protrudes into the lumen of the intestine on a stalk. **B.** The tumor is composed of uniform glands. The nuclei appear uniform but crowded.

Figure 8.30. Villous adenoma. A. Small tumor showing finger-like villi. **B.** The villi are lined by columnar mucinous cells.

Diagram 8.10. Neoplastic polyps. A. Tubular adenoma. **B.** Villous adenoma. **C.** Tubulovillous adenoma. **D.** Carcinoma in the stalk of tubular adenoma. **E.** Invasive carcinoma arising in a villous adenoma.

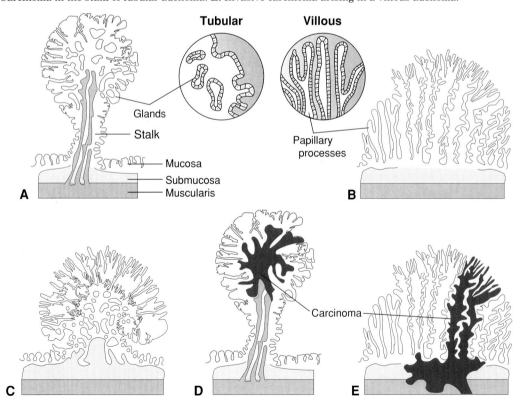

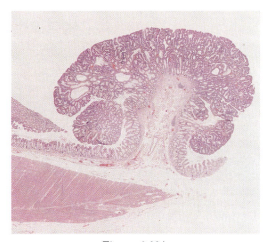

Figure 8.29A

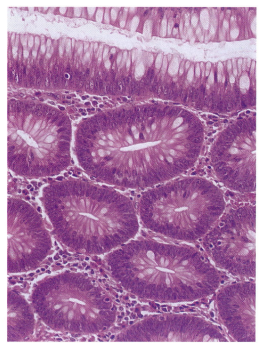

Figure 8.29B

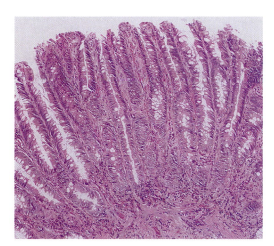

Figure 8.30A

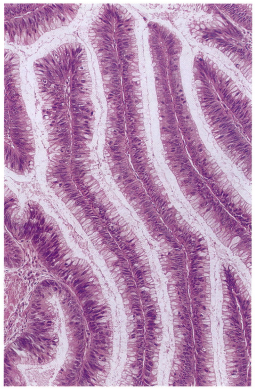

Figure 8.30B

PLATE 8.12. MALIGNANT NEOPLASMS

Figure 8.31. Adenocarcinoma of the colon. A. This tumor, composed of irregular gland-like structures, is arising in an adenoma. The benign glands are at the top. **B.** Carcinoembryonic antigen (CEA) appears as brown staining of the tumor cell membranes and intraluminal secretions in this photograph of immunohistochemically prepared tissue sections.

Figure 8.32. Carcinoid. A. The tumor is composed of small cells forming nests in the submucosa. **B.** The tumors cells have uniformly round nuclei and well developed eosinophilic cytoplasm. **C.** Electron microscopy of a carcinoid tumor. The cytoplasm contains membrane-bound, dense neuroendocrine granules. **D.** Carcinoid metastatic to the liver. This slow-growing tumor is separated from the liver cells by a fibrous capsule. At low magnification, one can appreciate nests of tumor cells separated from one another by connective tissue septa.

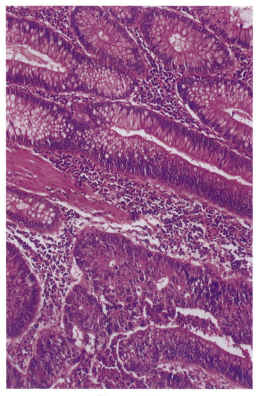
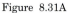

Figure 8.31A

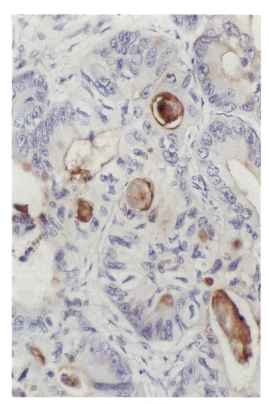

Figure 8.31B

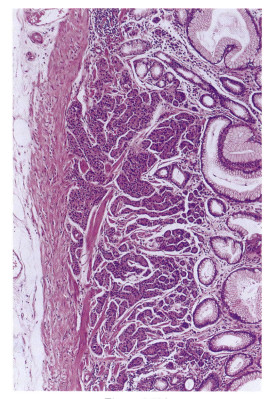

Figure 8.32A

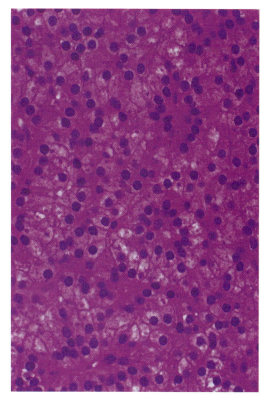

Figure 8.32B

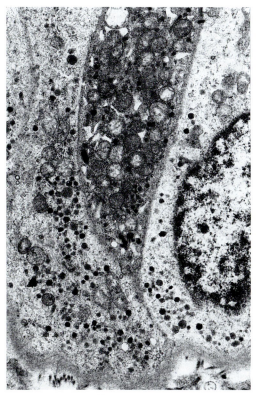

Figure 8.32C

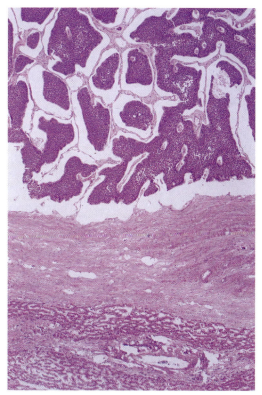

Figure 8.32D

NOTES

CHAPTER 9

Hepatobiliary System

NORMAL HISTOLOGY

The **liver** is a compact organ covered with a serosal layer of mesothelium, which forms the Glisson capsule (Diagram 9.1). Histologically, the liver is composed of several cell types, the most important of which are:

- **Hepatocytes.** These cells account for about 70% of all cells and for more than 90% of the total liver weight. Hepatocytes are arranged into functional units called acini, or lobules. Lobules have a central vein (terminal vein) and peripherally located portal tracts.
- **Bile ductal cells.** Bile ductal cells form ductules in the portal tract of the lobule. Ductules from adjacent lobules flow into ducts that extend toward the hilus of the liver, gradually increasing in size and diameter. Large intrahepatic bile ducts give rise to extrahepatic bile ducts that exit from the liver at the hepatic hilus (porta hepatis).
- **Vascular cells.** The liver has a dual blood supply; it receives arterial blood through the hepatic artery and venous blood through the portal vein. The hepatic artery and the portal vein enter the liver at the porta hepatitis and then branch into smaller vessels that run in parallel until they reach the portal tracts of the lobules. The small branches of the portal vein and hepatic artery together with the bile ducts are enclosed in the connective tissue of the portal tracts and are known as portal triads. From the portal tract, the venous and arterial blood enter into the sinusoids of the lobule and flow toward the terminal vein, which is the main effluent vessel of the lobule. The sinusoids are lined with Kupffer cells, which form a discontinuous "fenestrated" layer, incompletely separating the blood space from the liver cells. A narrow space of Disse separates the Kupffer cells from the liver cells.

The gall bladder and **extrahepatic bile ducts** are hollow organs with the general features of other parts of the gastrointestinal tube. On the luminal side they are lined by columnar epithelium. Underneath the epithelium lies a lamina propria and then a smooth muscle layer (*muscularis*). The external surface is partly covered with serosa and partly contiguous with the connective tissue of the liver capsule and/or hepatic hilus.

OVERVIEW OF PATHOLOGY

The response of the liver to injury may take several forms and involve the hepatocytes, vascular cells, or the bile ducts. The most important diseases are:

- Biliary obstruction
- Metabolic lesions, caused by genetic diseases or exogenous substances, such as alcohol
- Inflammation, especially that caused by hepatitis viruses
- Cirrhosis, or end-stage liver disease caused by a variety of pre-existing diseases
- Neoplasia

The gall bladder is affected by fewer diseases than the liver. The most important diseases are:

- Gall stones and related chronic inflammation
- Acute bacterial cholecystitis
- Neoplasia

Biliary Obstruction

Bile flow obstruction results in *jaundice*. Obstructive jaundice is typically caused by lesions in the main extrahepatic bile duct, such as carcinoma, impacted bile stones, or sclerosing cholangitis (Diagram 9.2). Bile accumulates in dilated bile ducts, ductules, and intercellular biliary canaliculi (Fig. 9.1). Injury of liver cells by stagnant bile results in intracellular accumulation of bile and *"feathery degeneration"* of liver cells. *"Bile lakes"* and *"bile infarcts"* form as the liver cells disintegrate and the bile permeates the necrotic tissue. The damaged bile ducts and ductules tend to proliferate in an attempt to repair the disruption and reestablish biliary excretion. This abortive repair is usually accompanied by fibrosis. Prolonged bile duct obstruction may cause **secondary biliary cirrhosis**.

Metabolic Disorders

Metabolic disorders of the liver may be *hereditary (genetic)* or *acquired*. The liver is affected by many hereditary metabolic disorders, which are best diagnosed in the context of other clinical and biochemical findings typical for each disease. Representative hereditary hyperbilirubinemias and disorders involving intermediate metabolism of lipids, carbohydrates, proteins, and heavy metals are listed in Table 9.1.

Congenital Metabolic Disorders

Congenital hyperbilirubinemia occurs in several forms. The best known congenital jaundice syndromes are *Gilbert syndrome, Crigler-Najjar syndrome, Rotor syndrome,* and *Dubin-Johnson syndrome*. The liver, affected by these diseases, shows no morphological changes except in **Dubin-Johnson syndrome**. In this autosomal recessive syndrome, marked by conjugated hyperbilirubinemia, the liver cells contain brown granules resembling lipofuscin (Fig. 9.2). The nature of this pigment is not known, but biochemical analysis reveals that it does not contain bilirubin or iron, which is the hallmark of the brown pigment of hemosiderosis.

Table 9.1
Representative Hereditary Metabolic Disorders Affecting the Liver

Diseases	Liver Pathology
A. Hereditary hyperbilirubinemia	
• Gilbert syndrome	−
• Crigler-Najjar syndrome	−
• Rotor syndrome	−
• Dubin-Johnson syndrome	+
B. Storage diseases	
Glycogenoses	
• von Gierke disease	+
• Galactosemia	+[a]
Lipidoses	
• Wolman disease	+
Mucopolysaycharidoses	
• Hurler disease	+
Sphingolipidoses	
• Gaucher disease	+[b]
• Niemann-Pick disease	+
C. Defects of Catabolic or anabolic and regulatory proteins	
• Alpha-1-antitrypsin deficiency	+[a]
• Tyrosinemia	+
D. Heavy metal disorders	
• Hemochromatosis (iron)	+[a]
• Wilson disease (copper)	+[a]
E. Defects of heme synthesis	
• Porphyria	+

[a] Progress to cirrhosis.

[b] Only Kupffer cells are affects.

Diagram 9.1.   Normal hepatobiliary system.

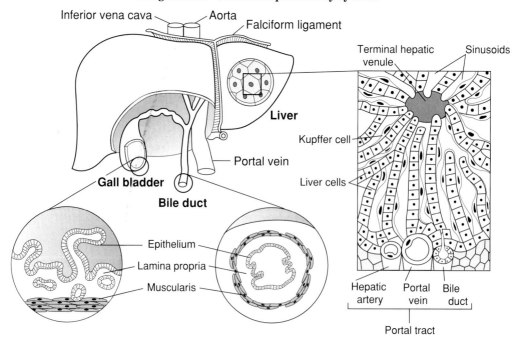

Storage diseases due to genetic defects involving specific enzymes often cause hepatomegaly, which is typical of lipidoses, glycogenoses, and mucopolysaccharidoses. The intermediate metabolites that cannot be processed accumulate in the liver cells or the Kupffer cells. In lipidoses, such as **Wolman disease** (*congenital lipase deficiency*), the hepatocytes have microvesicular cytoplasms due to lipid accumulation (Fig. 9.3). In **glycogenosis**, the liver cells appear enlarged and have clear cytoplasm rich in glycogen. In routinely stained slides, the cytoplasm appears hydropic because glycogen has been washed out. In some forms, such as glycogenosis type IV, fibrosis and cirrhosis develop early in life (Fig. 9.4). In **galactosemia**, an inborn error of galactose metabolism, accumulation of galactose and lipid in liver cells is accompanied by cholestasis and bile ductular proliferation. If untreated, the liver disease progresses to childhood cirrhosis.

Genetic enzyme deficiencies such as **alpha-1-antitrypsin deficiency** may also result in liver cell injury, which ultimately leads to cirrhosis. Histologically, the liver cells contain prominent eosinophilic, round, cytoplasmic globules, which stain red with PAS and are immunoreactive with antibodies to alpha-1-antitrypsin (Fig. 9.5). Deficiency of alpha-1-antitrypsin is an important cause of childhood cirrhosis.

Acquired Metabolic Disorders

Metabolic disorders can be induced in liver cells by a variety of ingested substances such as toxins, drugs, foods, and beverages.

Induced metabolic liver injury is best illustrated by the changes caused by alcohol. Ethyl alcohol is the most common cause of liver disease in the United States and Western Europe. **Alcohol** produces three types of liver disease (Fig. 9.6):

- **Fatty liver**. This change is predictable and dose-dependent and occurs within hours of ingestion of alcohol. Long-term alcohol intake results in massive hepatic steatosis and hepatomegaly. Fatty change is not associated with changes in liver function. It is reversible, and the accumulated fat disappears from liver cells upon cessation of drinking of alcohol.
- **Alcoholic hepatitis**. Alcoholic hepatitis develops in 15% of chronic alcoholics. Clinically, the disease presents as *hepatitis* of sudden onset. Symptoms include fever, leukocytosis, jaundice, nausea, and vomiting. Biochemical liver function tests are abnormal. Liver biopsy shows signs of liver cell injury and intralobular inflammation or fibrosis. Many hepatocytes are lipid-laden, and some of them contain cytoplasmic granular eosinophilic material known as *alcoholic* or *Mallory hyalin*.
- **Cirrhosis**. Cirrhosis develops in 15–20% of chronic alcoholics. As in other forms of cirrhosis, broad septa of connective tissue surround groups of liver cells. These nodules are usually smaller than 5 mm in diameter, and the cirrhosis is classified as micronodular. The liver cells contain fat and have a clear cytoplasm in routine histopathology sections. The hepatocytes may also contain alcoholic hyalin. These findings are, however, not pathognomonic, and several other, albeit rarer, liver diseases may show the same changes. The diagnosis of alcoholic cirrhosis should thus be made only in the context of clinical findings and documented intake of alcohol.

Viral Hepatitis

The term hepatitis is used to describe intralobular inflammation that may be due to *viral infection*, *autoimmune disease*, or *drugs*. Bacterial, parasitic, or fungal infections that may cause cholangitis or liver abscesses are traditionally not included under this heading. It is important to keep in mind that most histological features of viral hepatitis are indistinguishable from those of the autoimmune and drug-induced hepatitis, and that the final diagnosis of viral hepatitis often requires serological or immunochemical confirmation.

Viral hepatitis may be caused by one of the hepatotropic viruses (A, B, C, D, or E) or by viruses that infect the liver following systemic viremia. The latter group of viruses includes herpesvirus, cytomegalovirus, Epstein Barr virus, and several others. Most cases of viral hepatitis in clinical practice are caused by the hepatotropic viruses.

Hepatitis A virus (HAV) causes acute, self-limited disease that is transmitted orally. Hepatitis B virus (HBV) and hepatitis C virus (HCV) are transmitted by exchange of body fluids, such as through blood transfusion or sexual contact. These viruses can cause acute self-limited hepatitis but also chronic hepatitis if the virus infection persists. Hepatitis D virus (HDV) is a viroid that causes inflammation only in concert with HBV. Hepatitis E virus (HEV) is transmitted by the enteric route and causes a self-limited disease. HEV resembles HAV in that it does not cause chronic hepatitis and there is no carrier state.

Acute viral hepatitis caused by any one of the five hepatotropic viruses is histologically characterized by a set of histological changes (Fig. 9.7 and Diagram 9.3). These changes include:

- *Infiltrates of inflammatory cells*. The infiltrates are most prominent in the portal tracts but also "spill over" in a spotty manner into the lobules. Most of the cells in the infiltrate are lymphocytes and macrophages. Neutrophils are not evident except in the earliest stage of disease, which is rarely seen in biopsy or autopsy specimens. Plasma cells are usually not prominent except in some cases of HAV.
- *Hepatic cell injury*. Such injury includes *"ballooning degeneration"* marked by swelling and enlargement of the cytoplasm, which appears pale, and *acidophilic body formation*, a form of single cell death marked by loss of the nucleus and a prominently eosinophilic cytoplasm.
- *Kupffer cell hyperplasia and hypertrophy*. The Kupffer cells enlarge and become prominent early in the course of the disease. These phagocytic cells actively participate in the response to liver cell injury.

In addition to these cardinal histological signs, the liver may show cholestasis, which varies in intensity. In most uncomplicated cases, the lobular architecture is preserved although the cords may be distorted. There is no fibrosis and no ductular injury except in HCV. Regeneration of liver cells may be prominent in the periportal areas. The normal hepatic architecture is restored in most cases within weeks of the onset of infection.

Hepatitis virus infection usually is associated with reversible liver changes. Two important exceptions to this usual course are *massive hepatic necrosis* and *chronic hepatitis*.

Massive hepatic necrosis occurs in approximately 1% of HBV and HCV infections but extremely rarely in HAV and HEV infection. For unknown reasons, 20% of pregnant women acutely infected with HEV develop massive hepatic necrosis. Fulminant liver failure ensues within days of infection and is usually lethal unless an emergency liver transplantation is performed.

Massive hepatic necrosis is histologically characterized by widespread liver cell necrosis (Fig. 9.8). The necrotic liver cells disappear, leaving behind only the reticular connective tissue framework of the sinusoids and the Kupffer cells. The collapse of the lobule results in the narrowing of the normal distance between the portal tracts and the terminal vein. The area occupied previously by the lobule consists in such cases of connective tissue, remaining Kupffer cells, a few hepatocytes, and scattered lymphocytes and macrophages. Regeneration occurs relatively early in some cases, but in others it may not be evident. Bile ductular proliferation is common in patients who survive the acute attack of the disease. Nodules of regenerating liver cells are often surrounded by fibrous tissue replacing large areas of liver cell necrosis. This may lead to postnecrotic cirrhosis.

Chronic hepatitis (Fig. 9.9) is an uncommon, but important, complication of HBV and combined HBV-HDV infections. It does not develop in HAV and HEV infections. Many HCV infections, possibly even 50%, present with histological features of chronic hepatitis. Chronic hepatitis caused by drugs and autoimmune hepatitis may present with similar histological changes. The diagnosis of chronic hepatitis is based on an abnormal liver function test, which remains abnormal for at least 6 months following a bout of acute hepatitis. In many cases of chronic hepatitis, the acute episode is never documented. In all cases, the final diagnosis requires liver biopsy, which is also essential for the staging of the disease and grading of the extent of liver injury.

Histologically, chronic hepatitis is characterized by *hepatocellular changes*, *inflammation*, and, often, although not invariably, *fibrosis* (Fig. 9.6).

Hepatocellular changes resemble those in acute hepatitis and also include necrosis. Liver cell necrosis may occur in several forms:

- Single cell necrosis
- Foci of multicellular intralobular necrosis
- Periportal necrosis at the interface between liver parenchyma and the portal connective tissue that erodes the limiting plate, i.e., the demarcation line between the portal tract and the lobule (known as piecemeal necrosis)

- Confluent necrosis, often referred to as bridging necrosis because it extends from portal tracts to terminal veins

Inflammatory infiltrates consist of lymphocytes, macrophages, and plasma cells in varying ratios. The inflammatory cells may be found in the portal tracts and inside the lobules.

Fibrosis is a common and important feature of chronic hepatitis, although occasionally it may not be evident at all. Minimal fibrosis results in the expansion of portal tracts. In more advanced cases, the fibrosis extends from the portal tracts into the lobules, where it surrounds groups of liver cells. Extensive fibrosis leads to the formation of connective tissue bridges between portal area and central veins, or portal-to-portal fibrous strands. Massive liver cell loss and consequent fibrosis ultimately lead to *cirrhosis*, which is a frequent outcome of chronic hepatitis.

The viral cause of chronic hepatitis may be documented immunohistochemically, by staining the slides with specific antibodies to hepatitis viruses. Chronic hepatitis was previously classified as *chronic persistent* and *chronic active hepatitis*. This classification was found to be impractical and of limited clinical significance. It was replaced by a reporting system according to which chronic hepatitis is defined etiologically (e.g., chronic HBV or HCV); the activity of the disease is given in descriptive terms in liver biopsy (i.e., liver cell necrosis and inflammation); and the extent of fibrosis is graded as mild, moderate, or severe.

Bacterial and Parasitic Hepatitis

Liver infections caused by bacteria or parasites may be *hematogenous,* most often through the portal vein and less often through the hepatic artery, or *canalicular ascending* through the bile ducts from the intestine. Bacterial infections are typically caused by enteric bacteria. In the preantibiotic era, liver abscesses were a common complication of acute appendicitis. Bacterial infections of the liver today are most often complications of inflammatory bowel disease and cholecystitis. Parasitic infections of the liver are less common in the United States but are prevalent in the tropics.

Bacterial liver infections are classified as *cholangitic* if related to biliary tract infection, *pylephlebitic* if the infection has reached the liver through the portal vein, or *arterial* as in sepsis or due to infected emboli. Bacterial infection typically causes **abscesses** in the liver (Fig. 9.10). Histologically, venous and arterial abscesses cannot be distinguished from one another. Cholangitic abscesses are typically associated with purulent cholangitis.

Bacterial cholangitis is characterized by accumulation of neutrophils in the lumen of bile ducts and the periductal connective tissue (Fig. 9.11). These changes usually cause obstruction, which may be recognized as bile plugs and bile lakes in the lobule. Obstruction of the bile ducts results in the extension of purulent inflammation into the liver parenchyma and bile ductular proliferation. Cholangitic abscesses are yet another complication.

Parasitic infections may be caused by a variety of protozoa. *Entamoeba histolytica* is the most important parasitic pathogen affecting the liver. Amebae cause localized liver necrosis. The lesions caused by the spread of amebae from the intestine are colloquially called abscesses even though they contain few neutrophils and almost no pus (Fig. 9.12). *Clonorchis sinensis* and *Schistosoma mansoni* infections of the liver are associated with prominent fibrosis (Fig. 9.13). Such fibrosis is periportal and extends along the bile ducts ("pipe stem fibrosis").

Immunological Disorders

The most important immune disorders of the hepatobiliary system are:

- Primary biliary cirrhosis
- Autoimmune "lupoid" hepatitis
- Primary sclerosing cholangitis

Immune injury is also prominent in liver transplantation. Some histological evidence of graft rejection can be seen in most transplanted livers.

Primary biliary cirrhosis is an autoimmune disorder affecting mostly middle-aged women. It is often associated with other autoimmune disorders, such as atrophic gastritis and thyroiditis. It is diagnosed by typical symptoms inductive of slowly evolving biliary obstruction and serological abnormalities such as antimitochondrial antibodies, which are present in 90% of patients.

Bile duct destruction with infiltrating lymphocytes is considered the primary lesion (Fig. 9.14). Histologically, the earliest findings are the so-called *florid duct lesions* of medium size and large interlobular bile ducts, but the disease also involves the smaller bile ducts. The damaged bile ducts disappear, thus causing intrahepatic biliary obstruction in advanced disease. The portal tracts are devoid of bile ducts and infiltrated with lymphocytes. The branches of the portal artery and the vein are not affected. Chronic lesions are associated with fibrosis, which ultimately leads to cirrhosis.

Autoimmune (lupoid) hepatitis is a disease that also usually affects women. It is usually associated with other autoimmune disorders such as systemic lupus erythematosus. Histologically, this disease shows signs of portal tract and lobular inflammation and may resemble other forms of chronic hepatitis. The inflammatory infiltrates contain typically plasma cells (Fig. 9.15).

Primary sclerosing cholangitis is a disease of young men that typically affects the extrahepatic biliary ducts and causes progressive obstructive jaundice. The initial histological changes in the liver reflect biliary obstruction and are indistinguishable from other forms of bile stasis. As the disease extends from the extrahepatic to intrahepatic bile ducts, typical periductal fibrosis develops (Fig. 9.16). Progressive biliary obstruction ultimately leads to cirrhosis.

Cirrhosis

Cirrhosis is a chronic liver disease characterized by widespread fibrosis and regenerative nodules, which diffusely replace the normal liver parenchyma. This term is used as a synonym for irreversible end-stage liver disease that may have been preceded by a number of liver diseases such as alcoholic liver disease, viral hepatitis, or primary biliary cirrhosis. The major causes of cirrhosis are listed in Table 9.2.

Several morphological criteria have been used to classify cirrhosis. On the basis of the size and shape of nodules, cirrhosis may be

Table 9.2
Causes of Cirrhosis

1. Alcoholism
2. Viral hepatitis
   • HBV, HCV, HDV
3. Hereditary metabolic diseases:
   • Alpha-1-antitrypsin deficiency
   • Wilson's disease
   • Hemochromatosis
4. Drugs and toxins
5. Biliary disease
   • Primary biliary cirrhosis
   • Primary sclerosing cholangitis
   • Cholelithiasis and bacterial cholangitis
6. Parasites (schistosoma, clonorchis)
7. Venous outflow obstruction
   • Budd-Chiari syndrome
   • Veno-occlusive disease
8. Idiopathic (15–20%)

divided into *micronodular* or *macronodular* types. Alcoholic cirrhosis typically produces small uniform nodules that measure less than 5 mm in diameter, whereas posthepatic or postnecrotic cirrhosis tend to produce large scars and irregular nodules varying in size and shape. However, there are many exceptions to this rule.

The color of the liver may be useful in diagnosing some cases: yellow fatty liver is found in alcoholics; brown pigmentary cirrhosis is typical of hemochromatosis, but may also be found in secondary hemosiderosis. Many other forms of end-stage liver disease are characterized by accumulation of iron in the liver. Greenish-yellow discoloration is common in biliary cirrhosis, but may occur in other forms of portal cirrhosis that have caused cholestasis as well.

Histological features may also provide some clues about the etiology of cirrhosis. For example, fatty change and alcoholic hyaline are typically found in alcoholic cirrhosis (Fig. 9.6). Viral antigens and ground-glass cell hepatocytes can be demonstrated in posthepatic cirrhosis (Fig. 9.9). Globular round cytoplasmic bodies are found in alpha-1 antitrypsin deficiency (Fig. 9.5). Hemosiderin can be found in excessive amounts in hemochromatosis and copper in cirrhosis of Wilson disease. However, with a few exceptions, most histological findings are not pathognomonic. Etiologic or pathogenetic diagnosis of cirrhosis is thus made only by correlating the clinical and historical data with the morphological findings. Even so, approximately 15–20% of cirrhosis patients have no obvious cause for their liver failure, and the disease is classified as idiopathic.

The clinical diagnosis of cirrhosis may be made tentatively on the basis of symptoms indicative of liver failure and portal hypertension, but the final diagnosis can be made only be demonstrating cirrhosis in the liver biopsy or at autopsy. Typical histological features (Fig. 9.17) include:

- *Fibrosis.* Broad strands of connective tissue encircle groups of liver cells or transect the parenchyma into irregular fields. These connective tissue strands consist of dense collagenous fibers and fibroblasts and include blood vessels and bile ducts. There are variable amounts of chronic inflammation, mostly consisting of lymphocytes and macrophages. In most cases of cirrhosis, no particular pattern of fibrosis can be recognized.
- *Liver nodules.* Nodules of various sizes are composed of apparently normal hepatocytes arranged into regular or irregular cords, islands, and sheets that lack normal sinusoids.
- *Architectural distortion of hepatic parenchyma.* The fibrosis and the nodules distort the normal architecture of the liver. Nodules composed of regenerating cells are especially prone to compress adjacent liver cells. Fibrous strands may obliterate vascular spaces or obstruct the bile ducts. Damaged bile ducts regenerate, and this regeneration is histologically recognized as bile duct proliferation. Bile stasis may be prominent. The sinusoids are usually abnormal, and the normal proportions of cord to sinusoid are distorted. The blood supply to the nodules may be compromised, and foci of liver cell necrosis may be found.

Liver Tumors

Primary liver tumors may originate from liver cells, from bile ductules, and less often from Kupffer cells and connective tissue cells of the hepatic capsule and portal tracts. **Benign tumors** of the liver are rarely diagnosed clinically. They comprise *liver cell adenomas, benign cholangiocellular adenomas,* and *hemangiomas.* Most hemangiomas are incidentally found at the autopsy (Fig. 9.18). An increased incidence of hepatocellular adenomas has been reported in young women on oral contraceptives (Fig. 9.19).

Hepatocellular carcinoma, also known as *malignant hepatoma* or simply *hepatoma,* is the most common primary malignant liver tumor. It is derived from liver cells and usually occurs in cirrhotic livers. Chronic infection with HBV and HCV are the best documented risk factors. Other forms of cirrhosis are also associated with an increased incidence of liver tumors.

Histologically, hepatocellular carcinoma may present in several forms that somewhat mimic normal liver. The tumor cells may be well, moderately well, or poorly differentiated. In contrast to normal cells, tumor cells have irregularly shaped, atypical nuclei. In well differentiated tumors, the cells resemble normal hepatocytes and have a well developed cytoplasm. Some tumors may even secrete bile, which accumulates in the intercellular canaliculi (Fig. 9.20). Less differentiated tumors may resemble fetal hepatocytes or show no resemblance to liver cells at all. Fetal hepatocyte-like cells are a feature of **hepatoblastomas,** malignant liver cell tumors of childhood (Fig. 9.21).

Most hepatocellular carcinomas secrete alpha fetoprotein (AFP), which is detectable in the serum of patients with tumors. Immunohistochemically, AFP may be demonstrated in the cytoplasms of tumor cells, which is useful for the diagnosis of poorly differentiated hepatocellular carcinomas.

Cholangiocellular carcinoma is a malignant tumor of bile ducts. Histologically, it is a scirrhous adenocarcinoma. These tumors consist of small cuboidal cells arranged into gland-like structures embedded into dense connective tissue (Fig. 9.22). Tumors of the extrahepatic bile ducts have the same histological features.

Metastases are the most common liver tumors in United States and the Western world. Most of these are carcinomas originating from the gastrointestinal tract, the lung, and the female breast (Fig. 9.23).

Gallbladder Diseases

Cholelithiasis, or gallstone formation, is the most common disease of the gallbladder. Gallstones may mechanically irritate the mucosa and cause nonspecific chronic inflammation or ulcerations. In patients with hypercholesterolemia, the underlying mucosa of the gallbladder may be infiltrated with cholesterol-laden macrophages. This condition, called **cholesterolosis** (Fig. 9.24), is morphological evidence of cholesterol uptake in the gallbladder mucosa. Besides that, it has no clinical significance.

Acute cholecystitis is typically caused by bacteria, and in most cases it is associated with gallstones. It appears histologically as suppurative fibrinopurulent or ulcerative inflammation. The surface epithelium of the mucosa may be ulcerated or intact. The mucosa is infiltrated with neutrophils (Fig. 9.25).

Chronic cholecystitis may be caused by infection or nonspecific irritation by gallstones. The mucosa is infiltrated with lymphocytes, macrophages, and a few plasma cells. The epithelium extends into deeper layers of the gallbladder wall, forming the so-called *Rokitansky-Aschoff sinuses* (Fig 9.26). The muscle layer of the gallbladder is usually thickened.

Benign tumors of the gallbladder have no clinical significance and are usually found accidentally in cholecystectomy specimens. Histologically, they appear as tubular and papillary adenomas, similar to intestinal polyps.

Malignant tumors are in 90% of cases *adenocarcinomas* (Fig. 9.27). The remaining 10% of tumors are *squamous cell carcinomas*. These tumors originate in foci of squamous metaplasia that sometimes develops in chronically irritated gallbladders. Irrespective of the tumor type, most gallbladder carcinomas have a poor prognosis.

NOTES

PLATE 9.1. OBSTRUCTIVE JAUNDICE

Figure 9.1.   Obstructive jaundice. A. Intercellular bile canaliculi are dilated and contain brown bile. **B.** The bile duct filled with bile has no epithelium, which was destroyed by bile stasis. **C.** Bile infarct consists of lysed hepatocytes and extravasated bile. **D.** In secondary biliary cirrhosis, fibrous strands surround groups of liver cells. The strands of connective tissue contain dilated bile ducts filled with bile.

Diagram 9.2.   Biliary obstruction. Obstruction leads to dilatation of the ducts, which are filled with bile. Extravasation of bile leads to formation of bile lakes and proliferation of biliary ductules. Intercellular biliary canaliculi are distended with stagnant bile.

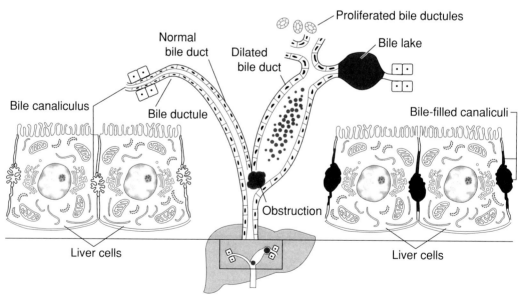

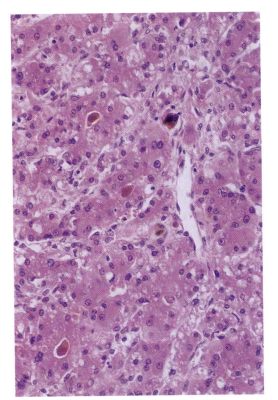

Figure 9.1A

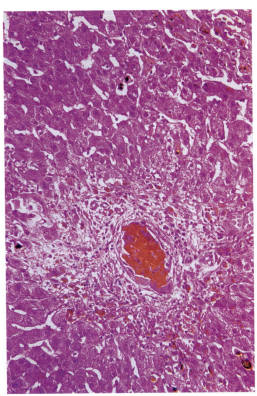

Figure 9.1B

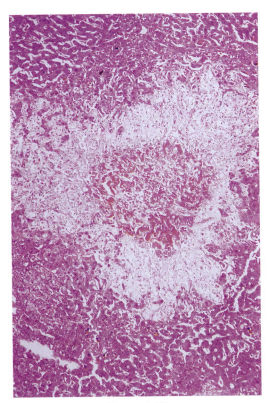

Figure 9.1C

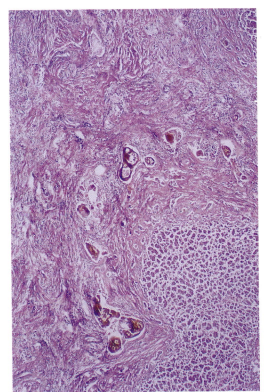

Figure 9.1D

PLATE 9.2. METABOLIC DISORDERS

Figure 9.2. Dubin-Johnson syndrome. The hepatocytes contain brown cytoplasmic granules.

Figure 9.3. Lipidosis (Wolman disease). The hepatocytes show microvesicular steatosis.

Figure 9.4. Carbohydrate storage diseases. A. Glycogenosis type IV leads to childhood cirrhosis, characterized by fibrous strands surrounding groups of liver cells. Liver cells have pale cytoplasm due to accumulation of fat and galactose. **B.** Galactosemia. The liver shows cholestasis and bile ductular proliferation.

Figure 9.5. Alpha-1-antitrypsin deficiency. A. The liver cells contain typical round cytoplasmic globules composed of alpha-1-antitrypsin. **B.** The cytoplasmic globules stain red with PAS. The disease progresses to cirrhosis evidenced by strands of fibrous tissue.

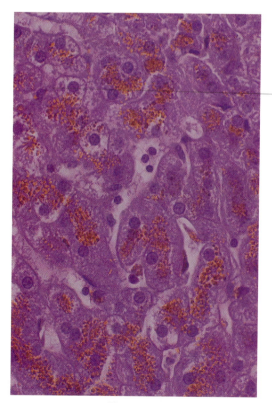

Figure 9.2

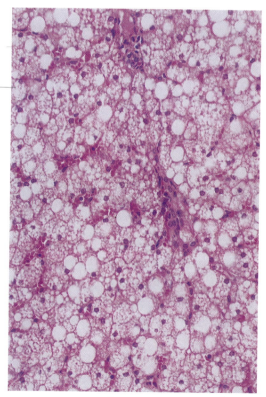

Figure 9.3

COLOR ATLAS OF HISTOPATHOLOGY

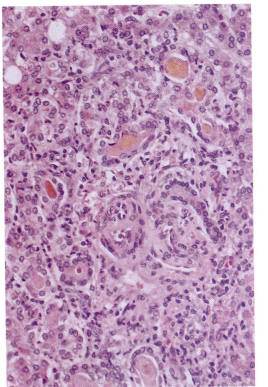

Figure 9.4A

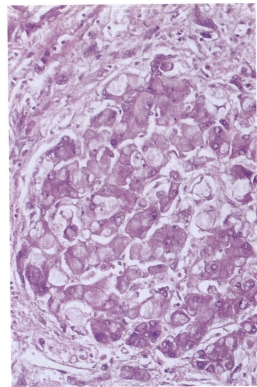

Figure 9.4B

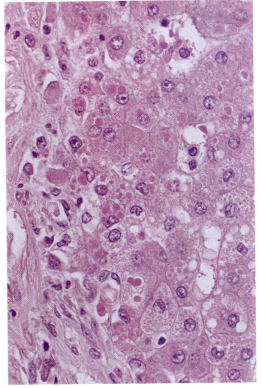

Figure 9.5A

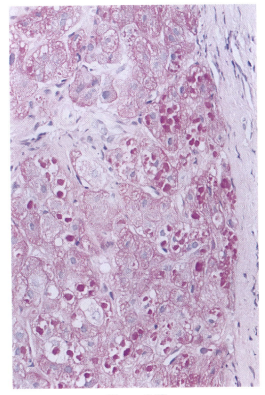

Figure 9.5B

PLATE 9.3. ALCOHOL–INDUCED LIVER CHANGES

Figure 9.6. **Alcoholic liver disease. A.** Fatty change. All the liver cells appear vacuolated since the fat has been dissolved during histological processing. **B.** Alcoholic hepatitis. There is intralobular inflammation. Some liver cells appear vacuolated and some contain alcoholic hyaline. **C.** Prolonged alcohol abuse leads to intralobular fibrosis. Mallory body formation and fatty change of hepatocytes. **D.** Fibrosis is most prominent around the terminal hepatic venule as shown by reticulin stain. **E.** Early cirrhosis shows perilobular fibrosis. The portal vein branches appear dilated because of portal hypertension. **F.** Alcoholic cirrhosis shows prominent fibrous strands surrounding nodules of liver cells. Many liver cells contain fat and are vacuolated.

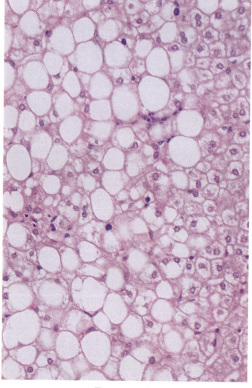

Figure 9.6A

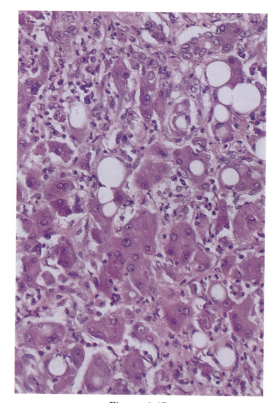

Figure 9.6B

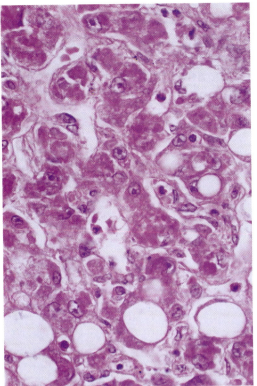

Figure 9.6C

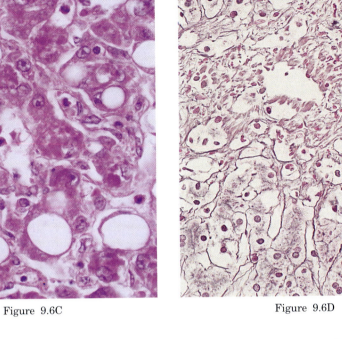

Figure 9.6D

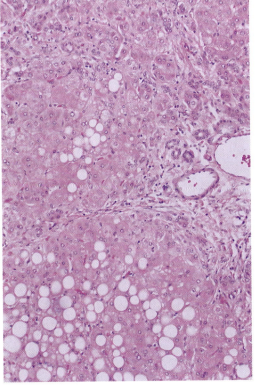

Figure 9.6E

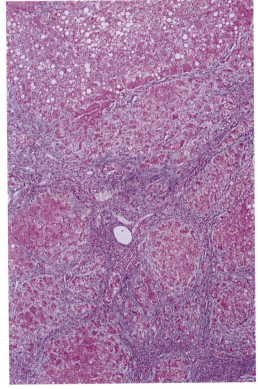

Figure 9.6F

PLATE 9.4.   ACUTE VIRAL HEPATITIS

Figure 9.7.   Acute viral hepatitis. A. The overall architecture of the lobule is obscured by intralobular inflammation and hepatocellular reaction to viral infection. **B.** The periportal hepatocytes show reactive changes and are surrounded by inflammatory cells and enlarged Kupffer cells. **C.** Intralobular inflammation with enlarged Kupffer cells and acidophilic bodies (*arrow*). **D.** Ballooning of liver cells. The arrow points to an acidophilic body.

Diagram 9.3.   Viral hepatitis. A. Normal hepatic lobule. **B.** Acute hepatitis shows portal and intralobular inflammation, liver cell injury, and Kupffer cell reaction. **C.** Massive hepatic necrosis. The collapse of the lobule caused by widespread liver cell necrosis leads to the narrowing of the space between the portal tract and the terminal hepatic venule. **D.** Chronic hepatitis. The inflammation involves the portal tract and the lobule and disrupts the limiting plate. There is also intralobular fibrosis and bile ductular proliferation.

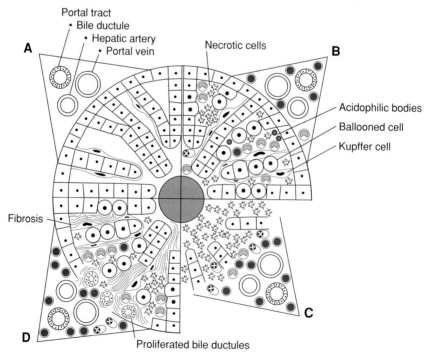

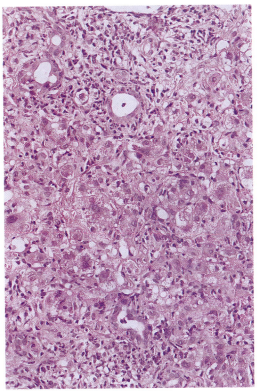

Figure 9.7A

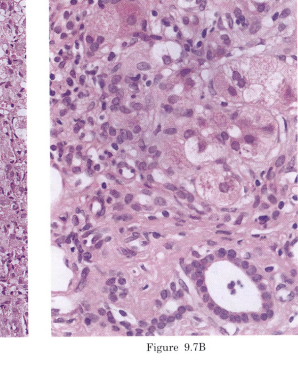

Figure 9.7B

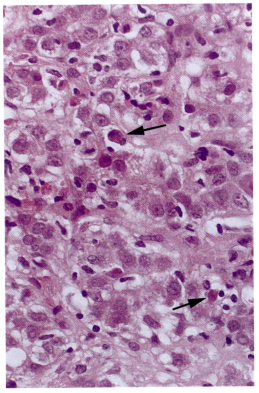

Figure 9.7C

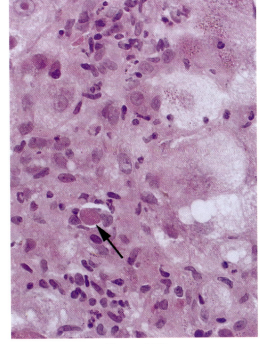

Figure 9.7D

PLATE 9.5. MASSIVE HEPATIC NECROSIS

Figure 9.8. Massive hepatic necrosis. A. The space between the terminal vein and portal tract is collapsed and contains connective tissue, few hydropic hepatocytes, and blood. **B.** Dissociated liver cells are surrounded by loosely arranged Kupffer cells and inflammatory cells filling the space previously occupied by liver cells. **C.** Regeneration following liver cell necrosis is characterized by bile ductular proliferation. **D.** Postnecrotic fibrous scar surrounding the nodule composed of regenerated liver cells.

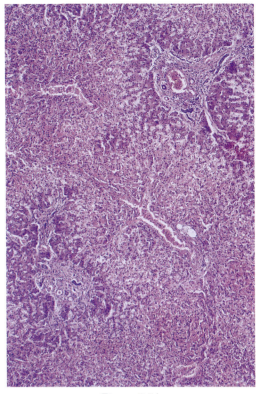

Figure 9.8A

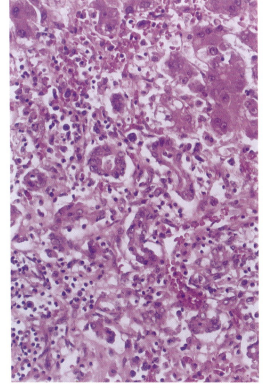

Figure 9.8C

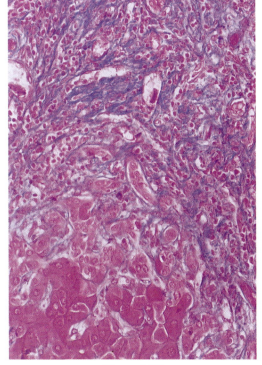

Figure 9.8D

PLATE 9.6. CHRONIC HEPATITIS

Figure 9.9. Chronic hepatitis. A. Mild persistent inflammation evidenced by a lymphocytic infiltrate in the portal tract. The limiting plate of the portal tract is sharp. **B.** Chronic hepatitis extending into the lobule. The limiting plate is indistinct. **C.** Intralobular inflammation with disruption of cords. Some hepatocytes appear swollen. **D.** "Ground-glass" appearance of hepatocytes in HBV infection. The cytoplasm appears smooth, like finely ground glass. **E.** Electron microscopy shows that the rough endoplasmic reticulum contains filamentous HBsAg. **F.** HBsAg can be demonstrated in liver cell nuclei by immunohistochemistry. The virus containing nuclei of liver cells appear dark brown. **G.** HBsAg is demonstrated immunohistochemically in the cytoplasm of liver cells.

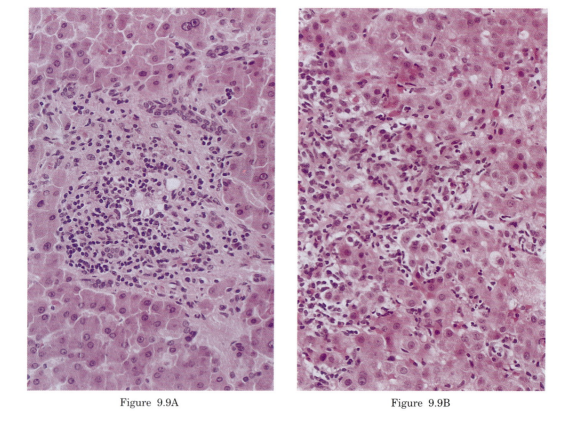

Figure 9.9A   Figure 9.9B

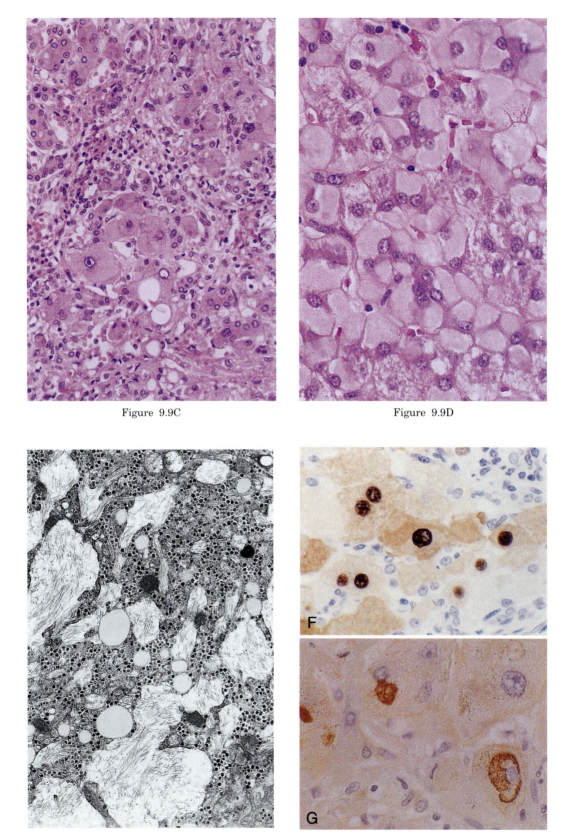

Figure 9.9C

Figure 9.9D

Figure 9.9E

Figure 9.9FG

PLATE 9.7. BACTERIAL AND PARASITIC HEPATITIS

Figure 9.10.   Liver abscess consists of aggregates of neutrophils.

Figure 9.12.   Amebic infection. The lesion has a fibrous capsule separating the amorphous material in the center of the ameboma from the surrounding liver.

Figure 9.11.   Bacterial cholangitis. A. Small bile duct contains neutrophils. There is periductal fibrosis. **B.** Bile ductal proliferation and infiltrates of neutrophils in the liver parenchyma are features of prolonged disease.

Figure 9.13.   Schistosomiasis of the liver. A. Ovum of the parasite in the liver parenchyma is surrounded by inflammatory cells and fibrous tissue. **B.** Periportal fibrosis appears prominent in this trichrome-stained tissue.

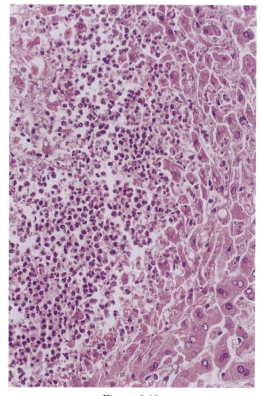

Figure 9.10

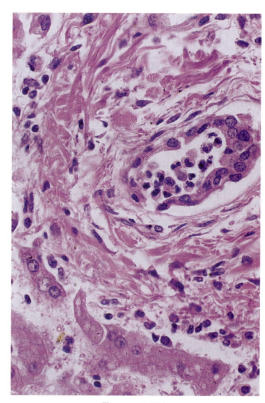

Figure 9.11A

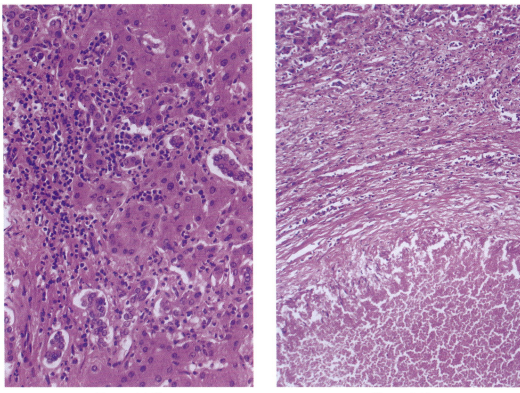

Figure 9.11B

Figure 9.12

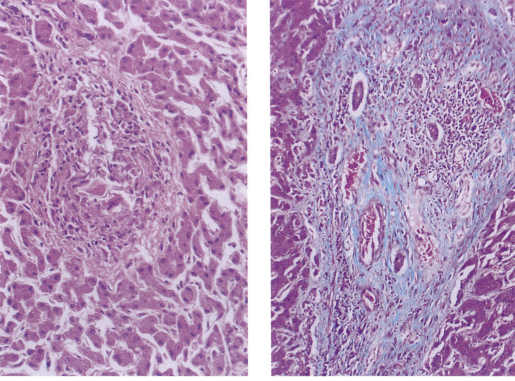

Figure 9.13A

Figure 9.13B

PLATE 9.8. IMMUNOLOGIC LIVER DISEASES

Figure 9.14.   Primary biliary cirrhosis. A. The bile ducts are destroyed by infiltrating lymphocytes. **B.** In later stages of primary biliary cirrhosis, the portal tract contains chronic inflammatory cells but no bile ducts. **C.** Advanced stage of biliary cirrhosis is characterized by broad fibrous strands surrounding nodules of liver cells.

Figure 9.15.   Autoimmune (lupoid) hepatitis. A. The infiltrates of inflammatory cells disrupt the normal lobular architecture. **B.** At higher magnification, one may see that the infiltrate consists of lymphocytes and plasma cells.

Figure 9.16.   Primary sclerosing cholangitis. Periductal fibrosis surrounds intrahepatic bile ducts.

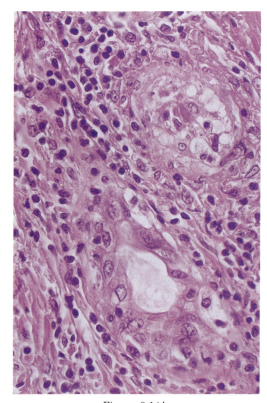

Figure 9.14A

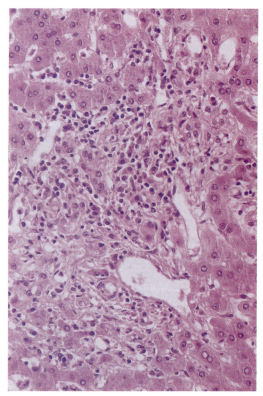

Figure 9.14B

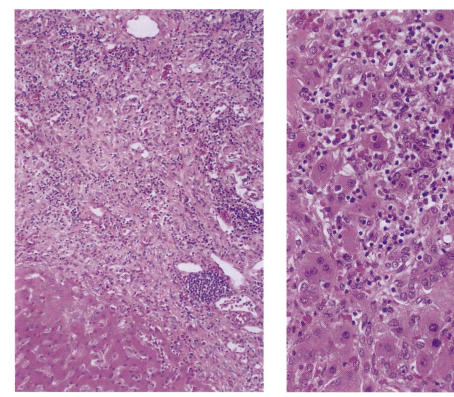

Figure 9.14C

Figure 9.15A

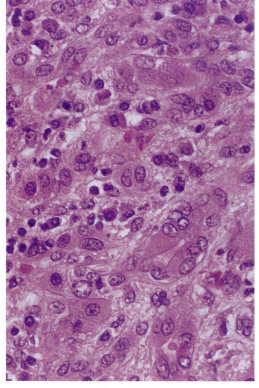

Figure 9.15B

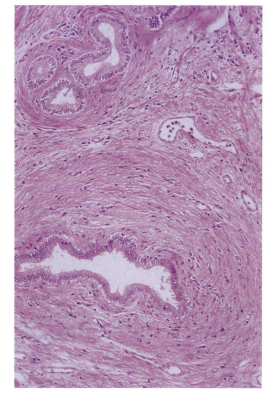

Figure 9.16

PLATE 9.9. CIRRHOSIS

Figure 9.17.   Cirrhosis. A. Fibrous septa of varying thickness divide the parenchyma into irregular nodules. **B.** Connective tissue stain shows that the bands consist of collagenous fibrous tissue (blue). **C.** Reticulin stain shows dense perinodular connective tissue extending into the nodules in the form of thin, but irregular, strands. **D.** Periphery of liver cell nodule. Liver cells do not show the usual cord-like arrangement, and the sinusoids are distorted. **E.** Fibrous septa of cirrhosis consist of connective tissue that contains lymphocytes and proliferating bile ducts. The small branches of portal vein are dilated because of portal hypertension.

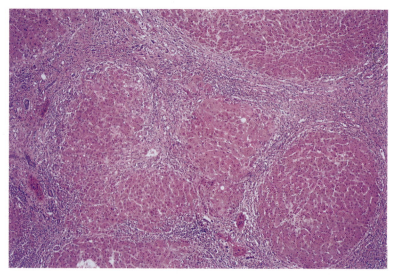

Figure 9.17A

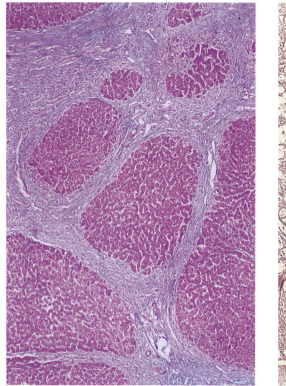

Figure 9.17B

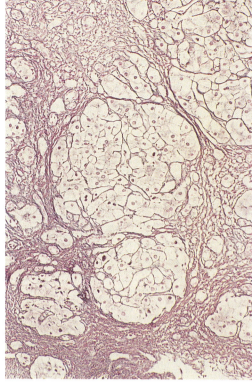

Figure 9.17C

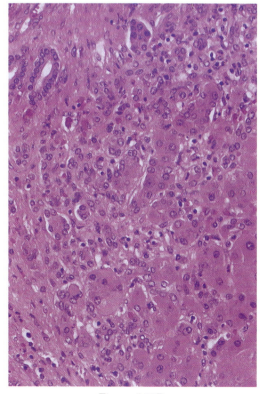

Figure 9.17D

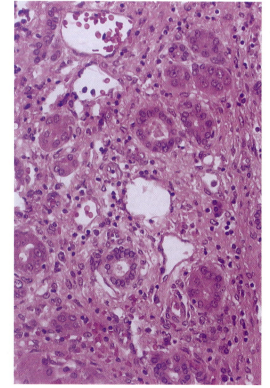

Figure 9.17E

PLATE 9.10. LIVER TUMORS

Figure 9.18. Hemangioma of the liver. The tumor consists of vascular spaces filled with blood.

Figure 9.19. Hepatocellular adenoma. This well differentiated tumor is composed of cells that resemble normal liver cells from which it is separated by a fibrous capsule.

Figure 9.20. Hepatocellular carcinoma. This well differentiated tumor is composed of cells resembling hepatocytes.

Figure 9.21. Hepatoblastoma. The tumor is composed of small cells that have round nuclei and well developed cytoplasm. The cells are arranged into tubules and acini.

Figure 9.22. Cholangiocellular carcinoma. The tumor is composed of atypical glands surrounded with dense connective tissue.

Figure 9.23. Metastatic adenocarcinoma. The tumor appears demarcated from adjacent liver cells.

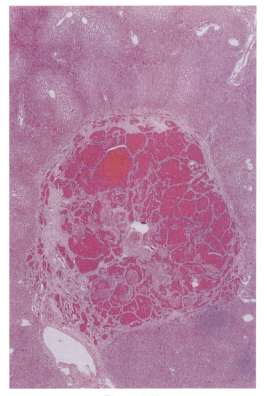

Figure 9.18

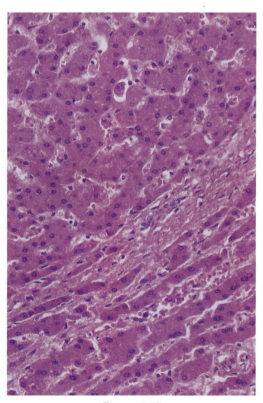

Figure 9.19

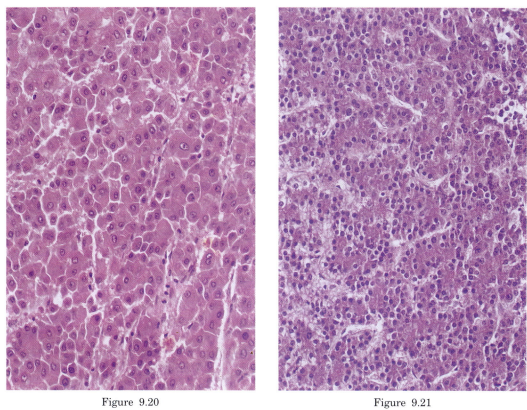

Figure 9.20

Figure 9.21

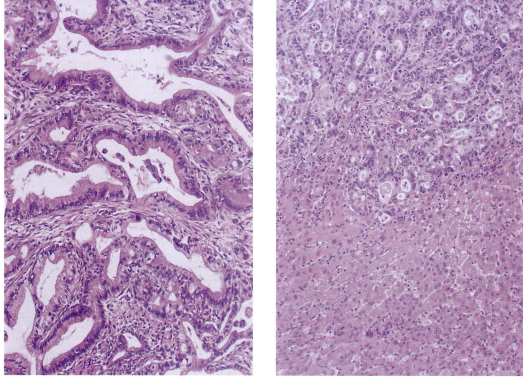

Figure 9.22

Figure 9.23

PLATE 9.11. GALLBLADDER DISEASES

Figure 9.24. Cholesterolosis. The lamina propria of the gallbladder mucosa contains lipid-laden macrophages.

Figure 9.26. Chronic cholecystitis. A. The mucosa consists of prominent folds and glands extending into the muscle layer. There are also scattered chronic inflammatory cells. **B.** The epithelium of glands forms Rokitansky-Aschoff sinuses that extend into the thickened muscle layer.

Figure 9.25. Acute cholecystitis. The mucosa is congested, edematous, and infiltrated with neutrophils. The surface epithelium has focally undergone necrosis, and the luminal side of the gallbladder is covered with fibrin.

Figure 9.27. Adenocarcinoma of the gallbladder.

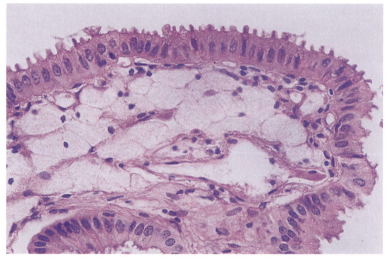

Figure 9.24

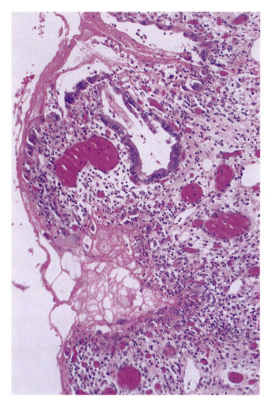

Figure 9.25

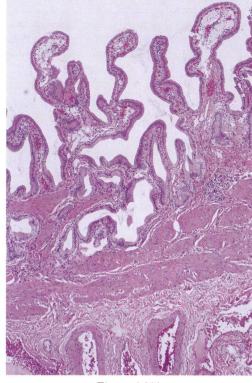

Figure 9.26A

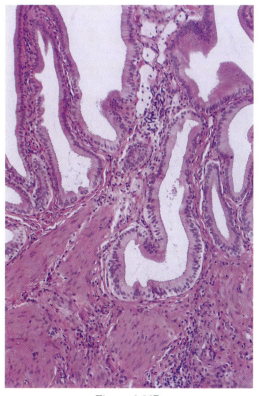

Figure 9.26B

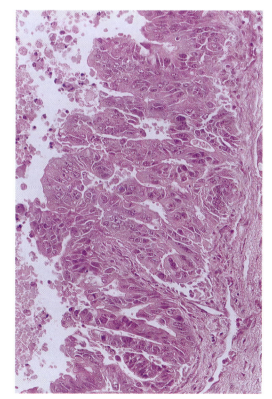

Figure 9.27

NOTES

CHAPTER 10

Pancreas

NORMAL HISTOLOGY

The pancreas is a mixed exocrine/endocrine gland connected to the duodenum and located in the retroperitoneal space of the upper abdomen (Diagram 10.1).

The **exocrine pancreas** forms more than 99% of the total gland and consists of lobules and ducts. The endocrine gland is composed of the *islets of Langerhans*. The exocrine cells of the lobules are arranged into acini, which are composed of trapezoid-shaped cells having granular cytoplasm and basally located nuclei. These cells surround a central lumen connected with the small ductules. The ductules merge and eventually form the main pancreatic duct that is the conduit for the exocrine pancreatic juices into the duodenum.

Islets of Langerhans consist of several cell types; the most numerous are the insulin-secreting beta cells, which account for

Diagram 10.1.   Pancreas. It is attached to the duodenum and has a head, body, and tail. It consists of an exocrine and an endocrine part. The exocrine secretory cells form acini attached to small ducts (inset). Small ducts form larger ducts, which lead into the main pancreatic duct or the accessory pancreatic duct. The endocrine pancreatic cells are grouped into islets of Langerhans.

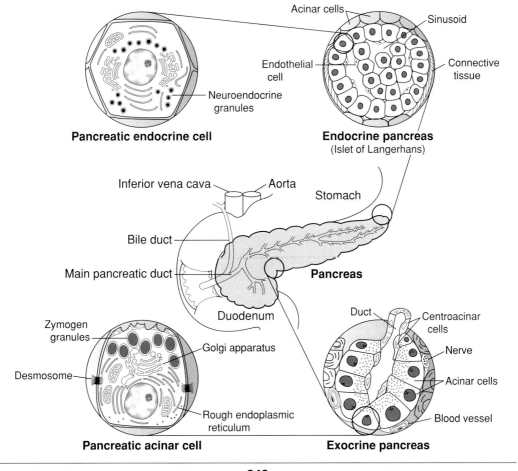

70% of the cell population. Alpha cells secrete glucagon; delta cells secrete somatostatin and vasoactive intestinal polypeptide (VIP); and PP cells pancreatic polypeptide.

In routine histology, sections of various endocrine cells cannot be distinguished from one another. However, this can be achieved by immunohistochemistry using specific antibodies to insulin, glucagon, and other hormones. Electron microscopy reveals that alpha, beta, and delta cells have unique neuroendocrine granules typical of each cell type.

OVERVIEW OF PATHOLOGY

The main diseases of the pancreas are related to the

- Premature activation of pancreatic proenzymes within the pancreas and consequent autodigestion of pancreas and adjacent tissues (e.g., acute pancreatis)
- Pancreatic exocrine insufficiency due to loss of acinar cells or obstruction of ducts (e.g., chronic pancreatitis)
- Functional insufficiency of the endocrine pancreas (e.g., diabetes mellitus)
- Neoplasia of exocrine or endocrine cells

ACUTE PANCREATITIS

Acute pancreatitis, also known as *acute pancreatic necrosis*, is a disease of sudden onset that leads to intrapancreatic activation of the proenzymes and autodigestion of the gland and adjacent tissues. It may result from several forms of chemical, physical, or infectious injury of the pancreas, as outlined in Diagram 10.2. All of these forms of injury result in premature activation of pancreatic proenzymes in the acini or intrapancreatic ducts, which represents the main pathogenetic event and accounts for the pathological changes in this disease. Activation of enzymes may be due to the obstruction of the main pancreatic duct with back pressure into the acini, spasm of the smooth muscles in the papilla of Vater induced by alcohol, or premature activation of proenzymes due to reflux of bile into the pancreatic duct. Infrequently, acute pancreatitis is related to direct injury of acinar tissue by viruses such as mumps, drugs such as thiazide, surgery, or direct blunt trauma.

Autodigestion of pancreatic parenchyma is histologically recognized as loss of pancreatic cell contours (Fig. 10.1). The necrotic cells are surrounded by neutrophils. Leakage of lipase and other enzymes into the surrounding fat tissue results in fat necrosis and formation of fat soaps, which usually contain calcium. The local destruction of blood vessels results in hemorrhage. Ultimately, the affected tissue is liquefied and transformed into an amorphous fluid enclosed by the remaining tissue of the pancreas. Since no epithelial lining is typical of cysts, this cavity is called a *pseudocyst* (Fig. 10.2). The wall of the pseudocyst consists of granulation tissue that gradually undergoes fibrosis.

CHRONIC PANCREATITIS

Chronic pancreatitis results in exocrine pancreatic insufficiency related to gradual destruction and loss of the pancreatic parenchyma. The destruction of acini is accompanied by fibrosis, mild chronic inflammation, and calcification. The destruction of the endocrine cells results in diabetes mellitus, which is encountered in one-third of all cases.

Histologically, the most prominent feature is fibrosis replacing the atrophic acini (Fig. 10.3). As the disease progresses, more and more acinar cells are replaced by fibrous tissue. Eventually, the acini are lost and only ducts surrounded with acellular fibrosis remain. The chronic inflammation is usually inconspicuous and consists of a few scattered lymphocytes. The islets of Langerhans may be spared for some time but ultimately disappear as well. Calcification may be present as aggregates of calcium salts in the connective tissue or intracanalicular calculi.

Cystic fibrosis is a multisystemic autosomal recessive disorder related to a mutation in the gene encoding the plasma membrane protein called cystic fibrosis transmembrane conductance regulator (CFTR). This protein is essential for transmembrane secretion of chloride. The mutation leads to the formation of viscid mucus in the pancreas, bronchi, bile ducts, and intestine. Proteinaceous mucous material may be recognized histologically in the dilated pancreatic ducts, which are lined by atrophic epithelium and are typically surrounded by atrophic acini and fibrous tissue (Fig. 10.4).

Obstruction of the neonatal fetal intestine with tenacious meconium may cause meconium ileus and, upon rupture, **meconium peritonitis** (Fig. 10.5). Meconium, i.e., the contents of fetal intestines, may be found throughout the peritoneal cavity and attached to peritoneal surfaces. If the baby survives, such meconium may calcify.

PANCREATIC NEOPLASMS

Tumors of the pancreas can originate from the ducts, acini, islet cells, and rarely the connective tissue components. Thus, the epithelial tumors can be classified as derived from the exocrine or the endocrine pancreas, and may be clinically benign or malignant. Benign exocrine tumors are rare and of limited significance. Malignant tumors originating from the ducts account for more than 95% of all neoplasms, the remainder comprising islet cell tumors, acinic cell carcinomas, and rare benign tumors such as cystadenoma.

Adenocarcinomas of the pancreas appear histologically as mucin-producing desmoplastic (scirrhous) tumors (Fig. 10.6). Pancreatic adenocarcinomas cannot be reliably distinguished from adenocarcinomas from other sites (e.g., breast or colon).

Islet cell tumors originate from the endocrine pancreatic cells and can be benign or malignant. The tumors are classified on the basis of their cellular composition and secretory activity, corresponding to the normal endocrine cells forming the islets of Langerhans (Table 10.1). The most common are insulin-secreting tumors. It should be noted that pancreas may give rise to gastrinomas, although normal islets of Langerhans do not contain gastrin-secreting G cells.

All endocrine pancreatic tumors have the same histological features and are indistinguishable from one another. They are typical neuroendocrine tumors and resemble carcinoid tumors of the intestine or the respiratory system. The final designation for each tumor depends on the immunohistochemical demonstration of the predominant secretory product. Thus, if a tumor secretes insulin, it is called *insulinoma*; if it secretes glucagon, it is a *glucagonoma*. Many islet cell tumors originate from developmentally pluripotent stem cells and contain several cell types. Such tumors are noncommittally designated "mixed endocrine tumors" or classified on the basis of the polypeptide hormone that dominates the clinical picture.

Light microscopy shows that the tumors are composed of small uniform cells arranged into trabeculae, cords, or nests surrounded by a delicate vascular network (Fig. 10.7). Nuclei are uniformly round and show little pleomorphism. Tumors may be locally invasive and multiple. Clinically, islet cell tumors may be benign or malignant, but such a diagnosis cannot be established on the basis of histological findings. Malignant tumors may show cellular pleomorphism and a higher mitotic rate, but even these morphological findings may be misleading. The only definitive evidence of malignancy are distant metastases.

The final diagnosis of cell specific tumor type is based on immunohistochemical analysis of polypeptide hormones contained in the tumor cell cytoplasm. Electron microscopy shows that islet cell tumors contain neuroendocrine granules which, however, do not necessarily resemble granules of normal islet cells. Electron microscopy of these lesions is, therefore, of limited diagnostic value.

Table 10.1
Endocrine Tumors of the Pancreas

Tumor	Equivalent Normal Cell Type	Secretory Product
Insulinoma	B (beta)	Insulin
Glucagonoma	A (alpha)	Glucagon
Somatostatinoma	D (delta)	Somatostatin
VIPoma	D_1 (delta-1)	Vasoactive intestinal polypeptide (VIP)
PPoma	PP	Pancreatic polypeptide
Gastrinoma	G	Gastrin
Nonfunctioning islet cell tumor	?	?

Note: Normal pancreas does not contain gastrin-secreting G cells. G cells are normally found in the stomach and duodenum.

DIABETES MELLITUS

Diabetes mellitus is a metabolic disorder characterized by hyperglycemia. It may be secondary to a deficiency or disturbances in secretion of insulin or to an abnormal response of peripheral tissues to insulin. The resulting metabolic derangement of the intermediary metabolism of carbohydrates, lipids, and proteins affects all organ systems but is most prominent in the arteries (macroangiopathy), arterioles, and capillaries (microangiopathy).

There are several forms of diabetes (Table 10.2). The most important are type I, also known as insulin-dependent diabetes mellitus (IDDM), and type II, or non-insulin-dependent diabetes mellitus (NIDDM).

IDDM is a disease that results from injury of islets of Langerhans and the destruction of insulin-producing beta cells. Hypoglycemia may be temporarily related to an acute viral disease. Autoimmune factors are thought to mediate the islet cell injury, but the exact pathogenesis of the disease remains unknown.

In early stages of the disease, the islets of Langerhans are infiltrated with lymphocytes. In late stages, the islets appear hypocellular and show fibrosis and hyalinization (Fig. 10.8). In some cases, the stroma of the islets may contain amyloid.

NIDDM is characterized by relative insulin deficiency, which can be compensated

Table 10.2
Classification of Diabetes Mellitus

Primary Insulin-dependent
1. Type I (IDDM)
2. Type II non-insulin-dependent (NIDDM)
3. Impaired glucose tolerance (IGT)
4. Gestational diabetes
Secondary
1. Pancreatic diseases
   - Chronic pancreatitis
   - Hemochromatosis
   - Cystic fibrosis
   - Tumors of pancreas
2. Endocrine disorders
   - Cushing disease
   - Acromegaly
   - Pheochromocytoma
3. Genetic disease
   - Glycogen storage disease
   - Down syndrome
4. Drug-induced
   - Diuretics (thiazide)
   - Psychoactive drugs (phenothiazine)

for by oral hypoglycemic agents, regulated diet, and weight loss. Histologically, the islets of Langerhans usually appear normal, and like normal islets, contain 60–70% insulin-producing beta cells and 20–30% glucagon-producing alpha cells (Fig. 10.9). These cells may be functionally normal or abnormal, but morphologically they appear normal.

NOTES

PLATE 10.1. ACUTE PANCREATITIS

Figure 10.1. Acute pancreatitis. Necrosis of pancreatic acini and adjacent fat tissue.

Figure 10.2. Pancreatic pseudocyst. The wall of treated cysts drained of its content consists of fibrous tissue and atrophic fibrosed pancreatic parenchyma.

Figure 10.3. Chronic pancreatitis. A. Fibrosis surrounds the ducts and replaces the acini. There are a few scattered chronic inflammatory cells. **B.** The wall of the pancreatic duct is fibrosed. The epithelium of this duct has been lost. The lumen contains amorphous material that is partially calcified and therefore appears bluish.

Diagram 10.2. Acute pancreatic necrosis. Autodigestion of parenchyma occurs because of the intrapancreatic activation of proenzymes. This could be due to (1) obstruction of common pancreatic and biliary duct and reflux of bile into the pancreatic duct under pressure, (2) alcohol, which acts as secretogogue and stimulates the sphincter of Oddi at the papilla of Vater, or (3) overeating, which increases the demand for pancreatic digestive juices. Various forms of direct tissue injury are less common causes of pancreatitis. They include (4) viruses, (5) drugs, and (6) trauma. Activated enzymes destroy pancreatic parenchyma, fat, and blood vessels. Consequences of enzymatic tissue destruction are fat necrosis and hemorrhage.

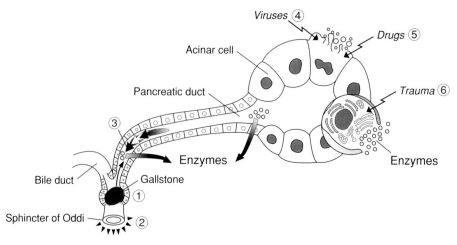

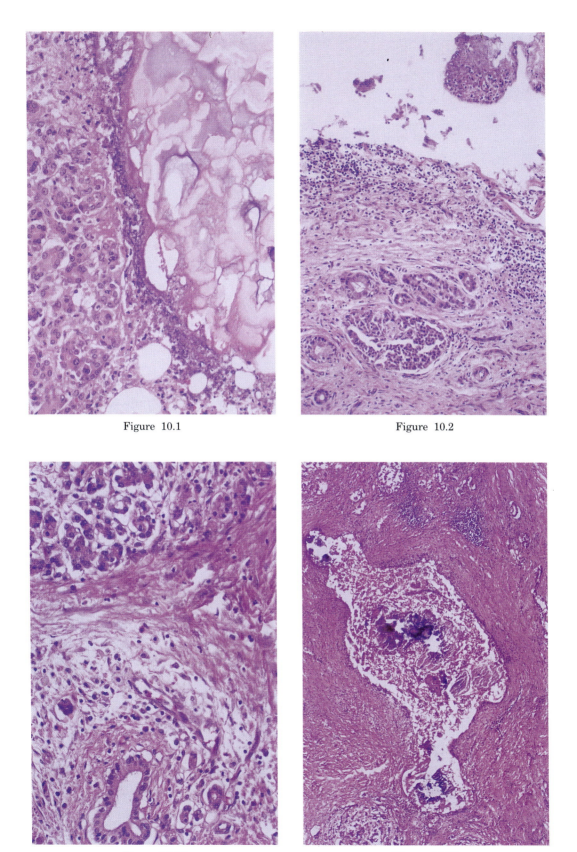

Figure 10.1

Figure 10.2

Figure 10.3A

Figure 10.3B

PLATE 10.2. CYSTIC FIBROSIS AND MECONIUM PERITONITIS

Figure 10.4.   Cystic fibrosis. A. The duct contains inspissated proteinaceous material. **B.** Prolonged disease shows dilatation of the obstructed ducts, periductal fibrosis, and atrophy of acini. **C.** Lungs show dilated bronchioles filled with pus (purulent bronchitis and bronchiolitis).

Figure 10.5.   Meconium peritonitis. A. The lumen of the small intestine contains meconium attached to the surface of the villi. **B.** Mucosal glands contain viscous mucus admixed to meconium. **C.** Subserosal calcifications resulting from the rupture of the intestine and dissipation of meconium across the peritoneal cavity.

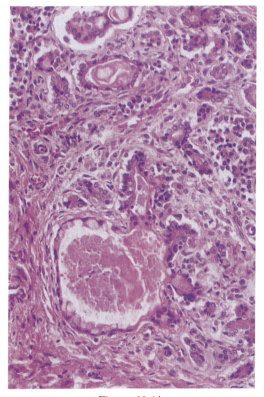

Figure 10.4A

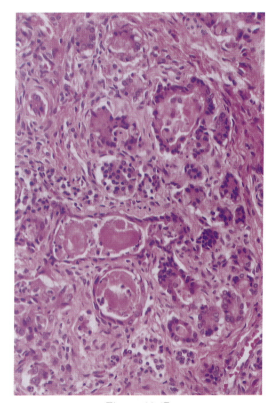

Figure 10.4B

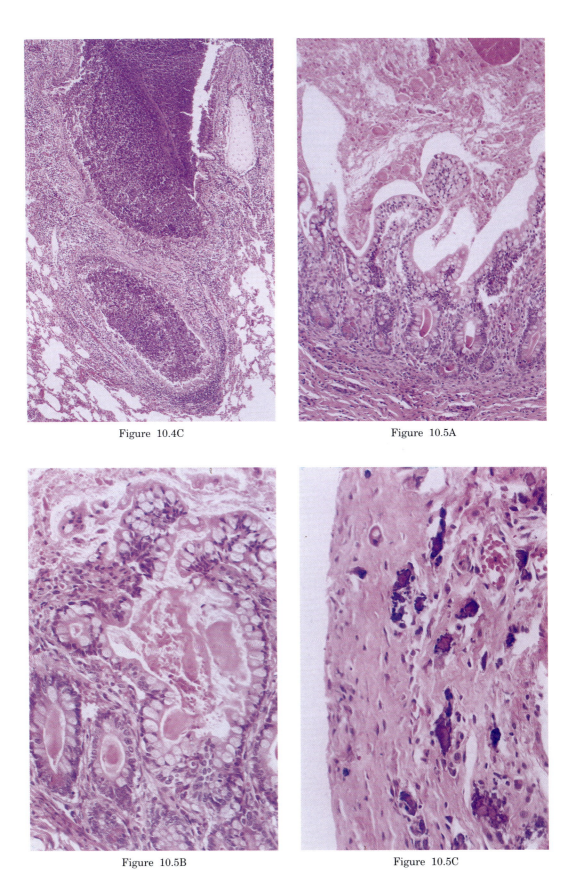

Figure 10.4C

Figure 10.5A

Figure 10.5B

Figure 10.5C

PLATE 10.3. PANCREATIC NEOPLASMS

Figure 10.6. **Adenocarcinoma of the pancreas. A.** Early adenocarcinoma consists of neoplastic cells adjacent to normal ducts from which it has arisen. **B.** This mucinous adenocarcinoma has no unique features that would suggest a pancreatic origin.

Figure 10.7. **Islet cell tumor. A.** The tumor is composed of small cells arranged into broad ribbons and cords. **B.** The tumor cells have uniform, round nuclei, typical of neuroendocrine neoplasms. **C.** Electron microscopy of a gastrinoma. The cytoplasm contains electron dense membrane-bound neuroendocrine granules. **D.** Malignant islet cell tumor metastatic to the liver shows nuclear pleomorphism.

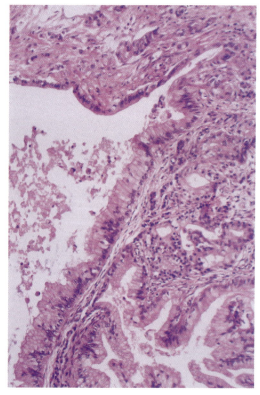

Figure 10.6A

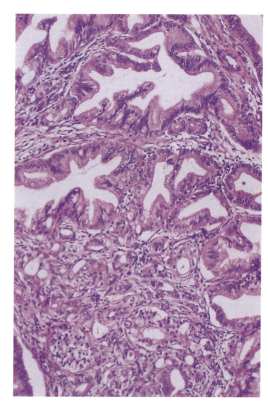

Figure 10.6B

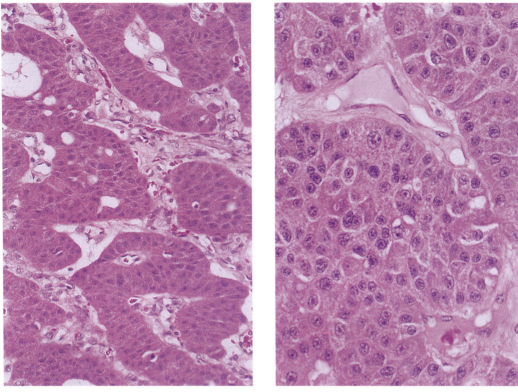

Figure 10.7A

Figure 10.7B

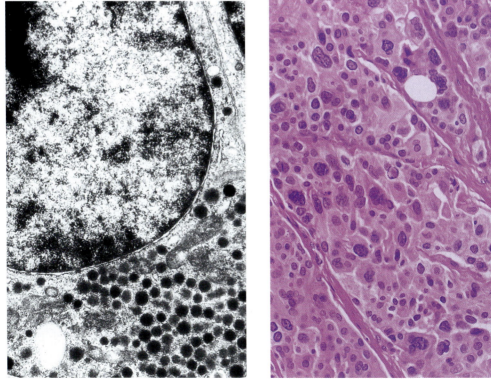

Figure 10.7C

Figure 10.7D

PLATE 10.4. DIABETES MELLITUS

Figure 10.8.   Insulin-dependent diabetes mellitus. A. The islet (*I*) surrounded by normal acini of the pancreas is small and partially hyalinized. **B.** High-magnification view of hyalinized interstitial connective tissue with a few lymphocytes replacing islet cells. **C.** Advanced IDDM with deposits of amyloid in the stroma.

Figure 10.9.   Non-insulin-dependent diabetes mellitus. A. The islet of Langerhans appears normal. Most patients with NIDDM have normal islets. **B.** Immunohistochemical reaction with antibodies to insulin shows that more than 70% of cells are immunoreactive (brown) and, thus, normal beta cells. **C.** Immunohistochemical reaction with antibodies to glucagon shows that the alpha cells (brown) are in the minority. Normally, alpha cells account for approximately 20% of islet cells.

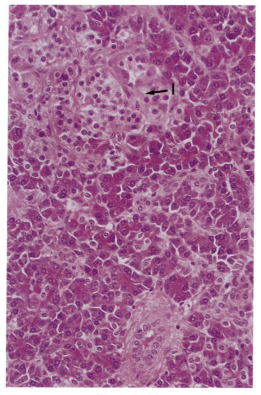

Figure 10.8A

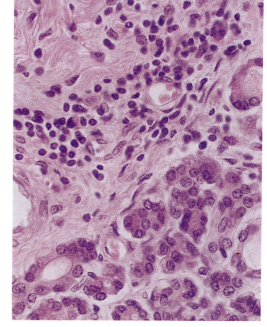

Figure 10.8B

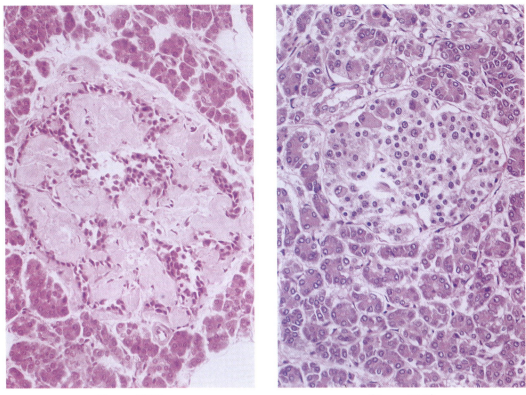

Figure 10.8C

Figure 10.9A

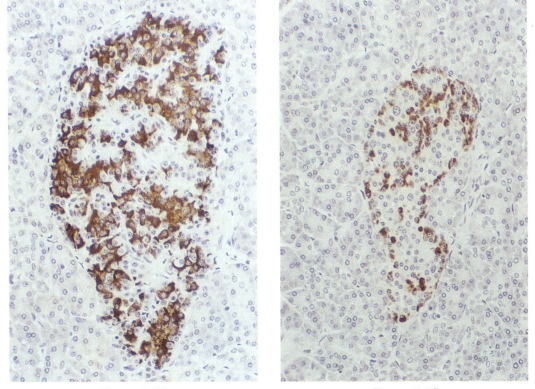

Figure 10.9B

Figure 10.9C

NOTES

CHAPTER 11

Urinary System

NORMAL HISTOLOGY

The urinary system comprises the kidneys with the urinary collecting system (calyces and renal pelvis), the ureters, the urinary bladder, and the urethra (Diagram 11.1).

The kidneys are histologically complex organs that have several functions. Each kidney is composed of several millions of nephrons, which are basic functional units of this organ. Each nephron consists of the glomerulus, tubules, and collecting ducts, all of which have unique anatomical and functional properties. For purposes of diagnostic histopathology, we shall not dwell on different segments of the nephron but shall consider the tubular and collecting ducts as one component, glomeruli as the second, blood vessels of the kidney as the third, and the interstitium as the fourth.

The histology of the **urinary collecting system**, **calices** and **pelvis**, the **ureters**, the **urinary bladder**, and the **urethra** is much simpler. These organs are hollow structures. Their luminal surfaces are lined by transitional epithelium, and they are encased in smooth muscle and connective tissue (adventitia or serosa). This simple architecture reflects their primary and only function, i.e., passage and storage of urine.

Electron microscopy is very important for the diagnosis of glomerular diseases, and thus we shall briefly review the main ultrastructural features of the glomerulus (Diagram 11.2).

The normal glomerulus consists of a *capillary tuft* enclosed in the space delimited by the *Bowman capsule*. The capillary loops are composed of basement membrane that has a dense central portion (*lamina densa*) and two less dense or lighter laminae (*lamina lucida interna* and *externa*).

The glomerular basement membrane (GBM) is lined on the internal side by **endothelial** cells, which have a discontinuously fenestrated cytoplasm. These fenestrae, or openings, facilitate filtration of

plasma. On the external side, the basement membrane is covered with foot process of the **epithelial** glomerular cells, which are called *podocytes* because of their "foot-like" cytoplasmic extensions. In response to hyperfiltration of proteins, these foot processes become broader. Since fewer can be seen, it is customary to describe this reactive change as "fusion of the foot processes."

Several glomerular capillary loops converge toward a common stalk area called the *mesangium*. The mesangium consists of basement membrane–like material enclosing one or two *mesangial cells*. Mesangial cells react to many forms of glomerular injury by altering their function or by multiplying. The mesangial matrix converges toward the hilus, where it merges with the wall of the afferent and efferent arterioles. The wall of the afferent arteriole contains the renin-secreting **juxtaglomerular cells**, which are essential for regulation of the blood pressure. The secretion of renin occurs in response to reduced arterial renal blood flow and the concentration of sodium in the specialized portion of distal tubule called *macula densa*, which is closely apposed to the glomerular hilus.

OVERVIEW OF PATHOLOGY

The most important diseases are

- Glomerular diseases, which are mostly immune-mediated
- Vascular renal diseases, such as those caused by hypertension or diabetes
- Infectious diseases, such as pyelonephritis and cystitis
- Tubulo-interstitial diseases
- Neoplasms

Glomerular Diseases

Glomeruli are affected primarily by immune, metabolic, and circulatory diseases. In many cases, such as in diabetic nephropathy, more than one mechanism contributes to disease. There are also important diseases of unknown pathogenesis. For example, *Alport syndrome* is probably caused by a genetic defect in the composition of the basement membrane.

Glomerular disease is evaluated morphologically by examining tissue obtained in renal biopsy or autopsy. The biopsy tissue is divided into three portions: one is prepared for light microscopic, the other for immunofluorescent microscopic, and the third for electron microscopic studies. These studies make it possible to classify the glomerular diseases into several clinicopathological entities, which are summarized in Table 11.1. Clinically, glomerular diseases present as *nephritic syndrome*, *nephrotic syndrome*, *acute renal failure*, *chronic renal failure*, or only with minor urinary findings such as *hematuria* or *proteinuria*.

Nephrotic Syndrome. The most important causes of nephrotic syndrome are lipoid nephrosis focal glomerulosclerosis with hyalinosis, membranous nephropathy, and diabetic glomerulosclerosis. The glomerular changes typical of these diseases as seen by electron microscopy are shown in Diagram 11.3.

Lipoid Nephrosis and Focal Glomerulosclerosis. Lipoid nephrosis, also known as *minimal change disease* or *nil disease*, is a disease of unknown pathogenesis

Diagram 11.1. The urinary tract comprises the kidney, calices and pelvis, ureters, urinary bladder, and urethra. The kidney consists of nephrons. A nephron is composed of glomeruli, tubules, and collecting ducts. The urinary collecting system and the lower urinary tract are lined by transitional epithelium that is encased with layers of smooth muscles.

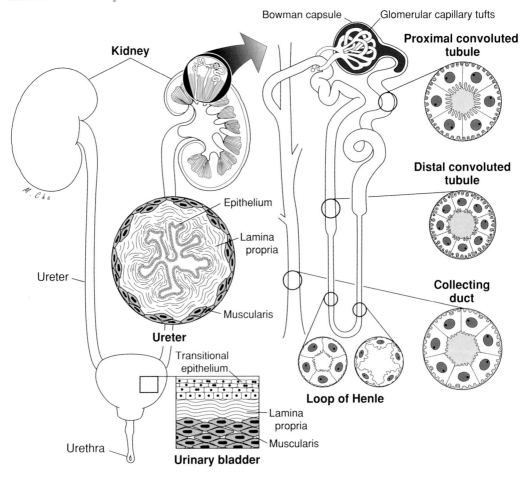

COLOR ATLAS OF HISTOPATHOLOGY

that clinically presents as a nephrotic syndrome—proteinuria, hypoproteinemia, edema, hyperlipidemia, and lipiduria. It occurs more often in children than adults, but does not spare any age group. It responds well to therapy with corticosteroids.

By light microscopy the glomeruli appear normal (hence the term "nil disease") (Fig. 11.1) or show only minimal reactive changes such as a slightly increased number of mesangial cells. Immunofluorescence microscopy findings are negative. By electron microscopy, GBMs appear unremarkable except for the fusion of epithelial cell foot processes. These epithelial cell changes are a nonspecific response to proteinuria.

Lipoid nephrosis is diagnosed in the context of nephrotic syndrome associated with normal light microscopic findings, negative immunofluorescence findings, and electron microscopic data indicative of proteinuria of glomerular origin.

Focal glomerulosclerosis (FGS) with hyalinosis is a disease that also presents as a nephrotic syndrome. Since FGS does not respond to corticosteroid treatment, it was proposed that it represents a form of lipoid nephrosis that has become steroid-resistant. It is more likely that FGS is a distinct disease entity that is unrelated to lipoid nephrosis and that it is resistant to steroids from the beginning. In the *primary form,* it occurs most often in children. *Secondary FGS* occurs mostly in adults; it is considered a "hyperfiltration injury." Any disease that destroys some glomeruli and results in hyperperfusion of the remaining glomeruli may induce FGS. The same morphological changes occur in AIDS and heroin-induced nephropathy.

In early stages of the disease, most glomeruli appear normal; less than 10% show the typical changes (Fig. 11.2). These include partial collapse of thickened capillary loops (*sclerosis*) and occlusion of the capillary lumen with a glossy, homogeneous eosinophilic material ("*hyalin*"). By electron microscopy, this hyalin is finely granular or homogeneous and resembles basement membranes, although it may also contain lipid droplets and proteinaceous inclusions. Intracapillary hyalin may contain im-

Diagram 11.2.   Normal glomerulus. The GBM is lined by fenestrated endothelial cells and covered with epithelial podocytes. The mesangial cells form their third glomerular cell components. The basement membrane and the mesangium separate the endocapillary space from the urinary space, which is continuous with the lumen of proximal tubules.

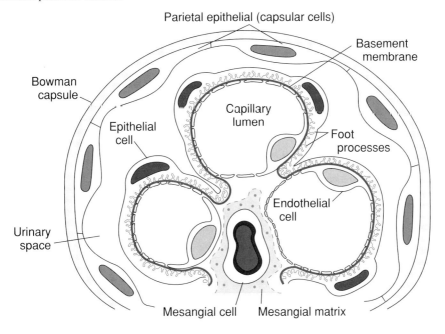

Table 11.1
The Most Important Glomerular Diseases

Disease	Symptoms	Morphology of Glomeruli		
		Light Microscopy	EM	IF
Lipoid nephrosis (minimal change disease)	Nephrotic syndrome	Normal	Fusion of foot processes	Negative
Focal segmental glomerulosclerosis	Nephrotic syndrome	Focal segmental sclerosis with hyalinization	Fusion of foot processes; hyaline lesions focally	Mostly negative; focal IgM, C3
Membranous nephropathy	Nephrotic syndrome	Thickened basement membrane	Subepithelial deposits	"Lumpy-bumpy" deposits IgG and C3
Poststreptococcal glomerulonephritis	Nephritic syndrome	Hypercellularity	Subepithelial deposits	Widespread deposits of all Ig and C3
Lupus nephritis	Mild proteinuria, hematuria	Mesangial hypercellularity	Mesangial deposits	All Ig, C3
	Nephritic syndrome	Focal or diffuse hypercellularity "wire loops"	Deposits in all parts of glomerulus; subendothelial deposits	All Ig, C3; fibrin
	Nephrotic syndrome	GBM thickening	Subepithelial deposits	All Ig, C3 ("lumpy-bumpy")
Focal necrotizing glomerulonephritis (Wegener granulomatosis)	Nephritic syndrome or acute renal failure	Focal fibrinoid necrosis and crescents	Not diagnostic	Not diagnostic "pauci-immune," focal fibrin; crescents also contain fibrin
Goodpasture syndrome	Acute renal failure	Crescents	Not diagnostic	Linear IgG in the GBM; crescents contain fibrin
Membranoproliferative glomerulonephritis		Mesangial hypercellularity	Subendothelial and intramembranous	IgG, C3; no C4 or C1
Type I	Nephritic syndrome	"lobulation";	deposits	IgG, C3, C4; properidin
Type II	Nephritic syndrome	reduplication of GBM	Dense deposits in the GBM	
IgA nephropathy (Berger disease)	Recurrent hematuria, proteinuria	Mesangial widening and hypercellularity	Mesangial dense deposits	IgA with or without IgG
Diabetic nephropathy	Nephrotic syndrome	Mesangial widening and GBM thickening	No deposits; increased BM material	Linear IgG

EM, electron microscopy; IF, immunofluorescence; GBM, glomerular basement membrane.

munoglobulin M (IgM) and complement (C3) as demonstrated by immunofluorescence microscopy. It is thought that the presence of IgM and C3 does not reflect an immune-mediated injury, but rather "trapping" of high-molecular-weight IgM followed by secondary binding of complement.

Membranous Nephropathy. Membranous nephropathy is an immune-mediated glomerular disease that presents as nephrotic syndrome. It may occur as an idiopathic primary kidney disease or secondary to another systemic, i.e., extrarenal,

disease (Table 11.2). The glomerular pathology results either from deposition of immune complexes circulating in blood or the formation of immune complexes in situ. Membranous nephropathy may occur at any age, but is most common is middle-aged adults. The nephrotic syndrome does not respond to steroid treatment. It can persist for 10–15 years, during which time many cases evolve into end-stage kidney disease requiring dialysis or kidney transplantation.

By light microscopy, the glomeruli appear normocellular but generally show basement membrane thickening due to deposits

Table 11.2
Membranous Nephropathy

Idiopathic (85%)
Secondary (15%)
- SLE
- Paraneoplastic (e.g., carcinoma of lung or colon)
- Post infections (e.g., viral hepatitis, malaria)
- Drug induced (e.g., penicillamine, organic gold)

of immune complexes (Fig. 11.3). By electron microscopy, the deposits are first seen on the subepithelial side. As the disease progresses, these deposits become incorporated into the basement membranes, which become gradually thicker. These deposits consist of immunoglobulins, usually IgG and complement (typically C3), which are best demonstrated by immunofluorescence microscopy. Granular deposits of immunoglobulins along the GBM are colloquially described as "lumpy-bumpy."

Nephritic Syndrome. Nephritic syndrome is caused by glomerulonephritis, a generic term used for all inflammatory diseases affecting the glomeruli. Glomerulonephritis may be acute or protracted (chronic) and include such entities as postinfectious (post-streptococcal) glomerulonephritis, lupus nephritis, and membranoproliferative glomerulonephritis (Diagram 11.4).

Poststreptococcal Glomerulonephritis. Glomerulonephritis is a complication of several acute infectious diseases, but it occurs most often 10–14 days after an upper respiratory infection with the so-called "nephritic" strains of beta hemolytic streptococcus. The disease results from immune complexes of streptococcal antigens and antibodies. These complexes either circulate in blood and are deposited "preformed" in the glomeruli, or they are formed "in situ" from "planted" bacterial antigens that have become imbedded in the glomeruli and that then bind antibodies.

The disease occurs mostly in children and presents as a nephritic syndrome. The typical symptoms and findings such as proteinuria, hematuria, hypoalbuminemia, edema, and hypertension last 2–3 weeks and disappear spontaneously in 95% of cases. The remaining few cases progress to renal failure, which may evolve slowly as chronic glomerulonephritis or fast as rapidly progressive glomerulonephritis (RPGN).

Histologically, poststreptococcal glomerulonephritis is characterized by an inflammation of the glomeruli (Fig. 11.4). All the capillaries of the glomeruli are involved, and the inflammation is thus labeled *diffuse* and *global*. The typical glomerulus is enlarged and hypercellular. This enlargement is partly due to the proliferation of mesangial cells and partly to an inflammatory infiltrate that consists of neutrophils and macrophages (Diagram 11.4). By electron microscopy, these inflammatory cells appear in the capillaries often attached to the basement membranes. Also present are osmiophilic dense deposits of immune complexes that typically form large discrete "humps" on the subepithelial side. Most of the immune deposits are not dense enough to be visible by electron microscopy. However, they are easily demonstrable by immunofluorescence microscopy. These immune deposits are found in the basement membranes and mesangial areas and are distributed in an uneven and irregular pattern. The distribution of immune deposits depends on the stage of the disease. Some deposits appear granular, some linear, comma-like, or confluent. As the disease wanes, the deposits disappear. Since the clearance of immune complexes is not even, the resolving acute glomerulonephritis may morphologically appear as a focal and segmental glomerular inflammation, or as mild mesangial hypercellularity.

Lupus Nephritis. Glomerulonephritis of systemic lupus erythematosus (SLE) is caused by deposits of circulating immune complexes in the glomeruli. Nephritis occurs in about 70–75% of all patients with SLE, but the intensity of the renal charges and their extent vary (Fig. 11.5). Glomerulonephritis of SLE may be classified into five categories:

1. Clinical SLE without morphological evidence of glomerular disease (class I)
2. Mesangial glomerulonephritis (class II), characterized by an increased number of mesangial cells and deposits of immunoglobulins and complement in the mesangium. The basement membranes appear normal under light microscopy.

3. Focal proliferative glomerulonephritis (class III), characterized by partial involvement of some glomeruli (focal and segmental glomerulonephritis). The segmental lesions include inflammatory cells and proliferation of mesangial and endothelial cells. Deposits of immune complexes may be associated with fibrinoid necrosis. By immunofluorescence microscopy and electron microscopy, immune complexes may be seen in the GBMs or on the subepithelial or subendothelial side of the basement membrane and in the mesangium.
4. Diffuse proliferative glomerulonephritis (class IV), characterized by increased glomerular cellularity. The glomeruli contain inflammatory cells and an increased number of mesangial and endothelial cells. Deposits of immune complexes can be seen with immunofluorescence microscopy and electron microscopy in all segments of the glomerulus. Massive deposits of immune complexes and other plasma proteins on the subendothelial side of the capillary loops cause typical thickening referred to as "wire loops" and may lead to formation of intracapillary "hyalin thrombi." These intracapillary deposits consist of immunoglobulins, but may also contain other serum proteins, including thrombin and fibrin.
5. Membranous SLE nephropathy (class V) resembles other forms of membranous nephropathy. Class V lesions show no inflammation and only minimal mesangial cell proliferation, if any. Deposits of immune complexes are arranged in a lumpy-bumpy pattern on the epithelial side of the basement membrane, but are also present in the mesangial areas.

Membranoproliferative Glomerulonephritis (MPGN). This term denotes two distinct clinicopathologic entities: MPGN-I and MPGN-II. MPGN-I is usually idiopathic. Morphologically similar changes may be found in association with a number of systemic diseases such as SLE, chronic viral hepatitis, sickle cell anemia, or such changes are secondary to drug-induced injury. MPGN-II, also known as *dense deposit disease*, is a unique pathological entity caused by nephritogenic complement proteins. In all these conditions, the glomeruli show mesangial hypercellularity, increased amounts of mesangial matrix (which contributes to "lobular" appearance of glomeruli), and thickening of basement membranes of the capillary loops (Fig. 11.6). This thickening reflects new basement membrane formation. The capillaries with the

newly formed basement membrane appear reduplicated ("tram track appearance") and are best seen in silver-impregnated slides. By electron microscopy, the basement membranes appear duplicated and the cytoplasm of mesangial cells appears interposed between the old and the newly formed membranes. In MPGN-I, dense deposits of immunoglobulins are on the subendothelial as well as the subepithelial side of the basement membrane and the widened mesangial areas. In MPGN-II, electron microscopy shows distinct changes, which include diffuse permeation of thickened basement membrane with dense material ("dense deposit disease"). These are composed of C3 immunoglobulin and also contain properdin due to the activation of the alternative complement pathway.

Crescentic Glomerulonephritis. Crescentic glomerulonephritis is found in several conditions that cause an RPGN, listed in Table 11.3. Crescents are evidence of severe glomerular injury and can occur in any glomerular disease. It is thought that the lesion ruptures the GBM. Macrophages pass through the hole in the glomerular capillary and accumulate in the urinary space underneath the Bowman capsule (Diagram 11.5). These macrophages and some proliferated Bowman capsular cells transform into epithelioid cells (as in granulomas), forming a crescent and compressing the capillary tufts. Involved glomeruli become afunctional, severely reducing the glomerular filtration rate and causing acute renal failure with oliguria or even anuria.

Crescentic glomerulonephritis typically begins as focal and segmental necrotizing glomerulitis (Fig. 11.7). These glomerular capillary loops appear collapsed and are permeated with fibrin. Rupture of capillaries is

Table 11.3
Crescentic Glomerulonephritis

Goodpasture syndrome
Pauci-immune glomerulonephritis
• Wegener granulomatosis
• Polyarteritis nodosa
Postinfectious glomerulonephritis (severe)
• Poststreptococcal glomerulonephritis
Systemic lupus erythematosus

followed by accumulation of cells in the glomerular urinary space and formation of crescents. As the disease progresses, the crescents become less cellular and more fibrotic. Ultimately, the entire glomerulus becomes obliterated.

Immunofluorescence microscopy findings vary, reflecting the different underlying causes of necrotizing glomerulonephritis and crescent formation. In non–immune-mediated glomerular injury, the foci of fibrinoid necrosis contain fibrin and trapped plasma proteins including immunoglobulins. Such *pauci-immune glomerulonephritis* is typical of **Wegener granulomatosis** and **polyarteritis nodosa**.

Immune-mediated crescentic glomerulonephritis is a typical feature of **Goodpasture syndrome**. This disease is characterized by pulmonary hemorrhage and RPGN. Goodpasture syndrome is an autoimmune disorder in which autoantibodies form type IV collagen of the glomerular and pulmonary capillary basement membranes. Kidney disease begins as a focal and segmental necrotizing glomerulonephritis, which within days progresses to crescent glomerulonephritis. By immunofluorescence microscopy, glomeruli show typically linear deposits of IgG with or without complement. Antibodies to type IV collagen are found in the blood of these patients.

IgA Nephropathy (Berger Disease). In many parts of the world, *Berger disease* is the most common glomerular disease observed in renal biopsies of adults. It is of unknown etiology, although the first symptoms often follow an infection. The disease has protean clinical features, but most often it presents with recurrent microscopic hematuria or mild proteinuria. Despite the benign and protracted course of the disease, renal failure ultimately occurs in more than 50% of patients. This occurs over a period of 10–20 years, but may be accelerated in some patients. Histologically, Berger disease is characterized by mesangial widening and mild mesangial hypercellularity (Fig. 11.8). Deposits of IgA are typically limited to mesangial areas and/or paramesangial portions of the GBMs. Long-lasting disease results in glomerular hyalinization that is indistinguishable from other forms of chronic glomerulonephritis.

Chronic Glomerulonephritis. The term *chronic glomerulonephritis* does not denote a single entity but is used as a synonym for end-stage kidney disease resulting from all or any glomerular diseases. Clinically, it presents with chronic renal failure and uremia. The nature of the pre-existing disease that has caused renal failure cannot usually be deciphered from the histological changes in the kidney. Most glomeruli are hyalinized and obliterated (Fig. 11.9). Because of the loss of glomerular capillaries, the tubules lose their function and blood supply and undergo atrophy.

Vascular Renal Diseases

The renal arteries and arterioles are often affected by systemic diseases, the most important of which are atherosclerosis, hypertension, and diabetes. The kidneys, which are clinically hypoperfused with blood because of vascular diseases, shrink (*nephrosclerosis*). **Benign nephrosclerosis** (or more correctly *nephroangiosclerosis*) is the term used to describe the changes in small arteries and arterioles caused by long-lasting hypertension. These blood vessels show thickening of their walls and narrowing of their lumina. *Hyaline arteriolosclerosis, i.e., homogeneous hyalinization* of the arteriolar wall, is the most typical lesion (see Fig. 5.28). The small arteries show fibroelastic hyperplasia, which comprises reduplication of the elastic lamina and fibrosis of the media. Ischemia of the kidneys leads to hyalinization of glomeruli and atrophy of the tubules. Severe nephroangiosclerosis (Fig. 11.10) may be indistinguishable from chronic pyelonephritis and other forms of end-stage kidney disease.

Malignant hypertension refers to vascular lesions caused by sudden onset of hypertension or acceleration of pre-existing hypertension. The typical lesions include *fibrinoid necrosis* of arterioles and hyperplastic arteriolitis (see Fig. 5.29). Fibrinoid necrosis may extend into the glomeruli (Fig. 11.11). Similar changes can be seen in **scleroderma** (systemic sclerosis), a disease of unknown etiology, which also affects small arteries (Fig. 11.12).

Intracapillary thrombi in the glomeruli are a feature of **hemolytic uremic syn-**

drome and **preeclampsia**. Such thrombi and an endothelial cell response, which they elicit, lead to obliteration of capillary lumina (Fig. 11.13).

Diabetes mellitus causes often renal vascular changes that are most prominent in the arterioles and glomeruli (Fig. 11.14). The arterioles show hyalinization. The glomeruli show diffuse basement membrane thickening, which may be combined with nodular widening of mesangial areas (*nodular glomerulosclerosis* or Kimmelstiel-Wilson disease).

Tubulo-Interstitial Diseases

Tubular and interstitial diseases include developmental disorders, immune-mediated inflammatory disorders, and various infections.

Developmental Disorders. Developmental disorders may affect the entire nephron, but more often the lesions are limited to a segment of the convoluted tubules and the collecting ducts (Diagram 11.6). These lesions interrupt the continuity of the tubules, causing cystic dilation of the proximal segment and atrophy of the afunctional portion of the nephron below the lesion. Accordingly, various forms of cystic renal disease develop, most of which are rare and of limited significance. The only exception is *autosomal dominant polycystic kidney disease*, which is an important cause of renal failure and accounts for approximately 10% of patients undergoing renal transplantation.

Autosomal dominant polycystic kidney disease is inherited as an autosomal dominant trait. Since symptoms usually begin around 30 years of age, it is also known as the adult polycystic kidney disease. The cystic transformation is typically bilateral and results in enormous enlargement of the kidneys, which may exceed 10–20 times their normal weight. This enlargement is partly due to an increased amount of fibrous tissue and dilatation of tubules, but mostly due to accumulation of fluid in the cysts.

Histologically, affected kidney consists of cysts lined by flattened epithelium (Fig. 11.15). It is thought that these cysts arise from either collecting tubules or collecting ducts, but their exact origin cannot be determined morphologically.

Autosomal recessive (childhood) polycystic disease is a rare cause of bilateral cystic transformation of kidneys. The renal lesions are present at birth and may cause early renal failure. The cysts, lined by various cells, are found in the cortex and the medulla. The renal lesions are invariably associated with cystic changes of intrahepatic bile ducts.

Nephronophthisis is a rare familial disease marked by medullary cysts at the corticomedullary junction (Fig. 11.16). The disease is progressive and accounts for about 10% of renal insufficiency in childhood.

Medullary sponge kidney occurs without any definitive inheritance pattern. It may cause hematuria but otherwise does not markedly limit renal function. The cysts are limited to the medulla.

Cystic dysplasia is a unilateral renal malformation. It is the most common abdominal mass in infants and children under the age of 1 year. Histologically, the enlarged kidney consists of solid parts that contain abnormally shaped glomeruli and tubules. The stroma may show nonspecific features or contain heterologous tissue not normally found in the kidneys, such as cartilage or striated muscle (Fig. 11.17).

Immune-Mediated Tubulo-Interstitial Nephritis. Immune injury of the renal tubules may be initiated by drugs and chemicals, viruses, and other pathogens, and is common in renal transplants. Tubular changes are usually associated with interstitial infiltrates of cells that typically participate in immune reactions (e.g., plasma cells and lymphocytes). However, since it is impossible to determine whether the tubular injury elicited the inflammation or whether the inflammation occurred first and the tubular changes are secondary, it is customary to use the term *tubulo-interstitial nephritis*. It is also important to note that this term does not include bacterial infections of the tubules and renal interstitium, which are by convention grouped under the term *pyelonephritis*.

Acute tubulo-interstitial nephritis is typically related to drug hypersensitivity. These drugs include sulfa drugs, penicillins, nonsteroidal anti-inflammatory drugs, and many others. The disease is characterized by sudden onset of acute renal failure and oliguria, often with systemic signs of allergy. Kidneys appear swollen, and the interstitium is infiltrated diffusely with lymphocytes and macrophages (Fig. 11.18). Eosinophils may be prominent in some cases, and plasma cells are typically present during recurrent episodes or in persistent disease. Focal tubular necrosis and tubular regeneration are also evident.

Renal transplant rejection typically presents as *chronic tubulointerstitial nephritis*. It is characterized by interstitial infiltrates, which consist of lymphocytes, macrophages, and plasma cells (Fig. 11.19). The tubules show signs of chronic injury and are often infiltrated with lymphocytes ("tubulitis"). In chronic transplant rejection, the interstitium contains increased amounts of collagenous fibrous tissue, and the tubules are typically atrophic. The older grafts also show arterial endothelial lesions, which ultimately lead to obliterative endarteritis and marked narrowing of arterial lumen.

Other Forms of Tubulo-Interstitial Nephritis. Tubular injury may be caused by various metabolic diseases and drugs. Drugs taken in large amounts, various *toxins* and *heavy metals* most commonly damage the proximal tubules, i.e., the first portion of the nephron. This results in typical coagulation necrosis of proximal tubules (Fig. 11.20). Necrosis of tubular cells elicits a reaction of scavenger cells: neutrophils appear within 1–2 days of injury and are then replaced by macrophages. Renal tubular cells may regenerate, and the lesion may be repaired completely in many cases (Fig. 11.21).

Pyelonephritis. Pyelonephritis is a term used for bacterial infections of the renal parenchyma. The infection may be ascendant from the lower urinary tract or hematogenous. The disease is often caused by bacterial flora with a predominance of *Escherichia coli, Proteus vulgaris,* and *Pseudomonas aeruginosa.*

Acute pyelonephritis is characterized by exudation of neutrophils into the renal parenchyma. Leukocytes may be found in the tubules and the interstitium (Fig.

11.22). Aggregates of neutrophils associated with destruction of tubules leads to the formation of microabscesses, which may become confluent. Pus may extend through the renal capsule (*perinephric abscess*) or accumulate in the collecting urinary system if there is obstruction of urinary flow. This results in *pyonephrosis*, marked by a widened pelvis that is filled with pus and rimmed by a partially destroyed kidney.

Chronic pyelonephritis is characterized by prolonged inflammation, resulting in interstitial fibrosis that replaces the destroyed renal tubules. The interstitial spaces are wide and contain lymphocytes, macrophages, and plasma cells (Fig. 11.23). The tubules are atrophic and lined by flattened cells that cannot be identified as belonging to the proximal or distal tubule. Such atrophic tubules often contain proteinaceous material (*hyaline casts*), and the entire parenchyma may histologically resemble the thyroid gland (*thyroidization*). Glomeruli attached to afunctioning or disrupted tubules undergo hyalinization and involute. The reduced need for blood, combined typically with hypertension, causes sclerosis and narrowing of renal arteries and arteriolosclerosis.

Renal Tumors

Renal tumors may originate from tubules, collecting ducts, and the epithelium of the calices and pelvis. These epithelial tumors, which are usually malignant, account for 98% of all renal neoplasms. There are no glomerular tumors. Other neoplasms, such as tumors of the juxtaglomerular apparatus, stromal fibroblasts, or fibrofatty tissue of renal capsule, are rare and of limited significance. Renal cell adenomas are small benign cortical tumors of no clinical significance.

Renal cell carcinoma, previously also called *hypernephroma*, accounts for the vast majority of malignant renal tumors in adults. The tumor has a propensity to invade the renal vein and metastasize hematogenously to the lungs or bones. Local extension and lymphatic spread are also common.

On gross examination, the tumors appear as solid yellow or brownish-tan masses on one of the poles of the kidney, separated by a fibrous tissue capsule from the compressed renal parenchyma. The yellow tumors are histologically composed of clear cells rich in glycogen and lipid. These substances are usually washed out during processing of tissue, and therefore the tumor cells appear clear (Fig. 11.24). The cells are arranged into solid sheets but also may form tubules reminiscent of normal renal tubules. Some renal cell carcinomas are papillary. The brownish-tan tumors consist of cells that have granular cytoplasm similar to the cytoplasm of normal tubular cells. These cells show the same histological arrangement as clear cell tumors. The distinction between the clear cell and the granular variant has no prognostic significance.

Wilms tumor or **nephroblastoma** is a malignant tumor of infancy and childhood. The tumor presents as an abdominal mass, which is usually one-sided except in 10% of cases, in which it is bilateral.

On gross examination, the tumor sometimes appears as a discrete mass but more often it invades, permeates, and replaces the entire kidney. On cross-section, the tumor appears grayish-white and has a solid fleshy or myxomatous and focally gritty structure. Histologically, several tissue components appear intermixed at random (Fig. 11.25). These include undifferentiated small blue cells arranged into nests without any pattern ("blastema") and surrounded by loose stroma, small epithelial cells forming tubules and abortive glomeruli, and strands of connective tissue that appear "sarcomatoid" as in leiomyosarcomas of fibrosarcomas. The tumor may contain various heterologous elements such as cartilage, striated and smooth muscle, and fat tissue. Areas of necrosis and hemorrhage also are common.

Transitional cell carcinoma of renal pelvis may be papillary or solid and is composed of transitional cells (Fig. 11.26). Such tumors resemble those in the ureters and the urinary bladder.

URETER, URINARY BLADDER, AND URETHRA

The most important diseases of the lower urinary tract are inflammation and tumors.

Urinary Tract Infection. Urinary tract infection (UTI) presents most often as *cystitis* or *urethritis*. The infection is typically caused by coliform bacteria such as *E. coli*, *P. mirabilis,* and *P. aeruginosa*. It is usually ascendant and more often occurs in females who have shorter urethras and are, thus, less protected from bacteria. Retention of urine in elderly men with prostatic hyperplasia or prostatic cancer and urinary calculi also predispose to infection.

Clinically, UTI presents as acute, chronic, or recurrent inflammation. Histologically, cystitis, urethritis, and ureteritis can be classified into several forms.

Acute cystitis is characterized by edema, hyperemia, and infiltrates of inflammatory cells. Polymorphonuclear leukocytes predominate (Fig. 11.27) (*suppurative cystitis*). The epithelium may be preserved or ulcerated (*ulcerative cystitis*).

Chronic cystitis results from recurrence of acute cystitis or incompletely cured acute cystitis (Fig. 11.28). It occurs in many morphological variants. Pseudomembranes are formed in cystitis secondary to cytotoxic drugs (*pseudomembranous cystitis*). Edema and chronic inflammation may cause mucosal protrusions (*polypoid cystitis*). Other forms of cystitis include eosinophilic, follicular cystitis, interstitial cystitis, and emphysematous cystitis. Histological subtyping of cystitis has little practical significance.

Malakoplakia is a peculiar form of chronic cystitis characterized by formation of soft yellow plaques. Histologically, such plaques consist of macrophages that have prominent eosinophilic cytoplasm and round cytoplasmic inclusions. These Michaelis Gutmann bodies consist of a central core of calcified material surrounded by a peripheral ring, best seen by electron microscopy (Fig. 11.29).

Neoplasms. From the tips of the renal papillae to the external orifice of the urethra, the urinary system is lined by transitional epithelium. It is thus obvious that the tumors that originate in these locations will all have the same histological appearance and are predominantly transitional cell neoplasms.

Urinary tract tumors may be benign, which is rare, or malignant. Malignant tumors may be papillary exophytic or endophytic, i.e., invasive, or both papillary and invasive (Diagram 11.7).

Table 11.4
Histological Features of Transitional Cell Tumors

Tumor	Thickness	Cellular Differentiation	Clear Cytoplasm	Mitoses	Nuclear Pleomorphism	Nuclear Polarization	Nuclear Crowding
Papilloma	<7 cell layers	Superficial layer present	+ +	+ / −	−	+	−
TCC-I	>7 cell layers	Normal or focal loss of layering	+ / −	+ / −	+ / −	+ / −	+ / −
TCC-II	Multilayered	Lost to a large extent	+ / −	+	+	−	+
TCC-III	Multilayered	Not evident	−	+ +	+ +	− −	+

Modified from Murphy WM. Current topics in the pathology of bladder cancer. Pathol Annu 18:1, 1983.

Transitional cell papillomas are benign tumors accounting for less than 2% of tumors in the urinary tract. These tumors may be solitary or multiple and measure from a few millimeters to 2 cm in diameter. Typically, they project into the lumen from the surface of the urinary tract. The papillae that form the tumor consist of a vascular core that is lined by regular transitional epithelium less than seven cells thick, and essentially is indistinguishable from normal transitional epithelium (Fig. 11.30).

Transitional cell carcinomas account for 90% of all bladder tumors. Transitional cell carcinomas begin as carcinoma in situ, which is typically flat, or as papillomas, which protrude from the surface.

In **carcinoma in situ,** the entire thickness of the epithelium is occupied by neoplastic cells. These cells do not show typical polarization and lack signs of maturation that are normally seen in transitional epithelium. The malignant cells are separated from the stroma by the basement membrane, and although these lesions may be multiple, there is no invasion. If not removed surgically, carcinoma in situ will progress to invasive carcinoma in more than 50% of cases, usually over a period of 5–10 years.

Papillary transitional cell carcinomas may be histologically graded and divided into three groups (Table 11.4). Such grading has prognostic significance and is important clinically. *Grade I tumors* show minimal differences from normal epithelium. However, the tumor cells form papillae that are lined with epithelium usually more than seven layers thick (Fig. 11.31).

The papillae of *grade II tumors* are lined with epithelium more than seven layers thick and that focally shows no superficial layers ("umbrella cells"). The cells show greater nuclear pleomorphism, and the loss of polarity is more prominent than in grade I tumors. *Grade III tumors* are invasive neoplasms that have lost the typical features of transitional epithelium. The cells show pleomorphism and are arranged into solid nests with invasive margins. The cells of the superficial layers also show less cohesion and are often necrotic.

In addition to transitional cell carcinomas, the tumors of the lower urinary tract may give rise to squamous cell carcinomas, adenocarcinomas, and small cell ("oat cell") carcinomas. *Squamous cell carcinomas* arise in foci of carcinomas in situ or in transitional epithelium that has undergone squamous metaplasia due to chronic inflammation. For example, in Egypt and some tropical countries in which schistosomiasis of the urinary bladder is endemic, most bladder tumors are squamous cell carcinomas. *Adenocarcinomas* are usually located on the dome of the bladder and presumably originate from the remnants of the urachus, an embryonic structure connecting the fetal bladder and the umbilicus that is lined by columnar epithelium. The *oat cell carcinomas* probably originate from neuroendocrine cells in the bladder. *Sarcomas* of the bladder are rare, and the only one worth mentioning is the *rhabdomyosarcoma* of the bladder of infants and children. It presents as *sarcoma botryoides* forming grape-like protrusions. Histologically, it has the typical features of embryonal rhabdomyosarcoma.

PLATE 11.1. LIPOID NEPHROSIS AND FOCAL SEGMENTAL SCLEROSIS

Figure 11.1.   Lipoid nephrosis (minimal change disease). A. By light microscopy, the glomerulus appears normal. **B.** Electron microscopy of the glomerulus shows diffuse fusion of the epithelial foot processes. The basement membrane appears normal.

Figure 11.2.   Focal segmental glomerulosclerosis. A. Light microscopy overview. This lesion is called *focal*, since only a few glomeruli contain lesions, and *segmental*, since the lesion involves only a part of the capillary loops. **B.** Electron microscopy shows occlusion of the capillary loop by homogeneous material ("hyalin").

Diagram 11.3.   Glomerular changes in nephrotic syndrome. A. Lipoid nephrosis shows only fusion of foot processes. **B.** FGS shows focal obliteration of capillary loops by hyalin. **C.** Membranous nephropathy shows deposits of immune complex on the epithelial side of the basement membrane or inside the basement membrane. **D.** Diabetic glomerulosclerosis shows thickening of basement membranes and widening of mesangial areas.

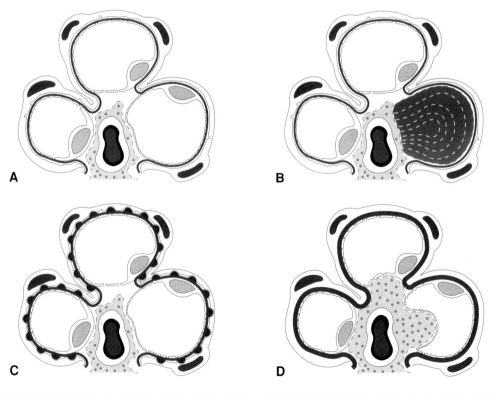

A

B

C

D

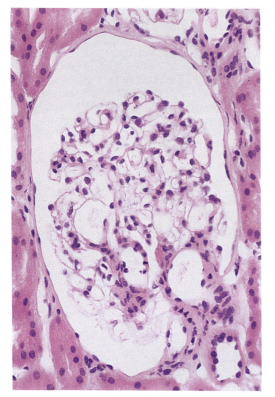

Figure 11.1A

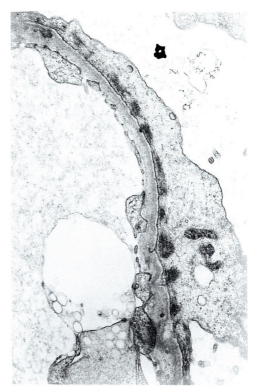

Figure 11.1B

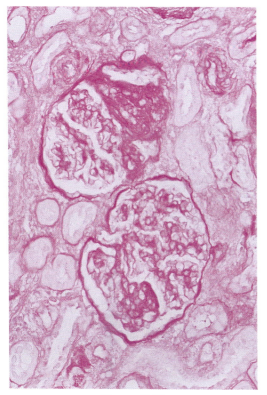

Figure 11.2A

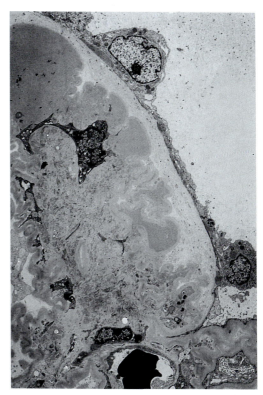

Figure 11.2B

PLATE 11.2. MEMBRANOUS NEPHROPATHY

Figure 11.3. **Membranous nephropathy. A.** By light microscopy, the glomeruli appear normocellular but have thickened basement membranes. **B.** Basement membranes stained with PAS appear unevenly thickened and porous. **C.** In silver-impregnated glomeruli, the thick basement membranes appear finely serrated and "moth-eaten." **D.** Immunofluorescence microscopy shows granular deposits along the GBM. **E.** Electron microscopy shows numerous deposits on the subepithelial side of the basement membrane. **F.** Electron microscopy of a more advanced case shows deposits located deeper in the central portions of the basement membrane.

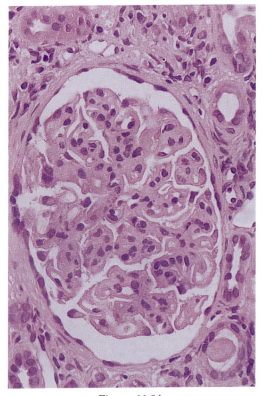

Figure 11.3A

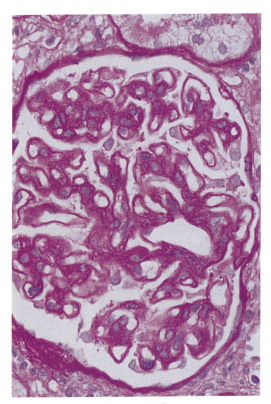

Figure 11.3B

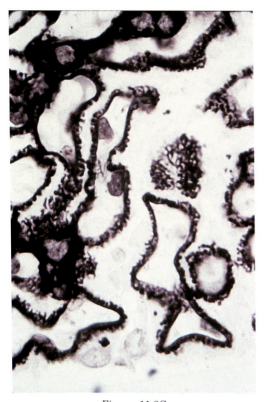

Figure 11.3C

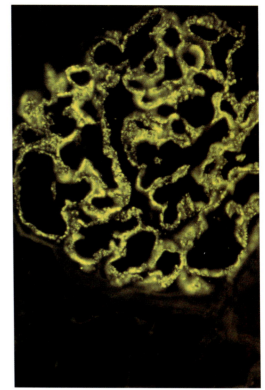

Figure 11.3D

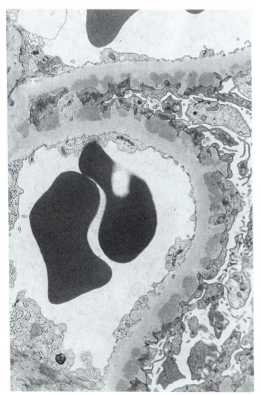

Figure 11.3E

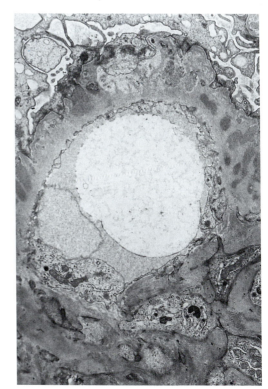

Figure 11.3F

PLATE 11.3. POSTSTREPTOCOCCAL GLOMERULONEPHRITIS

Figure 11.4.   Poststreptococcal glomerulonephritis. A. Light microscopy shows glomerular hypercellularity. This hypercellularity is due to inflammatory cells and proliferation of mesangial and endothelial cells. **B.** Immunofluorescence microscopy shows widespread granular and confluent deposits of immunoglobulin. **C.** Electron microscopy. Inflammatory cells are located in the capillaries and are, in part, attached to the basement membranes. Deposits of immune complexes are seen on the GBM (arrow). **D.** Higher-power view of a typical "hump" located on the subepithelial side of the basement membrane.

Diagram 11.4.   Glomerular changes in nephritic syndrome. A. Poststreptococcal glomerulonephritis shows subepithelial "humps" and acute inflammatory cells. **B.** Lupus nephritis may present in several forms. This diagram shows subendothelial deposits ("wire loops") and mesangial cell proliferation. **C.** MPGN-I shows deposits of immune complexes into the basement membrane, which is typically reduplicated because of new basement membrane formation and mesangial cell extension into the capillary lumen. **D.** MPGN-II shows dense deposits into the basement membrane.

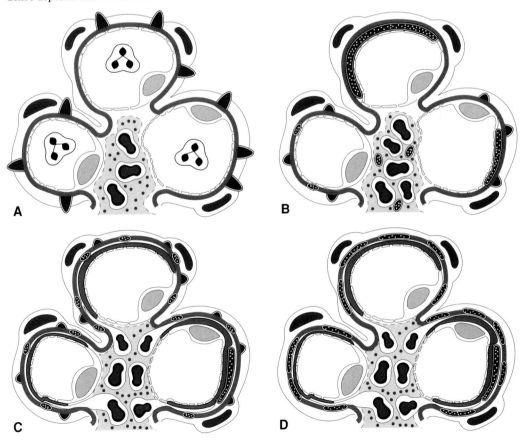

A

B

C

D

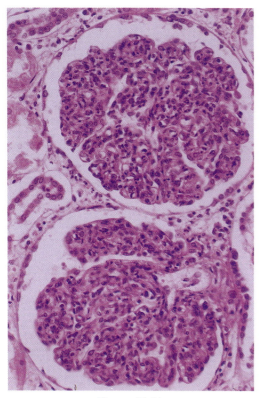

Figure 11.4A

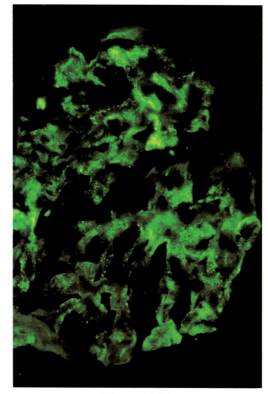

Figure 11.4B

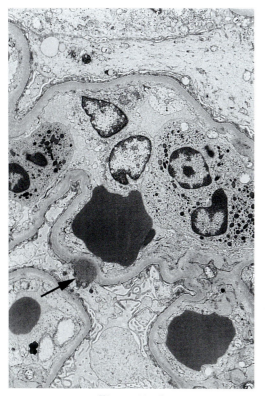

Figure 11.4C

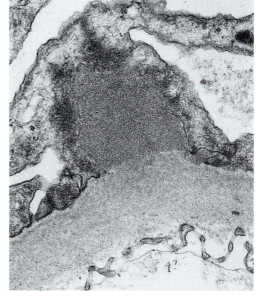

Figure 11.4D

PLATE 11.4. LUPUS NEPHRITIS

Figure 11.5. Lupus nephritis. The changes vary and may be classified into five categories. Class I glomeruli are normal by light microscopy (not shown). **A.** Class II lesions show mesangial hypercellularity. **B.** Class III lesions are focal and segmental, i.e., not all glomeruli are affected and those that are show lesions only in a portion of the glomerular tuft. **C.** Class IV lesions are characterized by diffuse glomerular involvement, intracapillary thrombi, and foci of fibrinoid necrosis. **D.** Wire loops are thickened basement membranes that appear dark red because of deposits of immunoglobulin and fibrin. This glomerulus also contains an intracapillary thrombus. **E.** By electron microscopy, there are typical subepithelial deposits, although the deposits may be seen in other locations as well. **F.** Immunofluorescence microscopy shows widespread deposits of all immunoglobulins ("full-house staining"). Class V lesions, which are indistinguishable from idiopathic membranous nephropathy. By light microscopy, such lesions resemble those illustrated in Figure 11.5D, but do not have intracapillary thrombi or subendothelial deposits on electron microscopy.

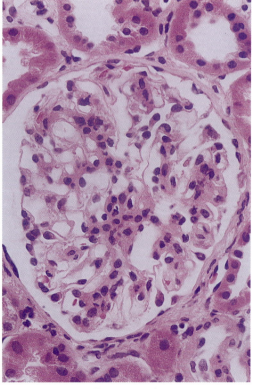

Figure 11.5A

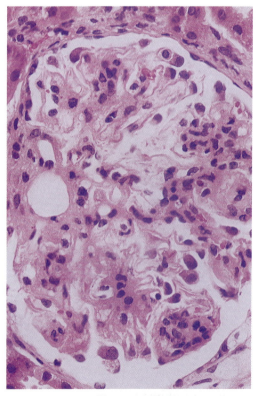

Figure 11.5B

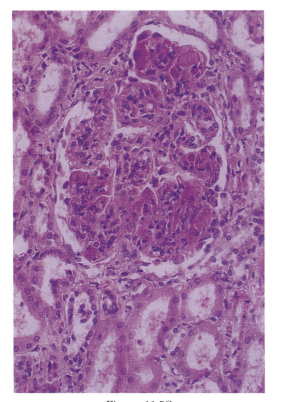

Figure 11.5C

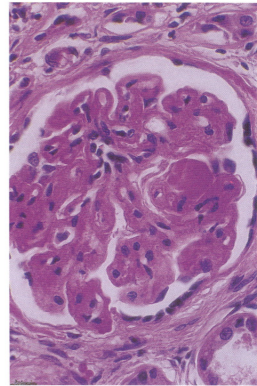

Figure 11.5D

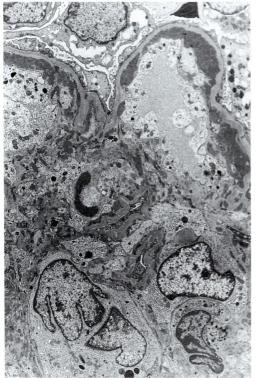

Figure 11.5E

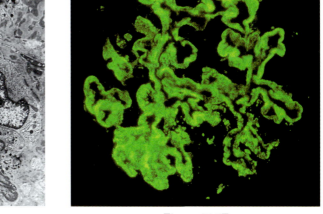

Figure 11.5F

PLATE 11.5. MEMBRANOPROLIFERATIVE GLOMERULONEPHRITIS

Figure 11.6.   Membranoproliferative glomerulonephritis (MPGN). A. Light microscopy shows lobular and hypercellular glomeruli and basement membrane thickening. **B.** Silver impregnation shows irregular thickening and reduplication of basement membranes. **C.** Immunofluorescence microscopy shows deposits of immunoglobulin in the mesangial areas and along basement membranes, which appear segmentally reduplicated. **D.** Type I MPGN. Electron microscopy shows dense deposits and interposition of cells between the original and newly formed basement membranes. **E.** In type II MPGN, there are "ribbon-like" diffuse dense deposits permeating the entire GBM.

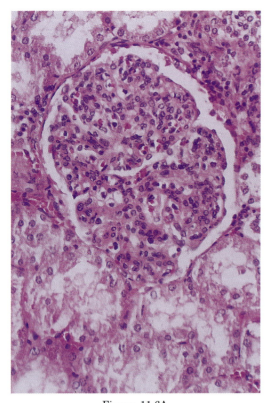

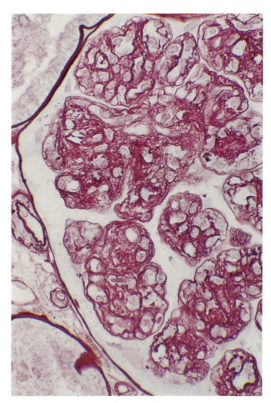

Figure 11.6A   Figure 11.6B

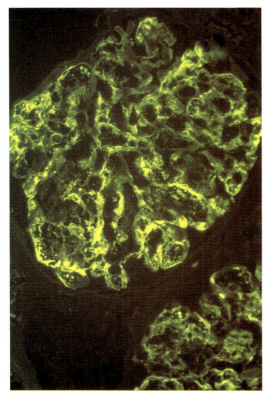

Figure 11.6C

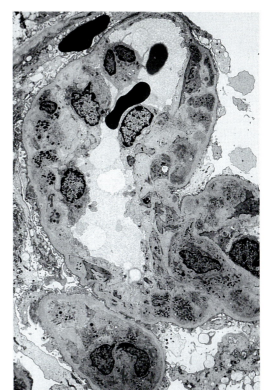

Figure 11.6D

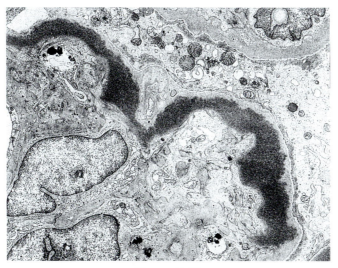

Figure 11.6E

PLATE 11.6.   CRESCENTIC GLOMERULONEPHRITIS

Figure 11.7.   Crescentic glomerulonephritis. A. Crescentic glomerulonephritis is typically preceded by focal-segmental necrotizing glomerular lesions. Segmental necrosis of capillary loops contains fibrin (fibrinoid necrosis). **B.** Early crescents are composed of cells filling the urinary space between the Bowman capsule and the capillary loops of the glomerulus. **C.** The fully developed crescents compress the capillary loops. In this PAS-stained slide, the crescent is between the PAS-positive Bowman capsule and the centrally located PAS-positive tuft of capillary loops. **D.** Goodpasture syndrome is characterized by linear deposits of immunoglobulins along the entire basement membrane.

Diagram 11.5.   Crescentic glomerulonephritis. A. The initial lesions is a focal necrosis of capillary loops. **B.** Macrophages exit from the capillaries into the urinary (Bowman capsular) space. **C.** Crescents are formed in the urinary space from macrophages and proliferated epithelial cells lining the Bowman capsule. **D.** Crescents and the compressed capillary loops of the glomerulus undergo hyalinization.

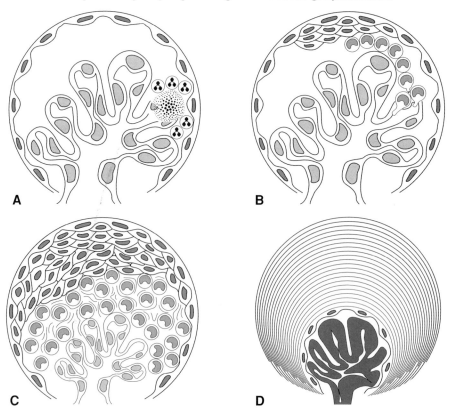

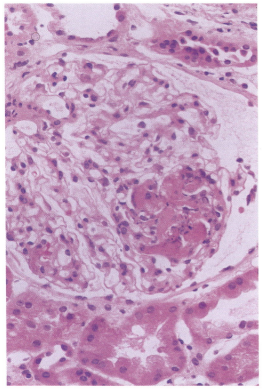

Figure 11.7A

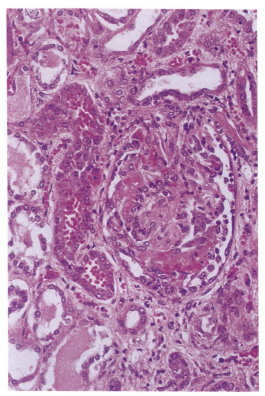

Figure 11.7B

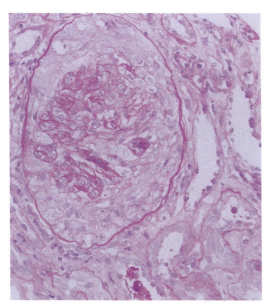

Figure 11.7C

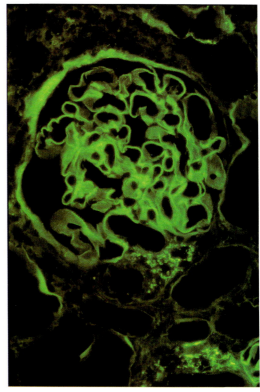

Figure 11.7D

PLATE 11.7. IGA NEPHROPATHY, CHRONIC GLOMERULONEPHRITIS

Figure 11.8.   IgA nephropathy. A. Light microscopy shows mesangial widening and a slightly increased number of mesangial cells. **B.** Immunofluorescence microscopy reveals that mesangial areas contain deposits if IgA. **C.** Electron microscopy shows dense deposits in the mesangial area.

Figure 11.9.   Chronic glomerulonephritis. The glomeruli are hyalinized and surrounded by atrophic tubules, vessels, and fibrous interstitium.

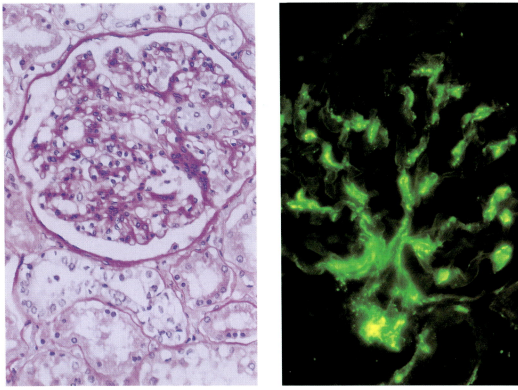

Figure 11.8A

Figure 11.8B

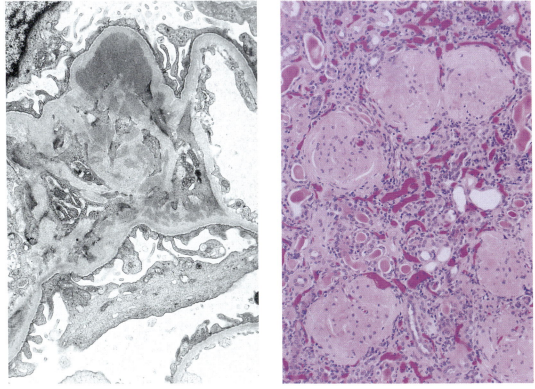

Figure 11.8C

Figure 11.9

PLATE 11.8. VASCULAR DISEASES

Figure 11.10. Nephroangiosclerosis. Chronic ischemia has caused marked atrophy of tubules and a loss of glomeruli. The remaining tubules are atrophic and contain protein casts. The interstitium contains infiltrates of lymphocytes.

Figure 11.12. Scleroderma. The small artery shows narrowing due to concentric proliferation of smooth muscle cells.

Figure 11.11. Malignant hypertension. Fibrinoid necrosis of arterioles and glomerular capillary loops. Fibrinoid appears as homogeneous magenta-red material.

Figure 11.13. Hemolytic uremic syndrome. The capillaries are narrowed because of endothelial cell swelling and incorporation of fibrin into the subendothelial basement membrane. The red blood cells inside the capillaries appear fragmented.

Figure 11.14. Diabetic glomerulosclerosis. A. The glomerulus shows diffuse widening of mesangial areas, basement membrane thickening, and arteriolar hyalinization. **B.** Nodular sclerosis is characterized by round hyaline masses in the mesangium.

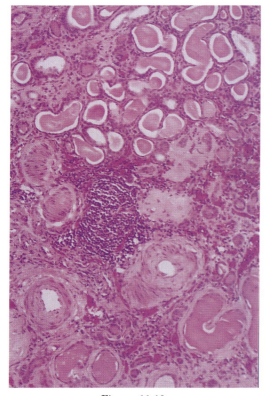

Figure 11.10

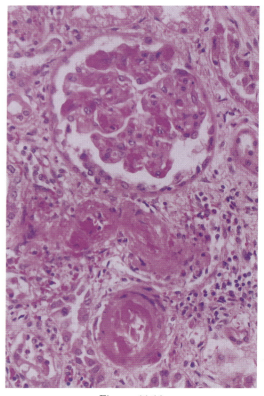

Figure 11.11

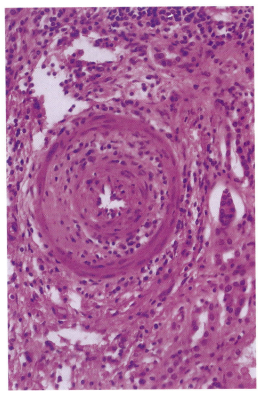

Figure 11.12

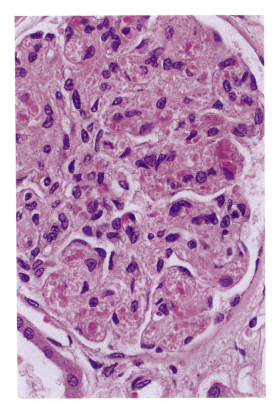

Figure 11.13

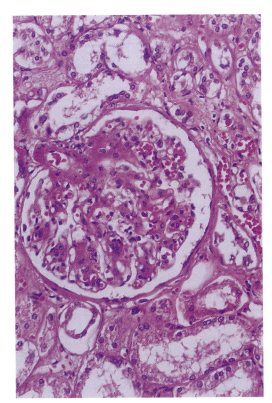

Figure 11.14A

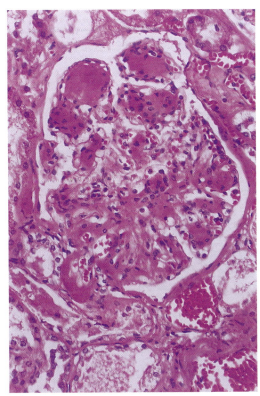

Figure 11.14B

PLATE 11.9. DEVELOPMENTAL KIDNEY DISEASES

Figure 11.15. Polycystic kidney diseases. A. Adult polycystic disease. The cysts are lined by nondescript, mostly flattened epithelium and contain proteinaceous eosinophilic material in their lumen. **B.** Childhood polycystic disease is characterized by cysts that are lined by flattened epithelium. Between the cysts there are tubules and immature (fetal) glomeruli.

Figure 11.16. Nephronophthisis. The medulla is fibrosed and contains cysts lined by cuboidal epithelium.

Figure 11.17. Cystic dysplasia of the kidney. The tubules have been replaced by solid areas that are composed of cartilage, smooth and striated muscle, and connective tissue.

Diagram 11.6. Developmental kidney diseases. A. Autosomal dominant polycystic kidney disease is characterized by widespread cystic dilatation of all parts of the nephron. **B.** Childhood polycystic disease is autosomal recessive, but also shows microcystic changes in all parts of the nephron. **C.** Medullary sponge kidney shows cystic dilatation of collecting ducts of the papillae. **D.** Nephronophthisis shows cystic dilatation of juxtacortical medullary tubules. **E.** Cystic dysplasia contains solid and cystic areas. The solid areas comprise homologous renal and heterologous (nonrenal) elements.

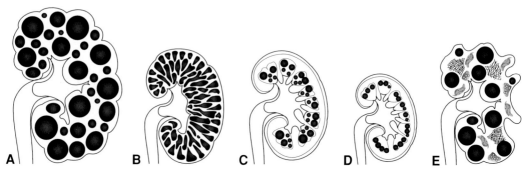

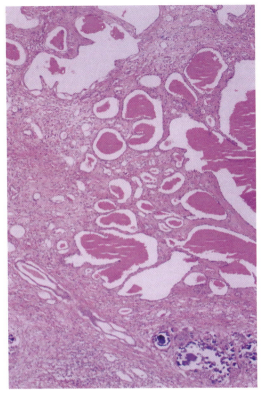

Figure 11.15A

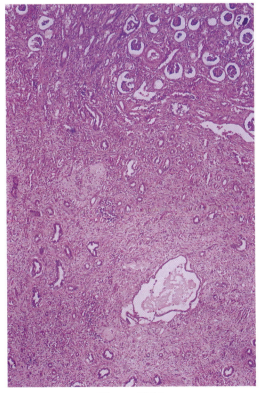

Figure 11.16

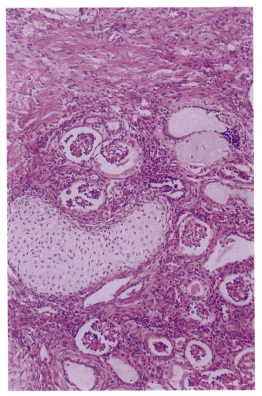

Figure 11.17

PLATE 11.10. TUBULOINTERSTITIAL NEPHRITIS AND TUBULAR NECROSIS

Figure 11.18. Drug-induced acute allergic tubulointerstitial nephritis. The interstitium is densely infiltrated with lymphocytes, eosinophils, and plasma cells. The infiltrate destroys tubules.

Figure 11.20. Tubular necrosis due to mercury poisoning. The proximal tubules have no nuclei, and their cytoplasm appears eosinophilic.

Figure 11.19. Renal transplantation. A. Cellular transplant rejection is characterized by interstitial infiltrates and a loss of tubules. Tubulitis is recognized by the invasion of tubules by lymphocytes. Round nuclei of the lymphocytes are included in the cytoplasm of the tubular cells. **B.** Vascular changes include endarteritis, which leads to progressive narrowing of the arterial lumina.

Figure 11.21. Tubular necrosis. A. Cortex contains dilated tubules lined by flattened cells. Some of these cells do not have nuclei; others have closely juxtaposed nuclei, which indicates that these cells have just been formed by mitosis. Such signs of regeneration are seen within 2–3 days after the onset of necrosis. **B.** Medullary tubules contain granular casts derived from the detritus sloughed off the necrotic cells of proximal tubules.

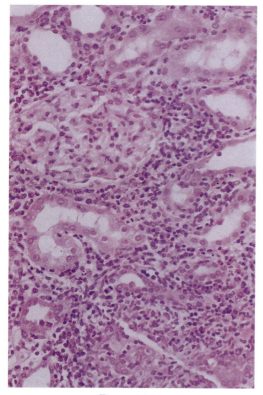

Figure 11.18

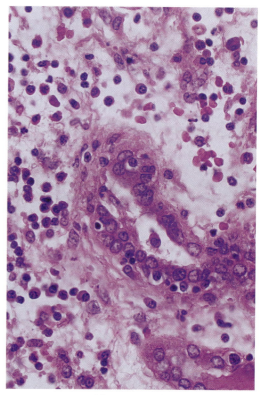

Figure 11.19A

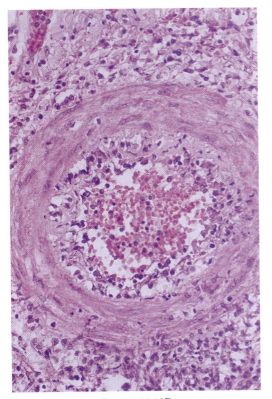

Figure 11.19B

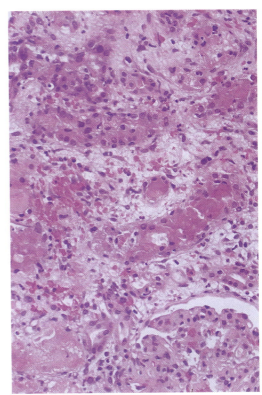

Figure 11.20

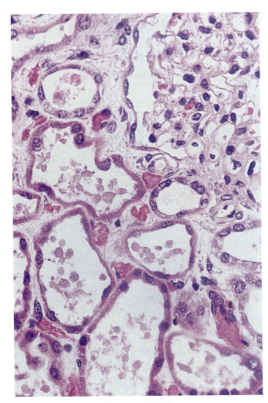

Figure 11.21A

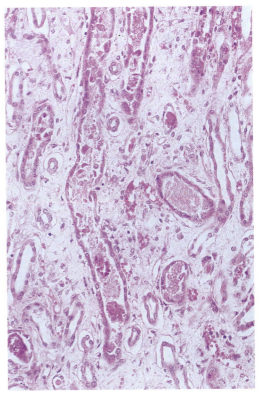

Figure 11.21B

PLATE 11.11. PYELONEPHRITIS

Figure 11.22. Acute pyelonephritis. A. The collecting tubules of the papilla contain neutrophils in this ascending infection. **B.** The tubules and interstitial spaces contain acute inflammatory cells.

Figure 11.23. Chronic pyelonephritis. A. Persistent inflammation is characterized by infiltrates composed of neutrophils as well as lymphocytes and plasma cells. **B.** Broad strands of interstitial fibrosis and chronic inflammation replace tubules. **C.** Atrophic tubules are filled with proteinaceous casts and resemble thyroid tissue. The interstitial spaces contain lymphocytes and plasma cells. **D.** Chronic inflammatory infiltrates consist of aggregates of lymphocytes and plasma cells.

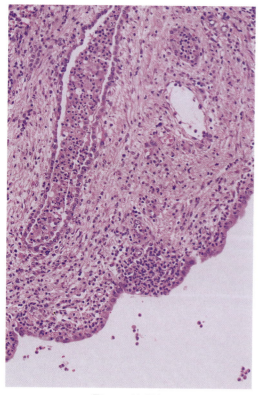

Figure 11.22A

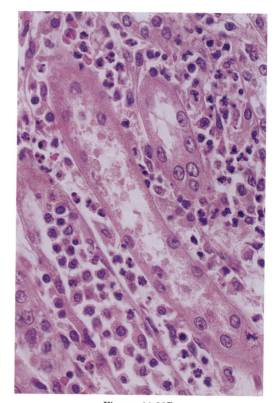

Figure 11.22B

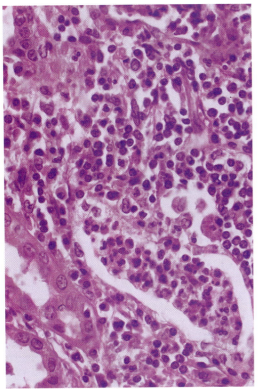

Figure 11.23A

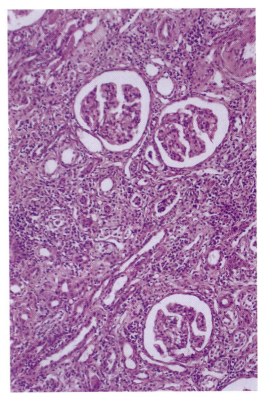

Figure 11.23B

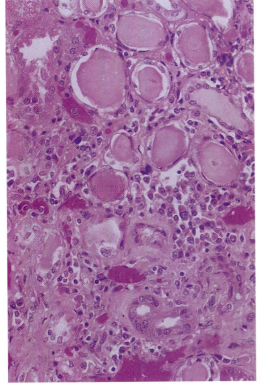

Figure 11.23C

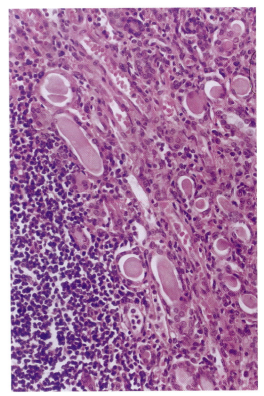

Figure 11.23D

PLATE 11.12. RENAL TUMORS

Figure 11.24.   Renal cell carcinoma. The tumor is composed of clear cuboidal cells arranged into tubules.

Figure 11.25.   Wilms tumor. A. The tumor is composed of small blue cells arranged in cords merging with the renal parenchyma. **B.** The tumor cells form tubules resembling fetal kidney.

Figure 11.26.   Transitional cell carcinoma of renal pelvis. The tumor is composed of nests of transitional epithelium.

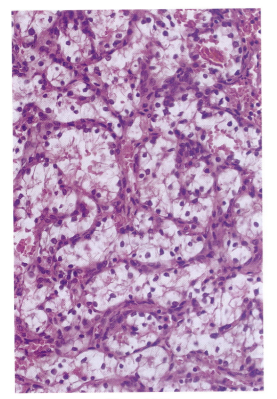

Figure 11.24

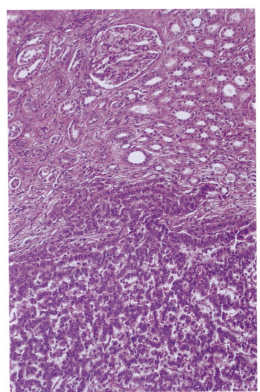

Figure 11.25A

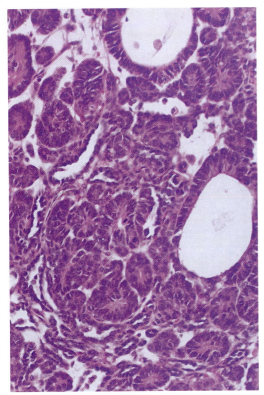

Figure 11.25B

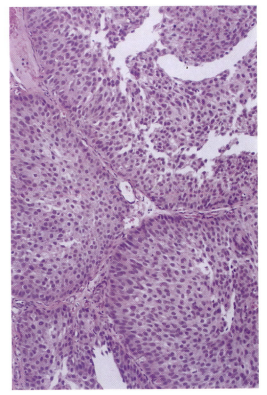

Figure 11.26

PLATE 11.13. CYSTITIS

Figure 11.27.   Acute cystitis. The wall of the bladder is infiltrated with leukocytes, some of which are also seen in the lumen of the bladder.

Figure 11.28.   Chronic cystitis. The urinary bladder is densely infiltrated with lymphocytes, scattered plasma cells, and macrophages.

Figure 11.29.   Malakoplakia of the urinary bladder. A. The infiltrate consists of macrophages that have prominent cytoplasm and often contain small round cytoplasmic inclusions (Michaelis-Gutmann bodies). **B.** By electron microscopy, the cytoplasmic inclusions appear as concentric targetoid structures rich in calcium salts (dark lines).

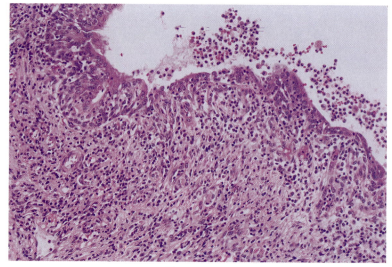

Figure 11.27

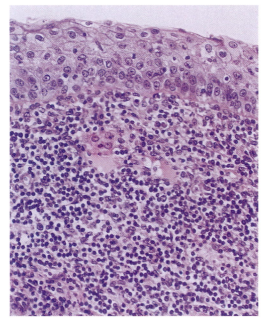

Figure 11.28

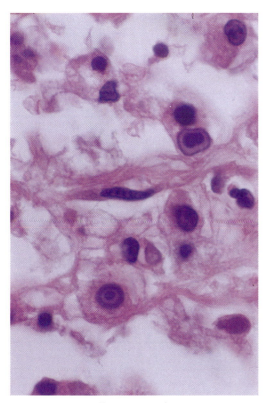

Figure 11.29A

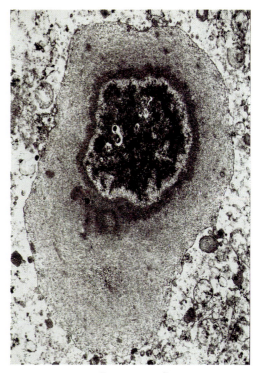

Figure 11.29B

PLATE 11.14. URINARY BLADDER TUMORS

**Figure 11.30. Transitional cell papilloma of
the urinary bladder.** The papillae are lined with
well differentiated transitional epithelium that is
less than seven cell layers thick.

Figure 11.31. Transitional cell carcinoma. A. In grade I carcinoma, the papillae are lined by a slightly
disorganized epithelium that is usually more than seven cells thick. **B.** Grade II tumors show more pleomorphism and less polarization. **C.** Grade III tumors are composed of cells that have retained few features of transitional epithelium, and form solid sheets and nests; cells show pleomorphism.

**Diagram 11.7. Urinary bladder cancer presents as flat or slightly raised plaque-like lesions or
papillary tumors. A.** Carcinoma in situ. **B.** Invasive carcinoma. **C.** Papillary carcinoma. **D.** Invasive papillary carcinoma.

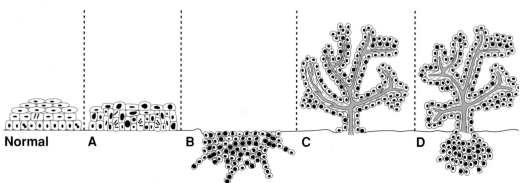

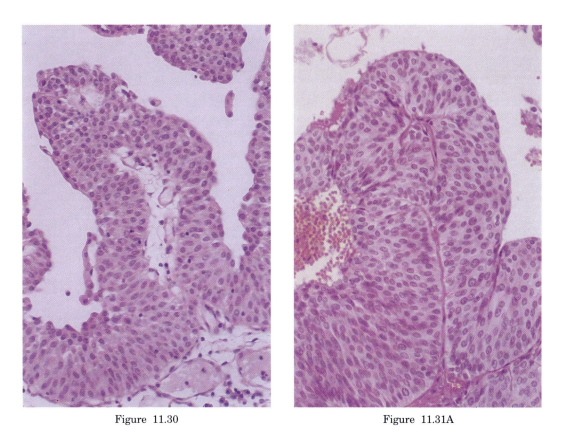

Figure 11.30

Figure 11.31A

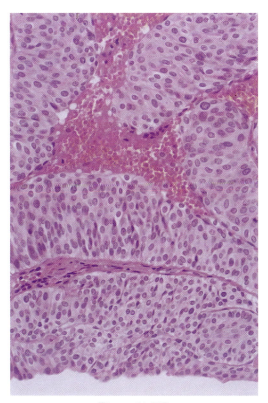

Figure 11.31B

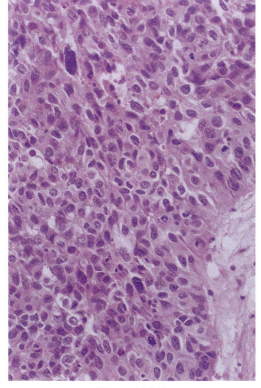

Figure 11.31C

NOTES

CHAPTER 12

Male Reproductive System

NORMAL HISTOLOGY

The male reproductive system consists of the testis, excretory ducts, and accessory glands (seminal vesicles and prostate) (Diagram 12.1). The penis, the copulatory organ, is also part of the urinary tract: the penile urethra serves as a conduit for both urine and the sperm.

The **testis** is predominantly composed of seminiferous tubules. These tubules are delimited by a basement membrane and contain germ cells in various stages of maturation (spermatogonia, spermatocytes, spermatids, and spermatozoa) and Sertoli cells. Leydig cells, the source of testosterone and related androgens, are located in the interstitial spaces between the tubules.

The excretory ducts of the testis, **epididymis**, and **vas deferens** are lined by tall columnar epithelium that is surrounded by smooth muscle cells of the muscularis. The accessory sex glands, the **seminal vesicles,** and the **prostate** are composed of glands and ducts embedded in fibromuscular stroma. The **urethra** is lined by transitional epithelium except for the terminal part, which is lined by squamous epithelium. The **penis** is covered with squamous epithelium.

OVERVIEW OF PATHOLOGY

The most important diseases are

- Developmental disorders, such as cryptorchidism and Klinefelter syndrome
- Infections, such as orchitis, epididymitis, and sexually transmitted diseases
- Hormone-induced lesions, such as benign prostatic hyperplasia
- Neoplasms

Developmental Disorders

Testes develop from the genital ridges, which are localized in the fetal abdominal cavity. To arrive at their normal scrotal position, the testes migrate causally and reach the scrotum through the inguinal canal. If the testis does not reach the scrotum, but remains hidden in the inguinal canal, the condition is called *cryptorchidism*.

Cryptorchid testes show focal atrophy of seminal epithelium, usually associated with thickening of the basement membranes, and often accompanied by interstitial fibrosis (Fig. 12.1). These changes may be associated with hypospermatogenesis and infertility.

The normal development of testes depends on the gene complex located on the Y chromosome known as the testis determining factor (TDF). Normal testicular development cannot occur without the Y chromosome or the TDF region. Similarly, testicular development is impeded in the presence of additional X chromosomes, as occurs in Klinefelter syndrome.

Klinefelter syndrome is characterized by a 47,XXY karyotype, small penis and testicles, eunuchoid body proportions, gynecomastia, and infertility. Histologically, the postpubertal testes in Klinefelter syndrome show diffuse tubular atrophy. The tubules contain only Sertoli cells, but with time even these are lost and the tubules undergo extensive hyalinization (Fig. 12.2). The interstitial spaces contain fibrous tissue and scattered Leydig cells, which although spared of atrophy are functionally inadequate and cannot produce enough testosterone to masculinize the body.

Male infertility may occur even without chromosomal anomalies. Such idiopathic or **primary testicular infertility** is characterized by *hypospermatogenesis* or *aspermatogenesis* if no sperm is found at all. Hypospermatogenesis results in *oligospermia* defined by convention as sperm count of less than 20 million per milliliter of ejaculate (normal is 60 million). In azoospermia, the ejaculate contains no sperm at all.

Histologically, aspermatogenesis is marked by a lack of spermatogonia and their descendants ("Sertoli cell only syndrome") or by a block in the spermatogenic

Diagram 12.1.   Male reproductive system consists of the gonad, excretory ducts, and accessory glands.

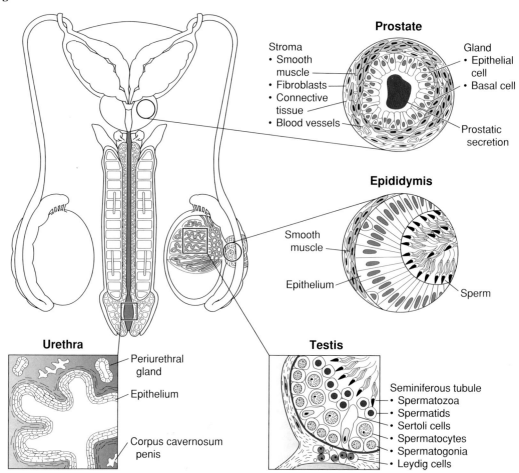

Prostate

Stroma
- Smooth muscle
- Fibroblasts
- Connective tissue
- Blood vessels

Gland
- Epithelial cell
- Basal cell

Prostatic secretion

Epididymis

Smooth muscle

Epithelium

Sperm

Urethra

Periurethral gland

Epithelium

Corpus cavernosum penis

Testis

Seminiferous tubule
- Spermatozoa
- Spermatids
- Sertoli cells
- Spermatocytes
- Spermatogonia
- Leydig cells

sequence (Fig. 12.3). This block can occur at any stage of spermatogenesis—for example, at the stage of spermatogonia, spermatocytes, or round spermatids. The lumina of such seminiferous tubules contain spermatogonia, spermatocytes, or round spermatids, but no mature sperm. Such tubules tend to undergo hyalinization.

In contrast to *primary testicular infertility,* **secondary testicular infertility** may occur because of the obstruction of seminiferous tubules or a deficiency of gonadotropins or gonadotropin-releasing factor in the pituitary or hypothalamus, respectively. The testes of patients suffering from such **hypogonadotropic hypogonadism** are small and immature. Histologically, the seminiferous tubules resemble those in the immature prepubertal testes

and contain more Sertoli cells than gonocytes (Fig. 12.4). There is no spermatogenesis, and the Leydig cells are inconspicuous.

Infections

Testis and epididymis are usually infected jointly; therefore, it is commonplace to call these infections **epididymo-orchitis**. Obviously, isolated orchitis or epididymitis may also occur, but less often. The former is typical of viral infections and syphilis, and the latter of bacterial infections ascending from the lower urinogenital tract. Epididymo-orchitis may be associated with other urogenital lesions such as balanitis, urethritis, or prostatitis (Diagram 12.2).

Infections reach the scrotum either by an ascending route from the urethra and the urinary bladder, or by hematogenous spread from distant sites and/or systemic viremia or bacteremia (Diagram 12.2). Ascending infections are caused by gram-negative bacteria typically causing cystitis or pyelonephritis (e.g., *Escherichia coli, Proteus vulgaris*). The same route of infection is followed by sexually transmitted pathogens (e.g., *Neisseria gonorrhoeae, Chlamydia*). Syphilis of the testis is usually due to hematogenous infection. Pyogenic cocci (*Streptococcus* and *Staphylococcus*) most often reach the scrotum by a hematogenous route in septicemia. Viruses such as mumps virus are invariably hematogenous pathogens.

Mumps orchitis is the most common viral infection of the testis. Typically, orchitis follows initial inflammation of the salivary glands and occasionally is associated with pancreatitis. Histologically, the interstitial spaces of the testis are infiltrated with lymphocytes, macrophages, and plasma cells (Fig. 12.5). The inflammation inhibits normal spermatogenesis. The germinal epithelium appears in disarray and no sperm is formed. Infertility may result from the extensive destruction of seminiferous tubules that undergo hyalinization.

Syphilis of the testis presents in two forms: as an *interstitial orchitis* or as *gumma*. **Interstitial orchitis** caused by syphilis resembles viral orchitis, although in typical cases the infiltrates are located around the interstitial blood vessels and composed predominantly of plasma cells. **Gumma** consists of a central area of necrosis surrounded by mononuclear inflammatory cells, mostly plasma cells, lymphocytes, and macrophages (Fig. 12.6).

Ascending bacterial epididymitis may present as an acute or a chronic inflammation. In acute infection, bacteria such as urinary pathogens (*E. coli and Pseudomonas aeruginosa*) cause exudation of polymorphonuclear leukocytes into the lumen of the epididymal canaliculi (Fig. 12.7). Chronic infections may present as an encapsulated abscess, or as diffuse infiltrates of inflammatory cells associated with fibrosis and obliteration of epididymal ducts.

Granulomas of epididymis with central necrosis may occur in tuberculosis and fungal infections. Such granulomas should be distinguished from noninfectious, noncaseating granulomas of sarcoidosis or post-vasectomy granulomas caused by extravasated sperm or suture material.

Neoplasms

Primary tumors of the testis originate from germ cells in 95% of cases; the remaining 5% of cases are accounted for by tumors of specialized sex cord cells (Sertoli and Leydig cells). Testes may be secondarily involved by infiltrates of lymphoma-leukemia cells. Metastases to testis are rare and usually derived from tumors originating in the prostate or large intestine. The most important tumors of the testis are listed in Table 12.1.

Germ cell tumors originate from intratubular germ cells that have undergone malignant transformation. These cells can be recognized as *carcinoma in situ* (CIS), also known as intratubular testicular germ cell neoplasia (ITGCN).

Neoplastic cells forming CIS have large irregularly shaped nuclei (Fig. 12.8). Nuclei are centrally located and surrounded by abundant cytoplasm rich in glycogen that makes the cytoplasm of tumor cells appear clear. Tubules occupied by CIS have thickened basement membranes and show no spermatogenesis.

The invasive neoplasms develop from CIS through a mechanism that is not fully understood. Two basic types of invasive tumors are recognized: *seminomas*, composed of a single cell type, and *nonseminomatous germ cell tumors* (NSGCTs), which have several subtypes (Diagram 12.3). It is not

Table 12.1
Tumors of the Testis

Germ cell tumors
  Carcinoma in situ
  Seminoma
  Mixed tumor (seminoma and NSGCT)
  Nonseminomatous germ cell tumors (NSGCTs)
    • Embryonal carcinoma
    • Teratocarcinoma
    • Choriocarcinoma
    • Yolk sac carcinoma
  Benign teratoma
  Yolk sac tumor of childhood testis
Sex cord tumors
  Sertoli cell tumor
  Leydig cell tumor
Stromal tumors (e.g., fibroma, liposarcoma)

known whether NSGCTs arise directly from CIS or whether CIS first gives rise to seminomas that then progress to NSGCTs. Both of these histogenetic pathways may be operational. The view that seminomas represent a stage in the development of NSGCTs is supported by the finding of seminoma cells in approximately 15% of so-called mixed tumors composed of seminoma and NSGCT elements.

Seminomas (also known as classic or pure seminomas) form approximately 40% of all testicular germ cell tumors. Such seminomas are composed of a monomorphous tumor cell population (Fig. 12.9). These tumor cells have vesicular nuclei, clear cytoplasm filled with glycogen, and distinct cell borders. The cells are arranged into compact groups surrounded by connective tissue septa infiltrated with lymphocytes. Seminoma cells resemble germ cells such as spermatogonia or primordial fetal germ cells. Tumor cells do not differentiate into any other cells except occasional syncytiotrophoblastic cells, which may be seen focally in 20% of tumors. These giant cells synthesize human chorionic gonadotropin (hCG), which can be demonstrated in scattered cells by immunohistochemistry. The serum levels of hCG are very low, however, and usually not detectable by routine testing.

NSGCT is a term that encompasses all malignant testicular germ cell tumors besides seminoma. The prototype of malignant NSGCT is **teratocarcinoma** (Fig. 12.10). Teratocarcinoma is a malignant tumor composed of malignant stem cells known as **embryonal carcinoma (EC)** cells and various differentiated derivatives of these developmentally pluripotent cells. EC cells correspond developmentally, as their name implies, to early embryonic cells. Like the normal embryonic cells, EC cells give rise to embryonic germ layers: ectoderm, mesoderm, and endoderm, and the periembryonic membranes: the placenta and the yolk sac. The embryonic germ layers, in turn, give rise to all somatic tissues that normally occur in the human body. The *somatic* EC cell derivatives include *ectoderm*-derived structures such as neural elements, and epidermis; various *mesoderm*-derived connective tissue structures, such as bone, muscle, and

cartilage; and *endodermal* structures, such as bronchial or intestinal epithelium. *Extraembryonic components* of teratocarcinomas are yolk sac epithelium and chorionic cytotrophoblast and syncytiotrophoblast. *Yolk sac cells* secrete alpha fetoprotein (AFP), and the *trophoblastic cells* secrete hCG. These proteins serve as serological markers for NSGCTs and can be demonstrated by immunohistochemistry in the corresponding tumor cells.

EC cells, the malignant stem cells of teratocarcinoma, may also proliferate as a monomorphous cell population showing no tendency for differentiation. Such tumor are called **embryonal carcinomas** (Fig. 12.11). Clinically, embryonal carcinomas do not differ from teratocarcinomas, except that these tumors do not secrete AFP or hCG. Embryonal carcinomas account for the 15–20% of AFP- and hCG-negative NSGCTs.

NSGCTs can evolve in other tumors. Tumors in which the proliferation of trophoblastic cells (i.e., cytotrophoblastic and syncytiotrophoblastic cells) overshadows all other elements are called **choriocarcinomas** (Fig. 12.12). Choriocarcinomas are extremely rare, accounting for less than 1% of all testicular tumors. NSGCTs can also evolve into pure **yolk sac carcinomas** since yolk sac elements are common in teratocarcinomas. Pure-form yolk sac carcinomas are very rare in adult testes, however. Such tumors occur more often in the ovary.

Yolk sac tumors are the most common tumors in the testes of children under 5 years of age (Fig. 12.13). Histologically, these tumors resemble yolk sac elements of teratocarcinomas.

Benign teratomas, i.e., tumors composed of well differentiated somatic tissues, are rare in the testis in contrast to the ovary, in which they are the most common germ cell tumors. Benign teratomas are mostly tumors of young children, with a peak incidence at 10 years. Histologically, these tumors resemble the more common ovarian tumors and are composed of benign somatic tissues, such as skin, neural tissue, or cartilage. Most importantly, teratomas do not contain any malignant cells and are devoid of EC cells, yolk sac components, and trophoblastic cells.

Other Tumors

Beside the germ cell tumor, the testes harbor neoplasms originating from the Sertoli cells and Leydig cells, as well as tumors of nonspecific stroma, nerves, blood vessels. Metastases from tumors of other organs are rare but may occur.

Sertoli cells tumors form 2–3% of all testicular tumors. Most Sertoli cell tumors are benign, but some are malignant. Histologically, Sertoli cell tumors consist of cells resembling normal Sertoli cells. Such cells are arranged into membrane-bound tubules in well differentiated tumors (Fig. 12.14) and into nonstructured sheets and groups in the less well differentiated tumor variants. Sertoli cell tumors typically do not produce hormonal symptoms, although minor hormonal aberrations may occur in some patients.

Leydig cell tumors account for 2–3% of all testicular tumors. They occur in all age groups. Histologically, the tumors are composed of cells that resemble normal Leydig cells (Fig. 12.15). In well differentiated tumors, the cells have round nuclei and well developed eosinophilic cytoplasm that occasionally contains Reinke crystals typical of Leydig cells. In the less well differentiated tumors, which are of low-grade malignant potential, the cells are less differentiated. The benign tumors account for 70% and the malignant tumors for 30% of all Leydig cell tumors. Both the benign and the malignant tumors may be hormonally active and secrete male sex hormones, female sex hormones, or both.

Metastatic tumors to the testes stem from bone marrow, lymph nodes, or adjacent pelvic organs, usually the prostate and colon. Lymphomas and leukemias with testicular involvement may occur in any age group, but are most notable in very young or very old patients, those under 5 or over 60 years of age, respectively. Lymphoblastic lymphomas with infiltration of interstitial connective tissue occur typically in children (Fig. 12.16).

Tumors of Epididymis

Tumors of the epididymis are rare. Occasionally, epididymis may be involved by benign tumors of mesothelial origin. These tumors, called **adenomatoid tumors**, arise from the tunica vaginalis testis, which is an extension of peritoneal mesothelium. They are composed of flattened epithelial cells, forming slit-like spaces in the dense connective tissue stroma (Fig. 12.17). The epithelial cells are of mesothelial origin and this tumor is, therefore, called benign scrotal mesothelioma.

PROSTATE

The most important diseases of the prostate are benign prostatic hyperplasia and carcinoma.

Benign prostatic hyperplasia (BPH) is a very common cause of prostatic enlargement in men over 60. Some degree of BPH may be found in most men over 65 years of age. It typically occurs in the periurethral portion of the prostate (Diagram 12.4), which undergoes nodular enlargement (Fig. 12.18). The glands are lined by hyperplastic yet benign cuboidal epithelium and normal basal cells. The stroma shows an increased amount of smooth muscle cells and fibroblasts. The hyperplastic glands contain proteinaceous secretory material, which often cannot be discharged because the ducts are compressed and partially occluded by the myoglandular nodules.

Carcinoma of the prostate is one of the most common malignant tumors. Typically, it is a tumor of old age; it is uncommon in men younger than 50 years. Histological evidence of prostatic carcinoma may be found in 50% of men older than 60 years, and in more than 80% of those older than 80 years. Fortunately, invasive carcinomas are less common, and most these histologically recognizable prostatic carcinomas remain clinically latent.

Most prostatic carcinomas originate in the peripheral portions of the prostate ("posterior lobe") (Fig. 12.19). The tumors are histologically composed of small glands that infiltrate the normal tissue. Because of the abundant fibroblastic stroma, some tumors present histologically as *scirrhous carcinomas* and are hard on palpation. The tumor invades into lymphatics and perineural spaces. Distant metastases are commonly found in the bones, especially in the vertebrae of the lumbar spine.

PENIS

The penis is the copulatory organ that also serves for urination. Most infections of the penis are thus acquired sexually or as urinary tract diseases (Diagram 12.2).

Inflammation of the mucosa of the glans is called **balanitis**. Balanitis is typically caused by bacteria or viruses transmitted sexually or is due to substandard hygiene. The best known cause of viral balanitis is herpesvirus. Herpes infection is marked by vesicular mucosal lesions. Treponema pallidum causes ulcerative lesions (**chancre**), typical of syphilis (Fig. 12.20). Gonorrhea and chlamydial infections typically involve the urethra and the periurethral glands.

Gonorrheal urethritis is characterized by purulent discharge (Fig. 12.21).

Condyloma acuminatum, or genital warts, are tumor-like lesions on the glans penis caused by human papilloma virus (Fig. 11.22).

Carcinoma of the penis is rare in the United States but is one of the more common malignant tumors in South America. This tumor of older men typically originates from the glans and is either exophytic or invasive. Invasive carcinoma is usually preceded by a carcinoma in situ known as Bowen disease (Fig. 12.23). Histologically, invasive malignant tumors are squamous cell carcinomas.

NOTES

PLATE 12.1. DEVELOPMENTAL AND GENETIC DISORDERS

Figure 12.1.   Cryptorchid testis. There is no spermatogenesis. The seminiferous tubules show a lack of spermatogenesis and are surrounded by widened interstitial spaces that contain increased amounts of fibrous tissue.

Figure 12.3.   Aspermatogenesis. A. Sertoli cell only syndrome. The seminiferous tubules are lined exclusively by Sertoli cells. **B.** Spermatogenic arrest at the round spermatid stage. The seminiferous tubules contain Sertoli cells and spermatogonia, spermatocytes, and round spermatids, but no sperm. **C.** Spermatogenic arrest is associated with hyalinization of seminiferous tubules.

Figure 12.2.   Klinefelter syndrome. The tubules show atrophy and are lined almost exclusively by Sertoli cells. The basement membranes are thickened. In the widened interstitial spaces, the Leydig cells appear preserved.

Figure 12.4. Hypogonadotropic hypogonadism. The seminiferous tubules appear immature and resemble those in prepubertal boys. The seminiferous tubules contain mostly Sertoli cells and only scattered prepubertal spermatogonia. There is no spermatogenic differentiation into spermatocytes, spermatids, or sperm.

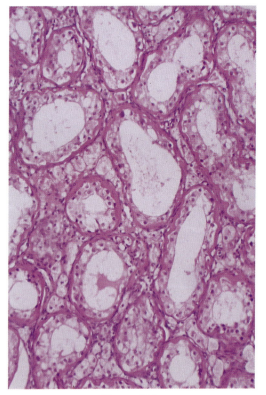

Figure 12.1

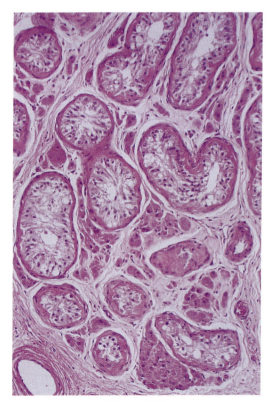

Figure 12.2

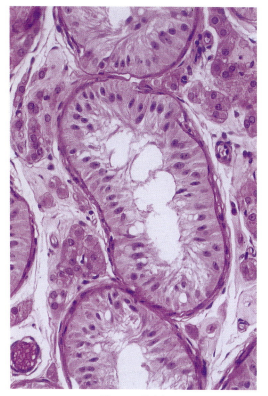

Figure 12.3A

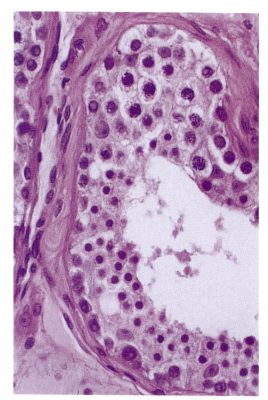

Figure 12.3B

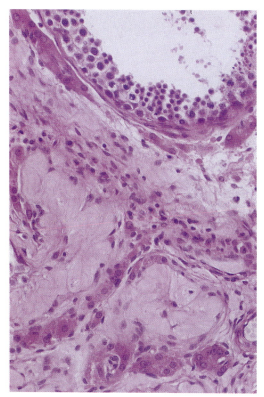

Figure 12.3C

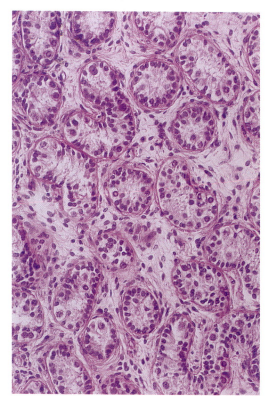

Figure 12.4

PLATE 12.2. INFECTIONS

Figure 12.5. Mumps orchitis. A. The interstitial spaces of the testis are infiltrated with mononuclear inflammatory cells. Some cells invade the tubules. There is disorganization of seminiferous epithelium. **B.** Late sequelae of orchitis. Most tubules are completely hyalinized and surrounded by interstitial fibrosis.

Figure 12.6. Syphilis. Gumma consists of a central area of necrosis surrounded by lymphocytes, plasma cells, and macrophages.

Figure 12.7. Acute epididymitis. The epididymal duct contains an exudate of polymorphonuclear leukocytes.

Diagram 12.2. Epididymo-orchitis. It may be due to an **(A)** ascending sexually transmitted infection, **(B)** urinary tract infection, or **(C)** blood-borne (septic) infection. Typical lesions include: (1) syphilitic chancre, (2) herpetic vesicles, (3) gonorrheal urethritis, (4) viral orchitis due to mumps, (5) epididymitis due to coliform bacilli, and (6) prostatitis due to coliform bacilli.

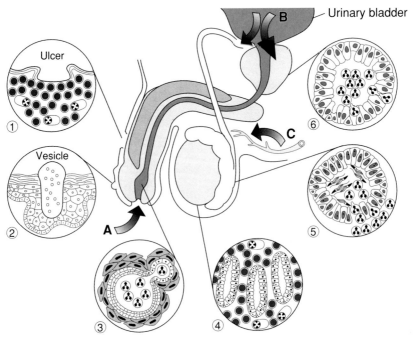

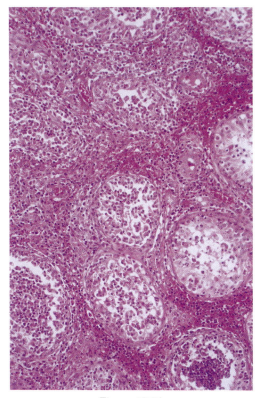

Figure 12.5A

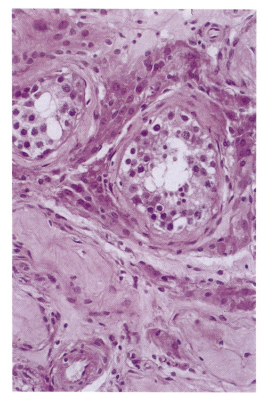

Figure 12.5B

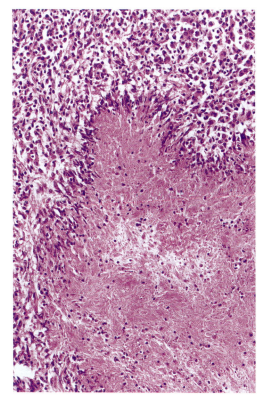

Figure 12.6

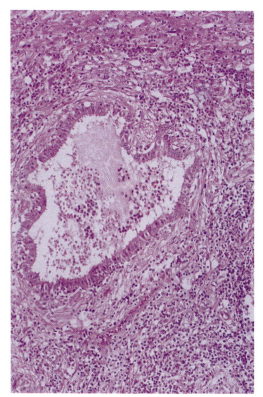

Figure 12.7

PLATE 12.3. CARCINOMA IN SITU AND SEMINOMA

Figure 12.8. CIS testis. A. Tubules with CIS adjacent to tubules that show normal spermatogenesis. **B.** The seminiferous tubule with CIS has a thickened basement membrane and contains large atypical cells. Neoplastic cells have centrally located nuclei that have irregular outlines and prominent nucleoli. The cytoplasm appears abundant and clear. There is no spermatogenesis.

Figure 12.9. Seminoma. A. The tumor is composed of uniform clear cells arranged into nests surrounded by fibrous strands that contain mononuclear inflammatory cells. **B.** Seminoma cells contain glycogen that stains red with the PAS reaction.

Diagram 12.3. Histogenesis of testicular germ cell tumors. All tumors originate from the transformed germ cells in the seminiferous tubules that form CIS. CIS gives rise to *seminoma*. Embryonal carcinoma probably arises from seminoma by progression or directly from CIS. EC cells can form monomorphous tumors composed of a single cell type that does not differentiate (*embryonal carcinoma*). If the EC cells differentiate into somatic and extraembryonic cells, complex tumors—*teratocarcinomas*—form. These are composed of malignant stem cells (EC cells) and differentiated cells. Secondary malignant tumors may also form in which the *yolk sac carcinoma* or *choriocarcinoma* elements overgrow all the other elements. Benign germ cell tumors composed of well differentiated somatic tissues (*teratomas*) can originate from parthenogenetically activated cells that have not undergone malignant transformation. Benign teratomas can also develop from teratocarcinomas in which the malignant stem cells have stopped proliferating and have differentiated into somatic tissues. Such "secondary" teratomas rarely form spontaneously, but have been found after chemotherapy, especially in metastatic sites.

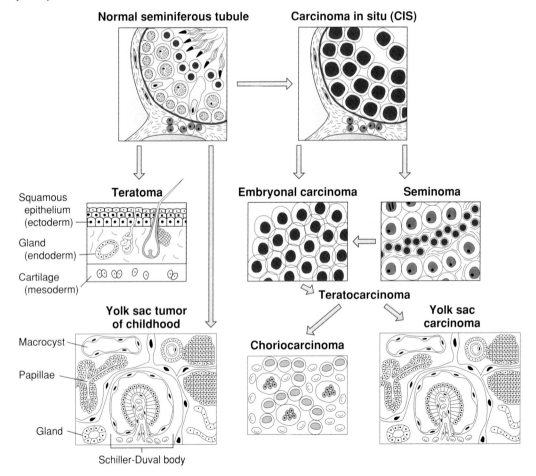

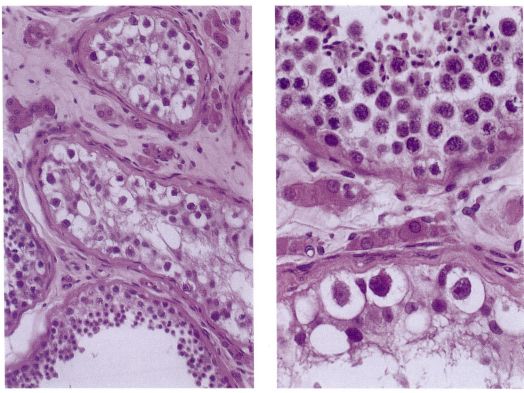

Figure 12.8A

Figure 12.8B

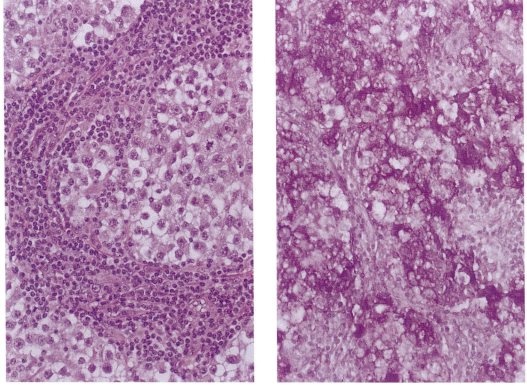

Figure 12.9A

Figure 12.9B

PLATE 12.4. NONSEMINOMATOUS GERM CELL TUMORS

Figure 12.10. **Teratocarcinoma. A.** Overview of the tumor at low magnification shows histological heterogeneity. This part of the tumor consists of mucinous epithelium pigmentary cells and immature neural cells. **B.** The undifferentiated stem cells, called EC cells, are adjacent to more differentiated tissues, such as cartilage. **C.** Human chorionic gonadotropin can be demonstrated immunohistochemically in scattered trophoblastic cells.

Figure 12.12. **Choriocarcinoma.** This tumor is composed of mononuclear cells with clear cytoplasm resembling cytotrophoblast and giant multinucleated and giant cells resembling syncytiotrophoblast. The latter cells secrete hCG. The tumor is highly invasive. It erodes and invades blood vessels and is, therefore, typically hemorrhagic.

Figure 12.11. **Embryonal carcinoma.** The tumor is composed of embryonal carcinoma cells that appear as undifferentiated cells with very little cytoplasm. The nuclei are clear, with finely distributed chromatin and small nucleoli. They overlap each other.

Figure 12.13. **Yolk sac tumor.** The tumor forms glands, papillae, and loosely arranged stroma similar to the yolk sac of the early embryo. The Schiller-Duval bodies, resembling glomeruli, are one of the histological hallmarks of these tumors.

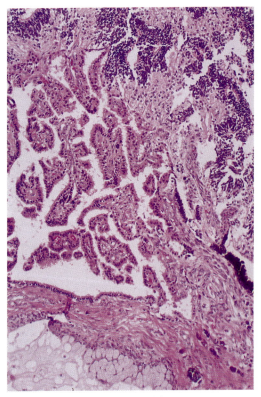

Figure 12.10A

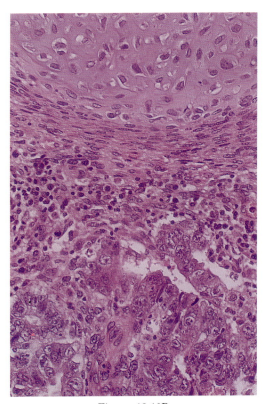

Figure 12.10B

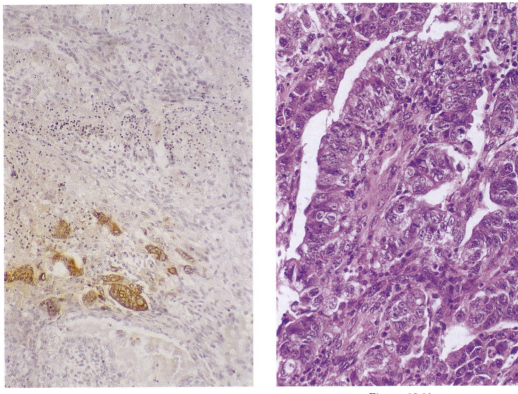

Figure 12.10C

Figure 12.11

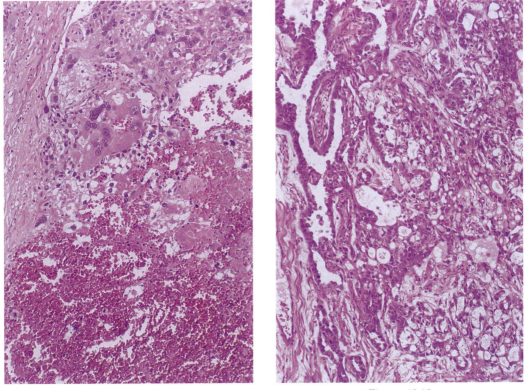

Figure 12.12

Figure 12.13

PLATE 12.5. SEX CORD TUMORS AND METASTASES

Figure 12.14.   Sertoli cell tumor. A. This well differentiated benign tumor is composed of tubules lined by Sertoli cells. It is also known as the "tubular adenoma of Pick." **B.** Less well differentiated Sertoli cell tumor consists of rows of cells.

Figure 12.15.   Leydig cell tumor. A. The tumor cells have round nuclei and prominent cytoplasm. The cells are grouped together without any obvious pattern. **B.** Reinke crystals (*arrows*), shown here in normal Leydig cells, are found rarely in tumors.

Figure 12.16.   Lymphoblastic lymphoma. The testis of this child is infiltrated densely with uniform lymphoid cells that have partially replaced the seminiferous tubules and surround the remaining ones.

Figure 12.17.   Adenomatoid tumor. The tumor is composed of flattened epithelial cells lining tissue spaces in a dense connective tissue stroma.

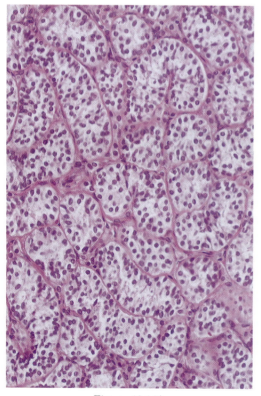

Figure 12.14A

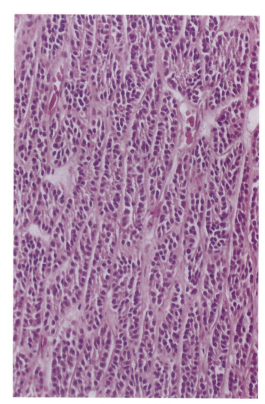

Figure 12.14B

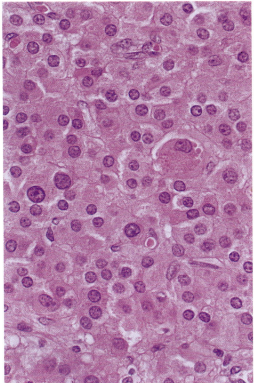

Figure 12.15A

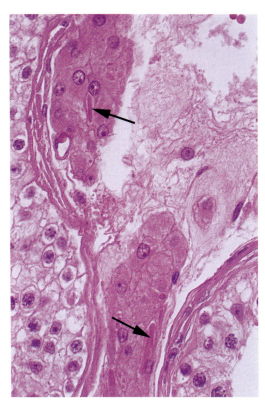

Figure 12.15B

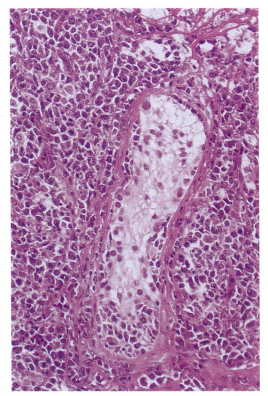

Figure 12.16

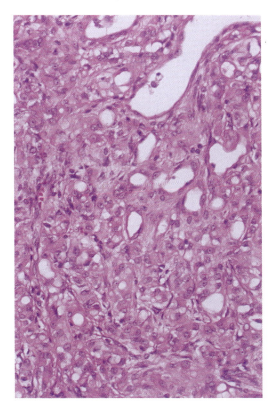

Figure 12.17

PLATE 12.6. PROSTATIC DISEASES

Figure 12.18. Prostatic hyperplasia. A. The prostate is enlarged because of nodules in the periurethral zone. **B.** Higher-magnification view of hyperplastic glands that still show the normal rim of basal cells like the normal prostatic glands. The glands are lined by cuboidal cells that have round regular nuclei and well developed clear cytoplasm.

Figure 12.19. Carcinoma of the prostate. A. The tumor is located in the peripheral parts (*P*) of the prostate ("posterior lobe"). The arrow points to adenocarcinoma, which is composed of clear cells and is therefore not too apparent. **B.** The carcinoma is composed of irregular small glands lined by low clear cuboidal cells, surrounded by connective tissue stroma. Three dilated nonneoplastic glands are seen in the left part of the photograph.

Diagram 12.4. Prostate. This fibromuscular gland has a periurethral part and a peripheral part, the former being the seat of BPH and the latter being the site of carcinomas.

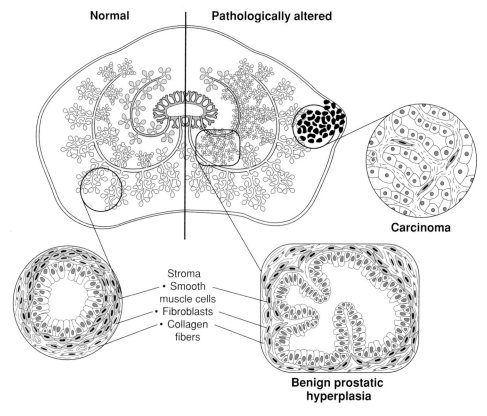

Normal | Pathologically altered

Carcinoma

Stroma
- Smooth muscle cells
- Fibroblasts
- Collagen fibers

Benign prostatic hyperplasia

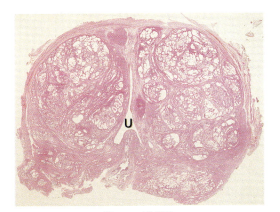

Figure 12.18A

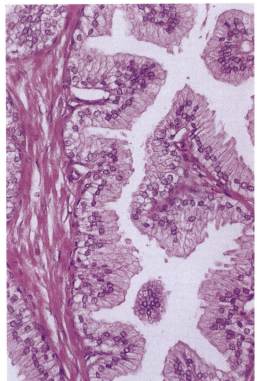

Figure 12.18B

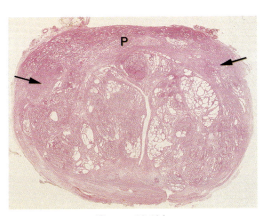

Figure 12.19A

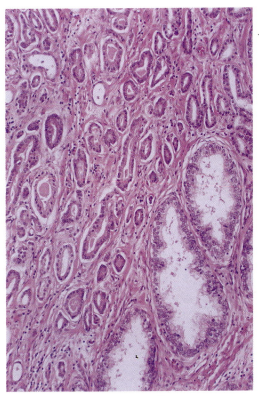

Figure 12.19B

PLATE 12.7. DISEASES OF PENIS

Figure 12.20.   Syphilitic chancre. A. The ulcer of the mucosa contains blood vessels and inflammatory cells. **B.** Higher magnification shows blood vessels surrounded by inflammatory cells, including lymphocytes and plasma cells.

Figure 12.21.   Gonorrhea. The pus discharged from the urethra consists of neutrophils containing diplococci.

Figure 12.22.   Condyloma acuminatum. This genital wart is a papillary excrescence lined by thickened squamous epithelium.

Figure 12.23.   Carcinoma of the penis. A. Carcinoma in situ shows irregular maturation of squamous epithelium. **B.** Invasive squamous cell carcinoma.

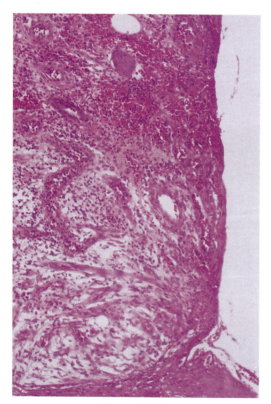

Figure 12.20A

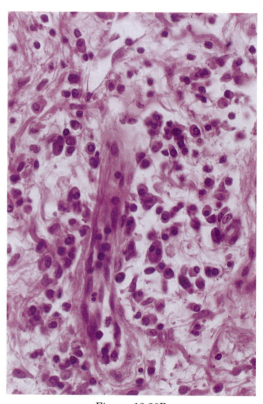

Figure 12.20B

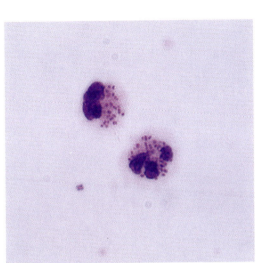

Figure 12.21

Figure 12.22

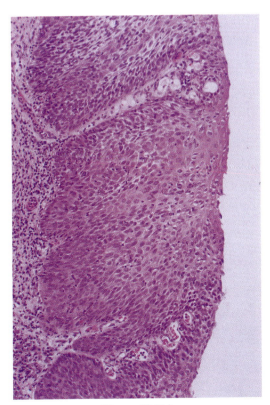

Figure 12.23A

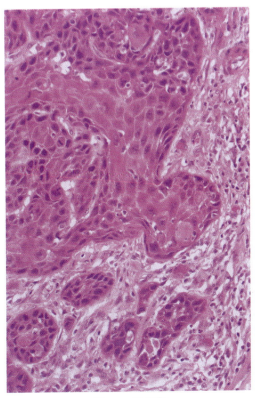

Figure 12.23B

NOTES

Female Genital System

NORMAL HISTOLOGY

The female genital system includes the vulva, vagina, uterus, fallopian tubes, and ovaries (Diagram 13.1). The *vulva,* the *vagina,* and the external surface of the *cervix* of the uterus (exocervix) are lined by squamous epithelium (Fig. 13.1). The cervical canal (*endocervix*) is lined by mucinous columnar epithelium. The border between the squamous epithelium of the exocervix and the mucous epithelium of endocervix is called the *transformation zone.* This region is important because it contains the proliferative stem cells, which repopulate damaged epithelium and also may give rise to neoplasms.

The **uterus** is composed of three layers: endometrium, myometrium, and serosa. The *endometrium* consists of glands and stroma that are hormone-sensitive and change during the menstrual cycle. The first

Diagram 13.1.   Female reproductive system. Vulva and vagina and exocervix are lined by squamous epithelium. The endocervical canal is lined by mucin-secreting cuboidal epithelium. The uterus and fallopian tubes have three layers: endometrium (or endosalpinx), muscularis, and serosa. The ovary is covered with serosa, also called ovarian surface epithelium or germinative epithelium. The ovary contains follicles composed of germ cells, granulosa, and theca cells (sex cord cells). The remainder of the ovary is composed predominantly of nonspecific stromal cells.

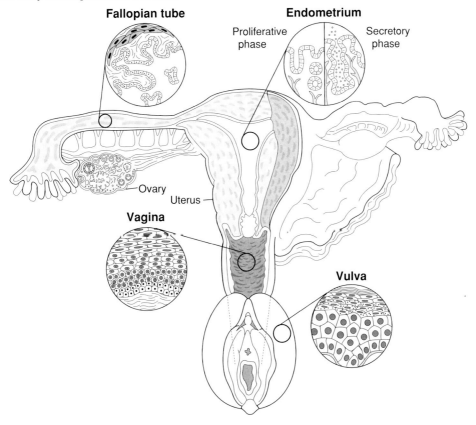

part of the menstrual cycle is governed by estrogen and is characterized by a proliferation of endometrial glands and stroma. After ovulation, the progesterone from the corpus luteum causes secretory transformation of glands and decidualization of stromal cells. These physiological changes prepare the uterus for implantation of the fertilized ovum. If fertilization and implantation do not occur, the secretory endometrium is sloughed, resulting in cyclic menstrual bleeding periods. The *myometrium* is composed of smooth muscle cells. The serosa is equivalent to the peritoneal mesothelium that covers other abdominal organs.

The **fallopian tubes**, like the uterus, are composed of three layers. The *endosalpinx* differs from endometrium in that it is much thinner, does not form glands, and contains less stroma. It is lined by serous cuboidal epithelium that changes only slightly during the menstrual cycle and does not slough off at the time of menses.

The **ovary** consist of multiple cell types. The surface epithelium, also known as germinative epithelium, is equivalent to peritoneal mesothelium. The ovary proper consists of germ cells, sex cord cells, and nonspecific stromal cells. Germ cells and sex cord cells form *follicles*. In response to the pituitary hormones follicle-stimulating hormone and luteinizing hormone, the follicles mature; at the time of ovulation, at least one follicle ruptures to discharge an ovum for fertilization. Preovulatory follicles are lined by *granulosa* and *theca cells*. These sex cord cells secrete estrogens. After ovulation, the ruptured follicle transforms into a *corpus luteum* that secretes progesterone. Corpora lutea involute and become fibrotic *corpora albicantia*.

OVERVIEW OF PATHOLOGY

The most important diseases of the female genital organs are:

- Infections (e.g., pelvic inflammatory disease)
- Hormonally induced lesions (e.g., endometrial hyperplasia)
- Tumors (e.g., carcinoma of the cervix, uterus, or the ovaries)
- Pathological lesions related to pregnancy (e.g., ectopic pregnancy or hydatidiform mole)

Infections

Infections of the female genital organs may be transmitted sexually or may be due to the spread of pathogens from adjacent or distant sites in the body. The infection may be limited to a part of the genital system and present as isolated vulvitis, vaginitis, cervicitis, endometritis, salpingitis, and oophoritis; or as a diffuse inflammation of internal genital organs known as pelvic inflammatory disease (Diagram 13.2).

Vulvitis. Infection of the vulva is most often caused by herpes virus, which leads to the formation of grouped vesicles indistinguishable from similar lesions on the lips or other anatomical sites (see Chapter 16). The vulva may be the site of primary syphilitic ulcer (*chancre*) or genital warts (*condyloma acuminatum*) caused by human papilloma virus (HPV).

Condyloma acuminatum is a wart-like papilloma that consists of folds of connective tissue covered with thickened epithelium (Fig. 13.1). The surface epithelium shows keratosis or parakeratosis. Epithelial vacuolization of middle and superficial layers (*koilocytic change*) is typical of HPV infection.

Vaginitis. In adult women, the vagina is lined by a multilayered squamous epithelium that is impenetrable to bacteria. **Bacterial vaginitis** is, therefore, uncommon during the reproductive age. **Bacterial vaginosis**, an intraluminal infection, is caused by *Gardnerella vaginalis*. This bacterium resides in the lumen of the vagina but is not invasive. *Gardnerella* infection is best recognized by the presence of typical "clue cells" in vaginal smears (Fig. 13.2). **Protozoal vaginitis** is caused by *Trichomonas vaginalis*. *T. vaginalis* lives in the lumen of the vagina (Fig. 13.3). It also causes exudation of inflammatory cells but does not penetrate into the vaginal epithelium.

Fungal vaginitis is most often caused by *Candida albicans*. *Candida* is a noninvasive pathogen that typically remains confined to the vaginal lumen. Fungal hyphae are found in vaginal smears (Fig. 13.4).

Atrophic vaginitis occurs typically after menopause. Without estrogen, the vaginal epithelium of postmenopausal women atrophies. This atrophy renders the vagina more susceptible to trauma during intercourse and bacterial infection (Fig. 13.5). Atrophic vaginitis also may occur in prepubertal girls whose epithelium has not yet been exposed to the maturation-promoting effects of ovarian estrogens or in women who have undergone bilateral oophorectomy. Without estrogen, the epithelium of the vagina cannot mature into squamous cells. The vaginal smear, therefore, lacks squamous cells and contains only parabasal or basal cells.

Cervicitis usually is due to ascending vaginal bacterial infection. Infections predominantly affect the glandular endocervix (Fig. 13.6) since the squamous epithelium of the exocervix is relatively resistant to bacterial invasion. On the other hand, viral infections such as those caused by HPV involve the squamous epithelium, causing wart-like protrusions or papillomas. This lesion can also be somewhat flat (*"flat papilloma"*). Squamous cells infected with HPV (*koilocytes*) are recognized by their clear cytoplasm and condensed "raisin-like" nuclei (Fig. 13.7). Viral particles can be demonstrated in the nuclei of koilocytes by immunohistochemistry or by in-situ hybridization. Koilocytes can also be identified in the routine pap smears as vacuolated cells.

Endometritis is a bacterial infection of the endometrium. Such infections are relatively rare during the reproductive life of a woman because the regular monthly shedding of the uterine mucosa usually removes the infected tissue. Bacterial endometritis may be secondary to sexually transmitted infections or nonsexual ascending infections (Fig. 13.8). Inflammation is typically limited to endometrium and does not extend into the myometrium. The inflamed endometrium does not respond adequately to estrogens and progesterone, and it cannot be "dated," i.e., classified as proliferative or secretory.

Salpingitis, an inflammation of the fallopian tubes, is most often caused by ascending infections from the lower female genital system. *Acute purulent salpingitis* is a typical manifestation of gonorrhea. Leukocytes infiltrate the villi of the fallopian tube and fill the lumen. In *chronic salpingitis*, which is often caused by mixed bacterial flora, the mucosa of the fallopian tube is infiltrated with lymphocytes and plasma cells (Fig. 13.9). *Granulomatous salpingitis*, caused by *Mycobacterium tuberculosis,* is rare in the United States and Western Europe.

Vulvar Dystrophy and Carcinoma

The term *vulvar dystrophy* is applied to benign lesions of unknown etiology. On external examination dystrophy may resemble early cancer, but histologically they are, nevertheless, distinct from carcinoma. Vulvar dystrophy occurs in two histological forms: the *atrophic form* known as **lichen sclerosus et atrophicus,** and the hyperplastic form known as **squamous hyperplasia** or **hyperplastic dystrophy** (Fig. 13.10). These two forms often concur in the same patient and such lesions are called **mixed dystrophy**. Both forms of dystrophy present with changes in the epithelium, which may be thickened or thinned. The epithelium does not show any evidence of malignancy.

Carcinoma of the vulva is of squamous cell type in the vast majority of cases. Typically, it begins as epithelial dysplasia that progresses to carcinoma in situ (CIS) and finally to invasive carcinoma (Fig. 13.11). Dysplasia and CIS are also known as **vulvar intraepithelial neoplasia** (VIN), which can be graded according to the severity of atypia as VIN I, VIN II, or VIN III. The criteria for grading VIN are similar to those applied to intraepithelial neoplasia of the cervix (see later). VIN III, or carcinoma in situ, also known as **Bowen disease**, is confined to the epithelium but occupies its full thickness. It occurs in two forms: as hyperkeratotic papillomas (*"Bowenoid form"*) or as flat epithelial lesions (*"basaloid form"*). Invasive carcinoma has the typical features of **squamous cell carcinoma** found in other sites.

The epithelium of vulva may be invaded by neoplastic cells originating in the underlying glands. The groups of malignant cells are seen in the epidermis. This form of cancer is called **"extramammary Paget disease"** (Fig. 13.12). Histologically, it resembles the better known Paget disease of the nipple.

Carcinoma of the Cervix

Carcinoma of the cervix originates from the epithelial reserve cells in the transformation zone that forms the border between the squamous epithelium of the exocervix and the glandular endocervical canal. The vast majority of cervical tumors are squamous cell carcinomas.

Carcinoma of the cervix is preceded by a preinvasive stage called **cervical intraepithelial neoplasia** (CIN) (Fig. 13.13). Early CIN, also known as mild dysplasia or CIN I, evolves into the more ominous moderate dysplasia (CIN II) and finally reaches the stage of severe dysplasia or carcinoma in situ (CIN III) (Diagram 13.3). The cells forming CIN III ultimately penetrate the underlying basement membrane and infiltrate the underlying stroma as microinvasive carcinoma. The invasive tumors are histologically classified as squamous cell carcinomas (Fig. 13.14). They may be well differentiated or undifferentiated, keratinizing or nonkeratinizing, and they are indistinguishable from squamous cell carcinomas in other sites. Carcinoma of the cervix often contains HPV type 16 and 18, which can be demonstrated immunohistochemically in tumor cell nuclei.

Endometrial Hormonal Lesions

The cyclic changes that occur during the reproductive life of a woman are hormonally regulated. Estrogens promote the proliferation of the endometrium during the first part of the menstrual cycle. Progesterone maintains the secretory activity of the endometrial glands during the second part of the menstrual cycle. Without proper hormonal stimulation, the endometrium of postmenopausal women atrophies, which is known as **postmenopausal endometrial atrophy** (Fig. 13.15). Prolonged estrogenic stimulation, as in anovulatory cycles or due to endogenous or exogenous hyperestrinism, results in endometrial hyperplasia. Histologically, three forms of endometrial hyperplasia are recognized:

- **Simple hyperplasia** (Fig. 13.16). This benign lesion is also known as cystic hyperplasia. The glands are dilated and lined by epithelium resembling proliferative stage endometrium or flattened epithelium. It is also known as Swiss cheese–type hyperplasia because, on low magnification, the glands resemble holes in Swiss cheese.
- **Complex hyperplasia without atypia** (Fig. 13.17). This benign lesion is composed of hyperplastic glands arranged in a complex manner, but without any evidence of cellular atypia.
- **Complex hyperplasia with atypia** (Fig. 13.18). This lesion is composed of glands that show varying degrees of nuclear atypia. Atypical hyperplasia may progress to adenocarcinoma.

Uterine Neoplasms

Uterine neoplasms may originate from glandular epithelium, endometrial stromal cells, or myometrial smooth muscle cells.

Adenocarcinoma of the endometrium is the most common malignant tumor of the uterus (Fig. 13.19). Histologically, adenocarcinoma of the endometrium has no features that would distinguish it from other adenocarcinomas.

Endometrial stromal sarcoma is a rare tumor derived from stromal cells of the endometrium. The tumor cells are elongated and arranged without any distinct pattern into nests and bands that extend into the myometrium, often invading the lymphatics (Fig. 13.20).

Mixed müllerian tumors are tumors composed of a malignant epithelial and a malignant stromal component (Fig. 13.21). The stromal component of these carcinosarcomas may include homologous cells or heterologous elements not formed normally in the uterus (e.g., rhabdomyosarcoma or chondrosarcoma cells).

Leiomyoma is the most common tumor of the uterus. This benign tumor is composed of smooth muscle cells arranged into intertwining bundles (Fig. 13.22). **Leiomyosarcoma**, the malignant smooth muscle cell tumor, is considerably less common. In contrast to benign leiomyomas, leiomyosarcomas show nuclear pleomorphism and numerous mitoses (Fig. 13.23).

Non-Neoplastic Ovarian Cysts

Ovarian cysts originate mostly from the follicles or corpora lutea.

Follicular cysts (Fig. 13.24) are the most common non-neoplastic ovarian cysts.

They are lined by granulosa cells similar to cells that form the normal follicles.

The wall of the **theca-lutein cyst** is composed of elongated theca cells that are usually laden with lipid and resemble luteinized sex cord cells.

Corpus luteum cysts are cystically dilated corpora lutea. The walls of these cysts consist of luteinized cells like those in the normal corpus luteum.

Polycystic ovary syndrome is characterized by numerous cysts (Fig. 13.25). Most of these are follicular or theca-lutein cysts and are surrounded by dense cortical fibrous tissue.

Paraovarian cysts are developmental remnants derived from embryonic structures such as mesonephros. Such cysts are lined by clear cells or cells that have a hobnail appearance (Fig. 13.26).

Endometriosis is characterized by the appearance of endometrial tissue outside the uterine cavity. It may involve any part of the peritoneum but most often affects the serosa of fallopian tubes. Ovarian endometriosis may form large blood-containing cysts (Fig. 13.27) that appear brown on inspection and are colloquially known as "chocolate cysts."

Ovarian Neoplasms

Primary ovarian neoplasms can be divided histogenetically into four groups: tumors of ovarian surface epithelium, germ cell tumors, sex cord cell tumors, and tumors of nonspecific ovarian stroma (Diagram 13.4).

Tumors of Ovarian Surface Epithelium

Ovarian surface epithelium gives rise to tumors that histologically resemble the epithelium derived from the embryonic müllerian ducts. Like the müllerian ductal epithelium, which can give rise to the *serous* epithelium of fallopian ducts, *mucinous* epithelium of endocervix, or *endometrial* glandular epithelium, the ovarian surface epithelium forms serous, mucinous, and endometrioid tumors. Less commonly it gives rise to other tumor types that are called *clear cell tumors* ("mesonephroid") or tumors of transitional epithelium called *Brenner tumors*. Serous and mucinous tumors are cystic, whereas other ovarian tumors are solid (Diagram 13.5).

Serous tumors are cystic tumors composed of tall cuboidal or columnar cells (Fig. 13.28). These cells secrete clear serous fluid. They are either benign or malignant. Since they are almost always cystic, they are called either *serous cystadenoma* or *serous cystadenocarcinoma*. Low-grade cystadenocarcinomas that show minimal stromal invasion are also known as *serous tumors of borderline malignancy* (Diagram 13.6).

Serous cystadenoma is composed of cysts lined by a uniform population of cuboidal or columnar cells. These cells have uniform round or oval nuclei and show no polymorphism or mitotic activity. The epithelium of **serous cystadenocarcinomas** is more pleomorphic and shows prominent nuclear atypia. The neoplastic cells also form papillae protruding into the lumen of the cysts (*papillary cystadenocarcinoma*) and invade into the connective tissue wall of the cysts. These tumors tend to spread by *peritoneal seeding* and often cause ascites that contains malignant cells.

Mucinous tumors are also cystic tumors but are lined by tall columnar cells secreting mucin (Fig. 13.29). These tumors are also classified as benign or malignant: mucinous cystadenoma or mucinous cystadenocarcinoma. Low-grade noninvasive cystadenocarcinomas are also called *mucinous tumors of borderline malignancy*.

Mucinous cystadenoma is composed of well differentiated, uniform mucin-secreting cells. The cells of **mucinous cystadenocarcinomas** are pleomorphic, and the glands that they form are more irregular. Tumor cells can invade the wall of the cysts, spread to the peritoneum, and cause *pseudomyxoma peritonei*, which is marked by abundant free mucus in the abdominal cavity.

Endometrioid carcinoma presents as a solid tumor. Histologically, this tumor is composed of neoplastic glands that do not seem to have secretory capacity and are similar to adenocarcinoma of the uterus (Fig. 13.30).

Some tumors have a more fibrous stroma and are considered to be *adenofibromas* of the ovary that have undergone malignant transformation. As the term implies, these tumors consist of neoplastic cuboidal or cylindrical epithelium surrounded by dense fibrous stroma (Fig. 13.31).

Clear cell carcinoma is composed of large cuboidal cells with clear cytoplasm. These cells form either glands or solid nests (Fig. 13.32).

Brenner tumor is composed of nests of transitional epithelium surrounded by fibrous stroma (Fig. 13.33). Most Brenner tumors are benign, but occasionally they are malignant.

Germ Cell Tumors

Germ cell tumors of the ovary are homologous to the germ cell tumors of the testis. In contrast to testicular germ cell tumors, which are predominantly malignant, ovarian germ cell tumors are more often benign. Benign teratomas are the most common germ cell tumor.

Teratoma, also known as *dermoid cyst*, is a benign tumor composed of various mature tissues derived from all three germ layers (Diagram 13.7). Ectoderm-derived skin and neural tissue are usually the most prominent components (Fig. 13.34). The tumors also may contain endodermal derivatives such as bronchial and intestinal epithelium and mesodermal derivatives such as striated muscle, bone, or cartilage.

Immature teratoma is a malignant tumor composed of immature, embryonic, and fetal cells, most often showing neural differentiation (Fig. 13.35).

Dysgerminoma is the ovarian equivalent of testicular seminoma. This tumor is composed of large cells with clear cytoplasm arranged into broad sheets and surrounded by scanty stroma that contains lymphocytes (Fig. 13.36).

Yolk sac carcinoma of the ovary is morphologically similar to the testicular yolk sac tumors, except that the ovarian tumors are always malignant. The tumor is histologically variegated and shows several patterns such as reticular, microglandular, polycystic (Fig. 13.37). Glomeruloid structures, called Schiller-Duval bodies, are often found.

Sex Cord Cell Tumors

Sex cord cells of the ovary comprise the granulosa, theca, and hilar lutein cells. Tumors originating from these cells are classified as (Diagram 13.8):

- Granulosa cell tumors
- Theca cell tumors
- Sertoli-Leydig cell tumors
- Hilar cell tumors

Granulosa cell tumors are either benign or low-grade malignant tumors composed of granulosa cells. Like their normal equivalents, neoplastic granulosa cells have elongated, oval, grooved ("coffee bean shaped") nuclei and scant cytoplasm. The cells are often arranged around an empty space as in the normal ovarian follicles. These structures are called *Call-Exner bodies* (Fig. 13.38).

Theca cell tumors are hormonally active benign tumors composed of elongated, lipid-rich cells arranged into bundles (Fig. 13.39).

Sertoli-Leydig cell tumors are hormonally active androgen-secreting tumors that may be either benign or malignant. Histologically, these tumors consist of Sertoli-like cells arranged into tubules or cords and Leydig cells forming small nests (Fig. 13.40).

Hilar cell tumors are rare. They present as small nodules composed of luteinized cells, a few of which are found normally in the hilus of each ovary. They are typically benign.

Tumors of Nonspecific Stroma

Fibroma is the most common tumor of the nonspecific stroma of the ovary. This benign tumor is composed of fibroblasts arranged into bundles. It is similar to theca cell tumors except that it does not contain lipid.

Metastases

Ovaries are occasionally involved by metastases. Most originate from the breast or the gastrointestinal tract. Mucin-producing adenocarcinoma of the stomach that diffusely infiltrates the ovaries is known as **Krukenberg tumor** (Fig. 13.41).

Pathology of Pregnancy

The most important pathological changes involving the placenta are ectopic pregnancy and trophoblastic gestational disease.

Ectopic pregnancy is the abnormal implantation of the fertilized ovum outside the uterus. The most common site of ectopic pregnancy is the fallopian tube (Fig. 13.42). The chorionic villi invade the wall of the fallopian tube. This condition is usually associated with profuse bleeding. The blood may accumulate in the lumen of the tube (*hematosalpinx*). Since there is little decidual reaction, the thin tubal wall ruptures to cause hemoperitoneum. If the fetus dies, the products of conception are aborted. The abortion is often incomplete. Retained fetal parts or placenta evoke an acute inflammation necessitating surgical removal of the affected fallopian tube.

Gestational trophoblastic disease is a term that comprises several proliferative and neoplastic placental lesions, the most important of which are:

• Complete hydatidiform mole
• Incomplete hydatidiform mole
• Choriocarcinoma

Hydatidiform mole is a developmental anomaly of the placenta related to abnormal fertilization. The complete form of mole develops through androgenesis, i.e., a process in which ova have acquired the paternal chromosomes from the fertilizing sperm but have lost all the maternal chromosomes. Complete mole typically has a 46, XX karyotype, which consists of two paternally derived sets of 23 chromosomes. The incomplete moles are triploid, i.e., they contain 69 chromosomes.

The *complete mole* consists of hydropically degenerated chorionic villi (Fig. 13.43). In addition to these abnormal villi, the *incomplete mole* also contains fetal parts and normal placental tissue.

Choriocarcinoma is a malignant tumor composed of chorionic cells: mononuclear cytotrophoblastic cells and multinucleated syncytiotrophoblastic cells (Fig. 13.44). Human chorionic gonadotropin can be demonstrated immunohistochemically in the syncytiotrophoblastic cells.

PLATE 13.1. VULVOVAGINITIS

Figure 13.1. Condyloma acuminatum. A. The lesion is a papilloma, i.e., it consists of finger-like protrusions of acanthotic squamous epithelium and cores of connective tissue stroma. **B.** Surface of papilloma shows parakeratosis. There is also vacuolization of epithelium.

Figure 13.2. Bacterial vaginosis. Infection with *Gardnerella vaginalis* is best recognized by typical "clue cells" in the vaginal smears. These squamous cells have clumped nuclei and folded cytoplasm that is covered with bacteria.

Figure 13.3. Infection caused by *Trichomonas vaginalis*. The protozoon can be recognized in vaginal smears (*arrow*). It produces reactive changes in the epithelial cells.

Figure 13.4. Fungal vaginitis. The infection is caused by *Candida albicans*. The vaginal smear contains fungal hyphae (*arrow*) and inflammatory cells.

Figure 13.5. Atrophic vaginitis. The squamous epithelium is thin. The underlying stroma contains a few mononuclear inflammatory cells.

Diagram 13.2. Infectious lesions of the female reproductive system include: **A.** Vulvitis. **B.** Vaginitis. **C.** Cervicitis and endometritis. **D.** Salpingitis. Common forms of vulvitis are: **A₁**. Herpesvirus infection. **A₂**. Condyloma acuminatum caused by HPV. **A₃**. Syphilitic chancre. Vaginitis may be caused by: **B₁**. *Gardnerella vaginalis*. **B₂**. *Trichomonas vaginalis*. **B₃**. Candida albicans **C, D**. Cervicitis, endometritis, and salpingitis present histologically as nonspecific acute or chronic inflammation.

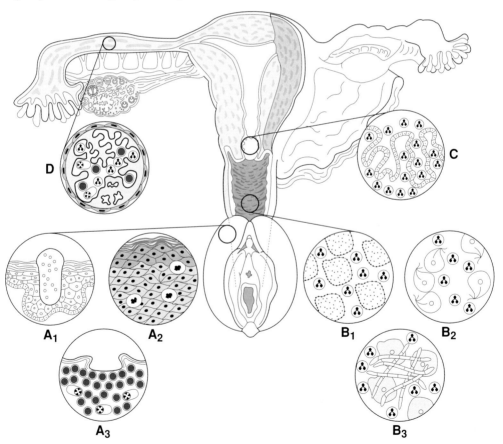

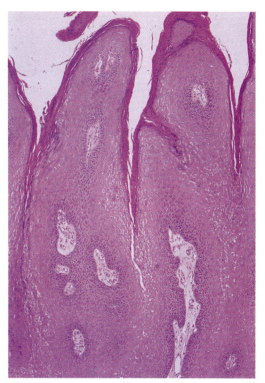

Figure 13.1A

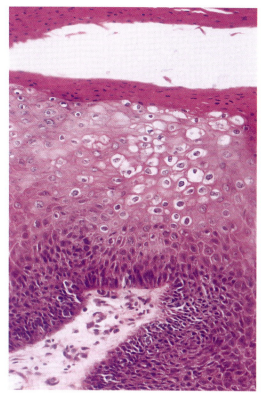

Figure 13.1B

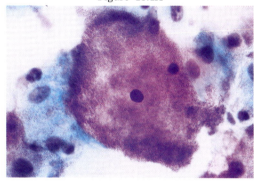

Figure 13.2

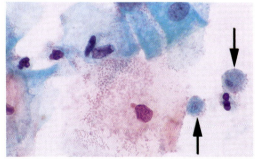

Figure 13.3

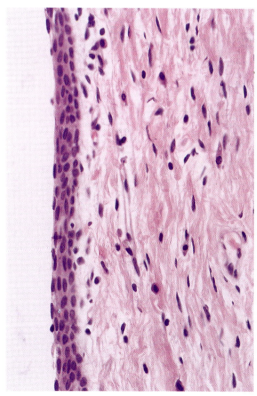

Figure 13.5

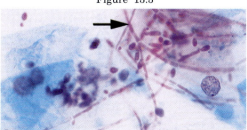

Figure 13.4

PLATE 13.2. INFLAMMATION OF UTERUS AND FALLOPIAN TUBES

Figure 13.6. Chronic bacterial cervicitis. The mucosa of the endocervix is infiltrated with inflammatory cells. The epithelium shows focal squamous metaplasia.

Figure 13.8. Chronic endometritis. The endometrium is infiltrated with lymphocytes, macrophages, and plasma cells.

Figure 13.7. HPV infection of the cervix. A. HPV invades the squamous epithelium, producing so-called koilocytic changes. **B.** Koilocytes have condensed nuclei and clear cytoplasm. **C.** HPV can be recognized in the nuclei of koilocytes by immunohistochemistry (red staining). **D.** Koilocytes can be recognized as cells that have clear cytoplasm in pap smears.

Figure 13.9. Chronic salpingitis. The mucosa of the fallopian tube is infiltrated with lymphocytes, macrophages, and plasma cells. The folds of the mucosa are broad and form adhesions that partially obliterate the lumen.

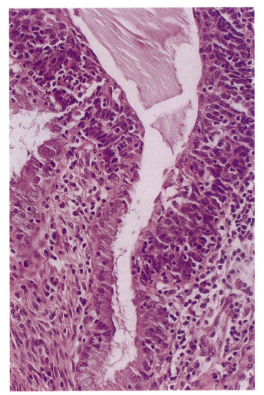

Figure 13.6

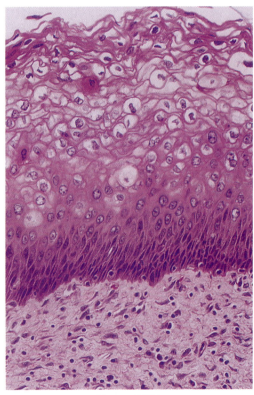

Figure 13.7A

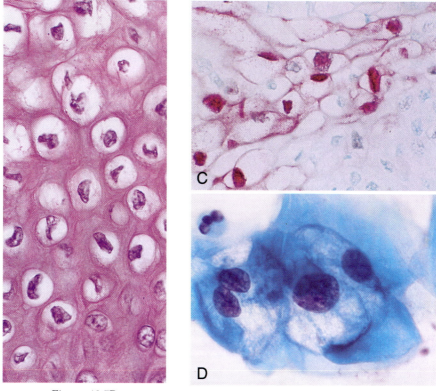

Figure 13.7B

Figure 13.7CD

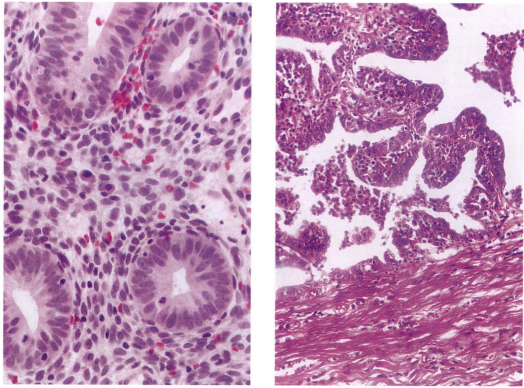

Figure 13.8

Figure 13.9

PLATE 13.3. VULVAR DYSTROPHY AND CARCINOMA

Figure 13.10.   Vulvar dystrophy. A. *Lichen sclerosus et atrophicus*, the squamous epithelium, is keratinized but atrophic. The underlying connective tissue appears sclerotic, i.e., condensed and hyalinized. **B.** *Squamous hyperplasia* is characterized by hyperkeratosis and epithelial thickening.

Figure 13.11.   Vulvar intraepithelial neoplasia (VIN) may have a bowenoid or a basaloid appearance. **A.** Bowen disease shows hyperkeratosis, papillomatosis acanthosis, and marked nuclear atypia. **B.** The basaloid VIN shows disorganized layering of atypical cells whose nuclei vary in size and shape. However, the basement membrane is intact, indicating that this is not an invasive carcinoma.

Figure 13.12.   Paget disease of vulva. The epidermis is infiltrated with groups of neoplastic cells.

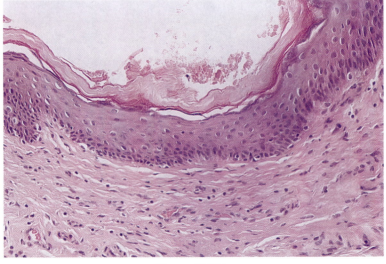

Figure 13.10A

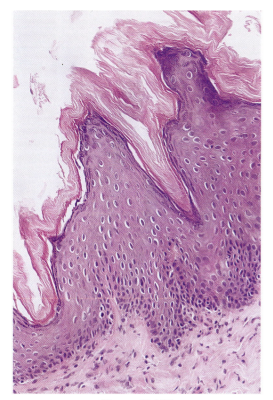

Figure 13.10B

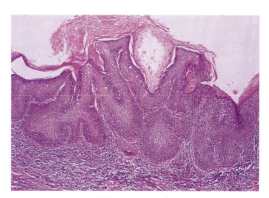

Figure 13.11A

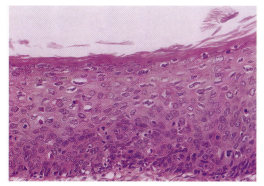

Figure 13.11B

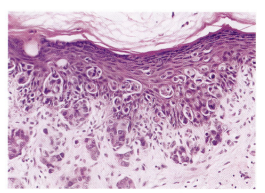

Figure 13.12

PLATE 13.4. CERVICAL NEOPLASIA

Figure 13.13.   Cervical intraepithelial neoplasia. A. Mild dysplasia, CIN I. The epithelium shows mildly disorganized layering (maturation) limited to the basal and suprabasal layer. **B.** Moderate dysplasia, CIN II. The epithelium shows almost complete disorganization, but the uppermost layer still shows maturation, i.e., flattening of the superficial squamous cells. **C.** Carcinoma in situ, CIN III. The epithelium shows complete loss of normal architecture. The atypical cells are found in all layers of the epithelium and there is no evidence of surface maturation.

Figure 13.14.   Invasive squamous cell carcinoma. Nests of carcinoma contain keratinized cores ("keratin pearls").

Diagram 13.3.   Carcinoma of the cervix evolves from CIN I (mild dysplasia) through CIN II (moderate dysplasia) and CIN III (carcinoma in situ).

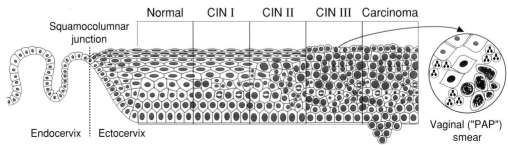

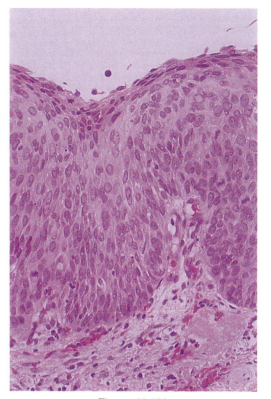

Figure 13.13A

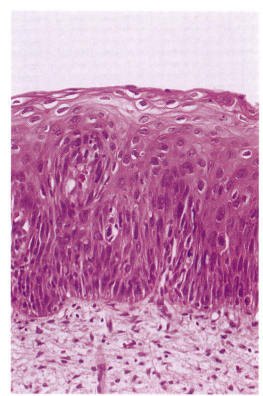

Figure 13.13B

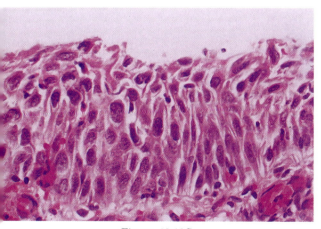

Figure 13.13C

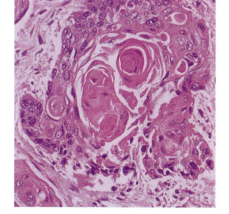

Figure 13.14

PLATE 13.5. ENDOMETRIAL HORMONAL CHANGES

Figure 13.15. Postmenopausal atrophy of the endometrium. The cystic glands are lined by atrophic, nondescript epithelium and surrounded by scant stroma.

Figure 13.17. Complex hyperplasia without atypia. A. The glands appear crowded and show budding and tufting. **B.** The glands are lined by tall proliferative epithelium but show no nuclear atypia.

Figure 13.16. Simple endometrial hyperplasia. A. The glands are irregularly dilated, giving the endometrium a "Swiss-cheese" appearance. **B.** The cells lining the dilated glands look like proliferative endometrium.

Figure 13.18. Complex hyperplasia with atypia. The glands are apposed to one another and show irregular layering of the nuclei with some atypia.

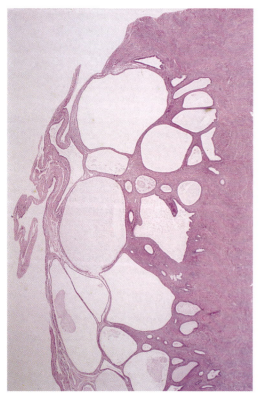

Figure 13.15

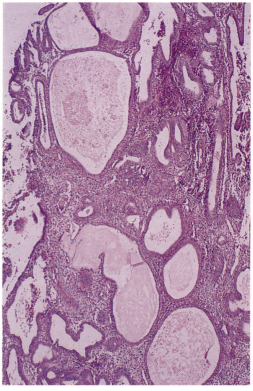

Figure 13.16A

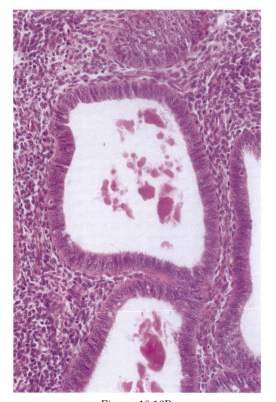

Figure 13.16B

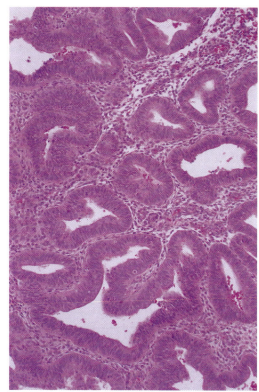

Figure 13.17A

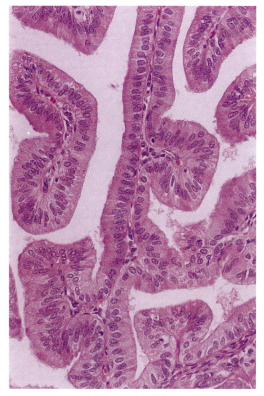

Figure 13.17B

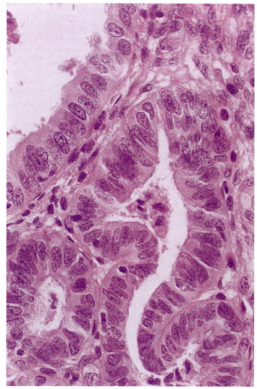

Figure 13.18

PLATE 13.6. NEOPLASMS OF THE UTERUS

Figure 13.19. Adenocarcinoma of the endometrium. A. In comparison with hyperplasia, there is more cellular atypia and the glands are much more irregular. **B.** Glands show "back to back" and "glands within glands" arrangement.

Figure 13.20. Endometrial stromal sarcoma. The tumor is composed of elongated stromal cells, which have less cytoplasm than myometrial cells and therefore appear bluish. The cells tend to invade the lymphatics.

Figure 13.22. Leiomyoma. The tumor is composed of uniform elongated smooth muscle cells arranged into bundles.

Figure 13.21. Mixed müllerian tumor. The tumor consists of a malignant epithelial and a malignant stromal cell.

Figure 13.23. Leiomyosarcoma. The tumor resembles leiomyoma. However, the nuclei vary in size and shape. Most importantly, there are numerous mitoses.

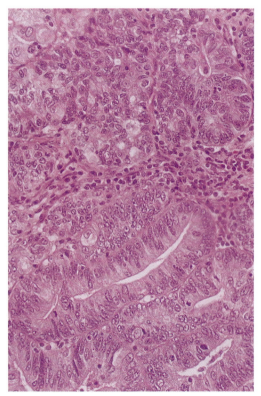

Figure 13.19A

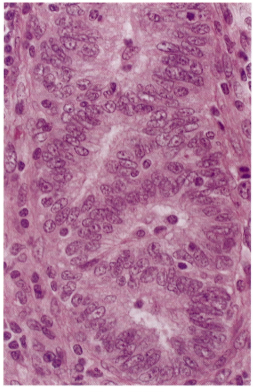

Figure 13.19B

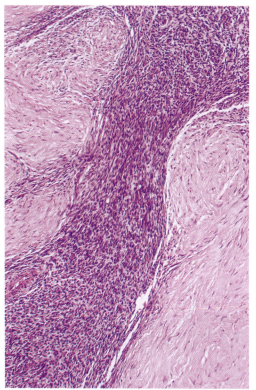

Figure 13.20

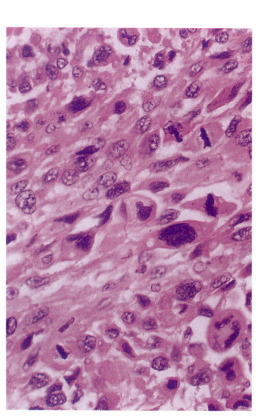

Figure 13.21

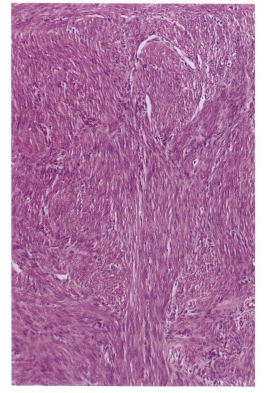

Figure 13.22

Figure 13.23

PLATE 13.7. OVARIAN CYSTS

Figure 13.24. Follicular cyst. The lumen of the cyst is surrounded by granulosa cells.

Figure 13.25. Polycystic ovary. The ovarian cortex contains numerous cysts.

Figure 13.26. Paraovarian cyst. The lumen is lined by cells that have a hobnail appearance.

Figure 13.27. Endometriosis. The lesion consists of endometrial glands and stroma.

Diagram 13.4. Ovarian neoplasms. The tumors may originate from the surface epithelium, germ cells, sex cord cells, or nonspecific ovarian stroma.

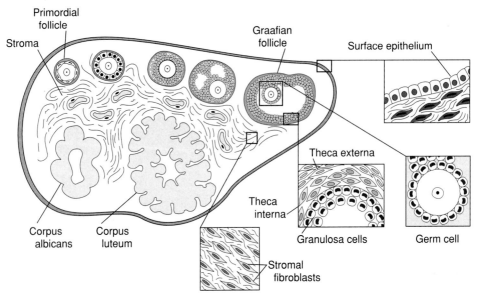

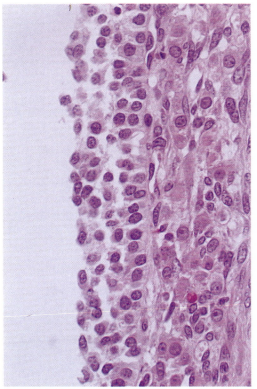

Figure 13.24

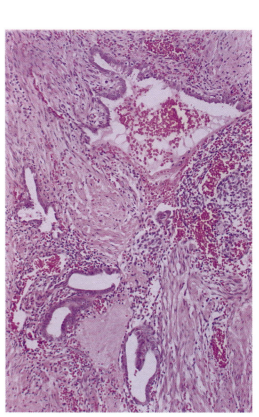

Figure 13.25

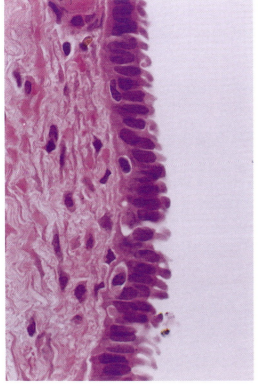

Figure 13.26

Figure 13.27

PLATE 13.8.   OVARIAN NEOPLASMS OF SURFACE EPITHELIUM

Figure 13.28.   Serous tumors. A. Papillary structures protrude into the lumen. **B.** Serous cystadenocarcinoma. The cuboidal cells show considerable pleomorphism. The tumor cell–lined papillae protrude into the lumen of the cysts. Tumor cells form glands that invade the stroma in the wall of the cyst.

Figure 13.29.   Mucinous tumors. A. Mucinous cystadenoma. The lining of the cysts is composed of columnar cells that have basally located nuclei and mucin-filled apical cytoplasm. The cells appear uniform. **B.** Mucinous cystadenocarcinoma. The mucin-secreting cells show considerable pleomorphism and form irregular layers.

Diagram 13.5.   The ovarian tumors of surface ("germinal") epithelium. The tumors may be classified as: **A.** Serous. **B.** Mucinous. **C.** Endometrioid. **D.** Clear cell. **E.** Brenner tumor. **F.** The serous and mucinous tumors may be cystic (unilocular or multilocular). **G.** The epithelium of cystic tumors may form papillae; such tumors are called papillary. **H.** Endometrioid, clear cell, and Brenner tumors do not form cysts but are solid.

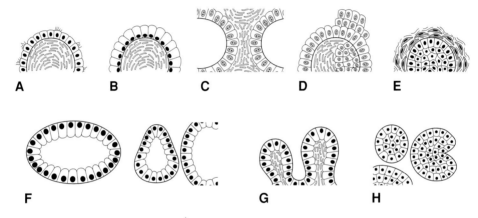

Diagram 13.6.   Serous tumor. A. Cystadenoma (benign). **B.** Serous tumor of borderline malignancy (low-grade malignant). **C.** Cystadenocarcinoma (malignant).

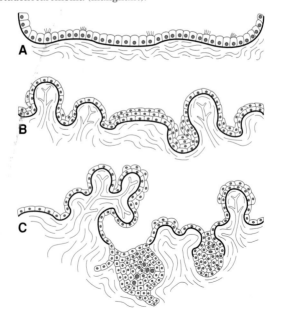

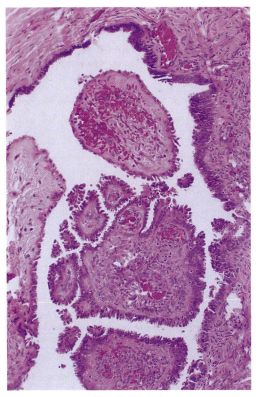

Figure 13.28A

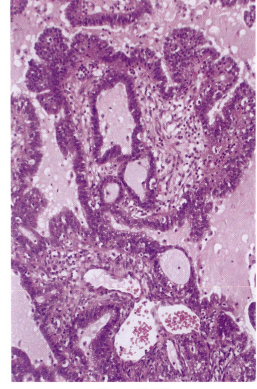

Figure 13.28B

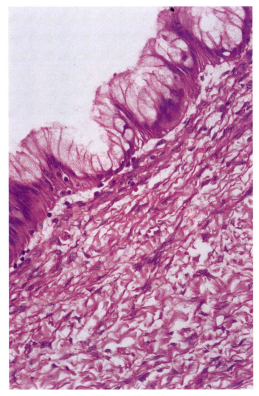

Figure 13.29A

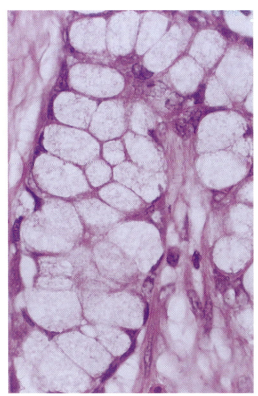

Figure 13.29B

PLATE 13.9. OVARIAN NEOPLASMS OF SURFACE EPITHELIUM

Figure 13.30. Endometrioid carcinoma. The tumor is composed of cuboidal cells forming glands of irregular size and shape. Histologically, this tumor is indistinguishable from endometrial adenocarcinoma of the uterus.

Figure 13.31. Adenocarcinoma with dense fibrous stroma (malignant adenofibroma). The glands lined by tall epithelium are separated from one another by dense stroma.

Figure 13.32. Clear cell carcinoma. A. The tumor cells have clear cytoplasm and are arranged in solid nests or abortive glands. **B.** Solid areas.

Figure 13.33. Brenner tumor. A. This benign tumor is composed of nests of transitional epithelium encased in nondescript fibrous stroma. **B.** Higher-power view of the benign transitional epithelium forming the epithelial tumor nests.

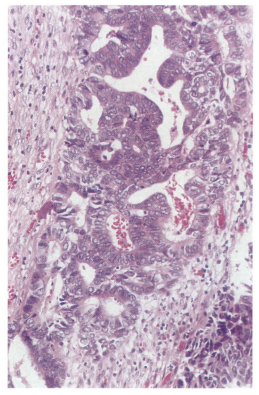

Figure 13.30

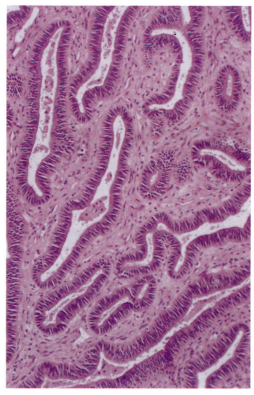

Figure 13.31

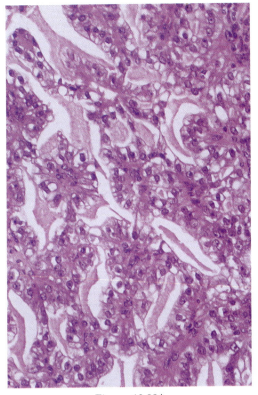

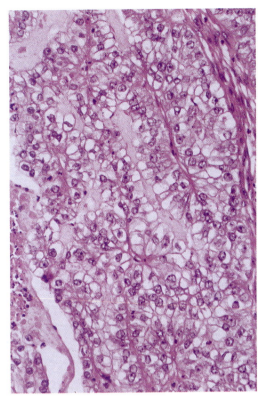

Figure 13.32A   Figure 13.32B

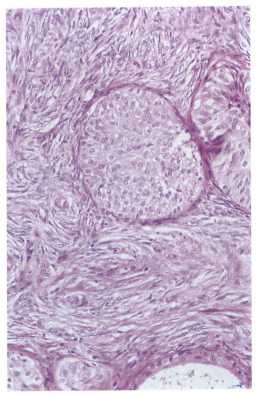

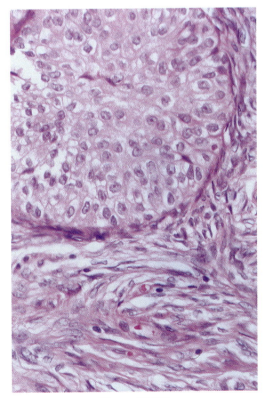

Figure 13.33A   Figure 13.33B

PLATE 13.10. GERM CELL TUMORS

Figure 13.34.   Teratoma. The surface of the cyst consists of skin and skin appendages.

Figure 13.36.   Dysgerminoma. The tumor is composed of a uniform population of cells that have clear cytoplasm. The intercellular spaces are focally infiltrated with lymphocytes.

Figure 13.35.   Immature teratoma. This tumor is composed predominantly of immature neural elements that resemble neuroblasts and are arranged into neural tubes.

Figure 13.37.   Yolk sac carcinoma. The tumor has a variegated appearance with a predominance of microglandular areas.

Diagram 13.7.   Germ cell tumors. A. Teratoma is composed of mature adult tissues. **B.** Immature teratoma is composed of immature neural tissue arranged into neural tube and rosette-like structures. **C.** Dysgerminoma is composed of clear germ cell–like cells surrounded by stroma that contains lymphocytes. **D.** Yolk sac carcinoma shows a variegated appearance—cysts, festoon-like columns, small glands, and loose reticular connective tissue zones.

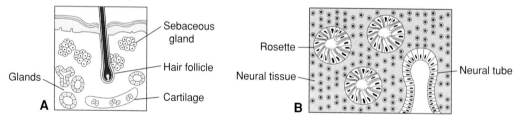

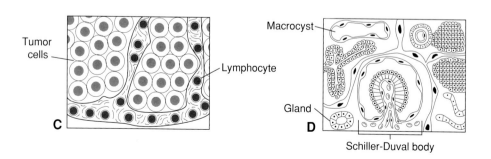

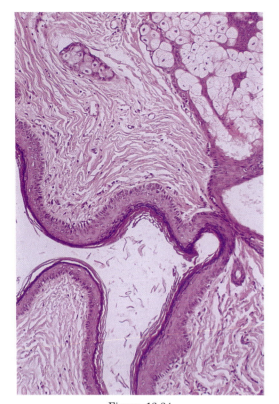

Figure 13.34

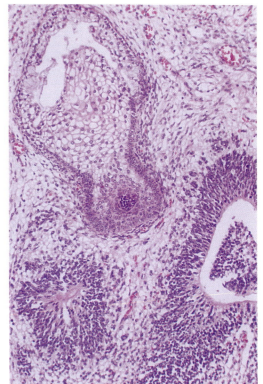

Figure 13.35

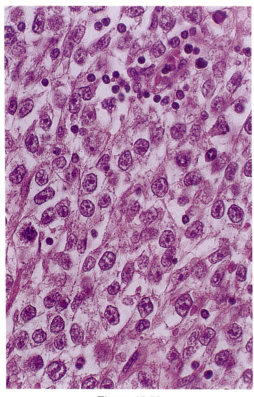

Figure 13.36

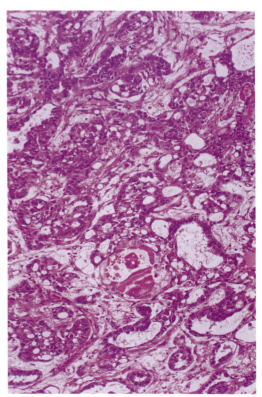

Figure 13.37

PLATE 13.11. SEX CORD CELL TUMORS, STROMAL CELLS AND METASTASES

Figure 13.38.   Granulosa cell tumor. The tumor cells have oval nuclei with a prominent central grove. The cells are arranged around a central space and form the so-called Call-Exner bodies.

Figure 13.40.   Sertoli-Leydig cell tumor. Tumor cells form tubules and cords.

Figure 13.39.   Theca cell tumor. A. Tumor is composed of elongated cells. **B.** The tumor cells contain lipid as demonstrated by this special stain (Oil red 0). Lipid appears in the form of red droplets.

Figure 13.41.   Krukenberg tumor. The ovary is infiltrated with tumor cells that have clear cytoplasm filled with mucin.

Diagram 13.8.   Sex cord cell tumors. A. Granulosa cell tumor is composed of cells with bean-shaped nuclei surrounding clear spaces ("Call-Exner bodies"). **B.** Theca cell tumor is composed of spindle-shaped cells arranged into bundles. **C.** Sertoli-Leydig cell tumors are composed cells resembling Sertoli cells, which form tubules, and cells resembling Leydig cells, which are arranged into groups.

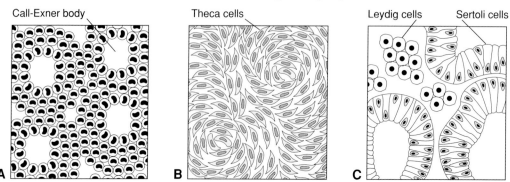

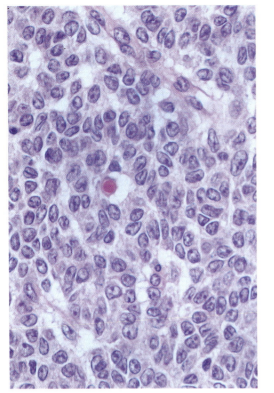

Figure 13.38

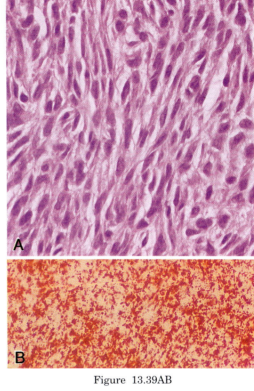

Figure 13.39AB

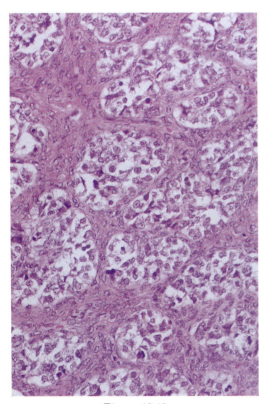

Figure 13.40

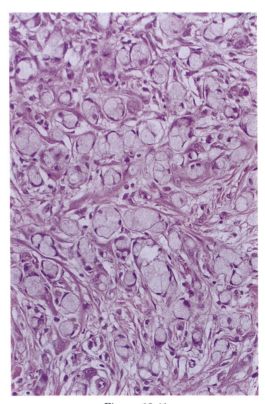

Figure 13.41

PLATE 13.12. PATHOLOGY OF PREGNANCY

Figure 13.42.   Ectopic pregnancy in the fallopian tube. A. The tube is distended and contains chorionic villi and extravasated blood. The fetal parts are not seen in this photograph. **B.** Higher-magnification view of chorionic villi. **C.** Necrotic villi surrounded by inflammatory cells following incomplete abortion.

Figure 13.43.   Hydatidiform mole. A. The chorionic villi are ballooned. The avascular core is composed of edematous loose connective tissue. **B.** The surface epithelium is composed of cytotrophoblastic and syncytiotrophoblastic cells that appear hyperplastic.

Figure 13.44.   Choriocarcinoma. The tumor is composed of mononuclear cytotrophoblastic cells and multinucleated syncytiotrophoblastic cells.

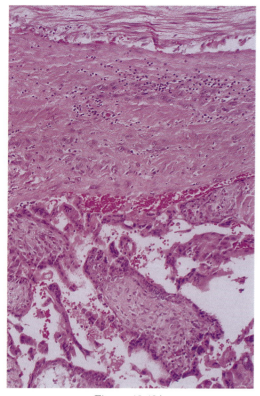

Figure 13.42A

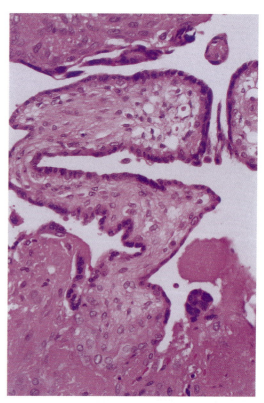

Figure 13.42B

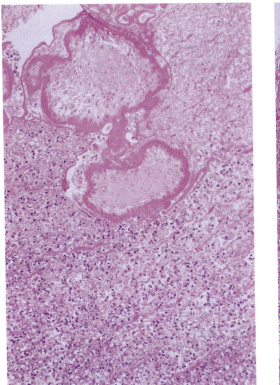

Figure 13.42C

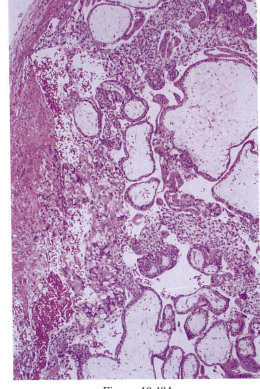

Figure 13.43A

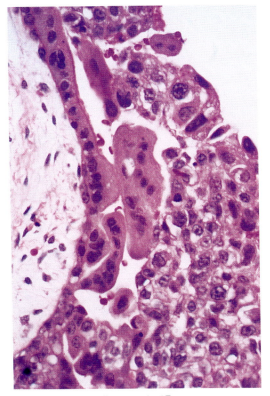

Figure 13.43B

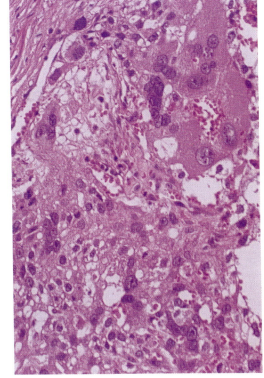

Figure 13.44

NOTES

CHAPTER 14

Breast

NORMAL HISTOLOGY

The breasts are modified apocrine glands arranged in several lobes and embedded into the fibroadipose tissue of the anterior chest wall. Breasts develop fully only in females at the time of puberty and realize their function only during lactation.

The principal parts of the adult female breast are: the *nipple*, the excretory duct system, the lobules, and the fibroadipose tissue (Diagram 14.1). The nipple is composed of convoluted epidermis with sebaceous units (Montgomery glands) and the orifices of excretory lactiferous ducts. The *lactifer-*

ous ducts are a confluence of the excretory ducts and have essentially the same structure as all other ducts.

The duct system of the breast consists of branching ducts, which extend from the nipple area into the fibroadipose tissue and terminate blindly in breast lobules. The *ducts* are lined by cuboidal epithelium enclosed by basement membrane and surrounded by a discontinuous layer of myoepithelial cells and fibrous connective tissue. The ducts branch into clusters of *terminal ductules*, which are enclosed in loose connective tissue stroma and form lobules. *Lobules*, the functional units of the female breast, are sur-

Diagram 14.1.   Normal breast. The nipple is covered with epidermis and contains the orifices of excretory lactiferous ducts. The excretory ducts are lined by cuboidal epithelium, a basement membrane, and a discontinuous layer of myoepithelial cells surrounded by connective tissue. The ducts branch into a cluster of terminal ductules, which are surrounded by loose intralobular connective tissue. The lobules are separated from one another by dense perilobular connective tissue and fat tissue that make up the bulk of normal female breasts.

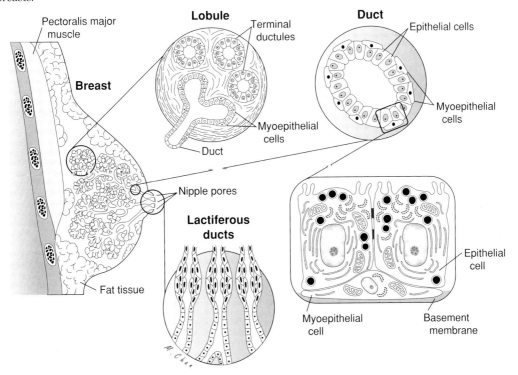

rounded by dense interlobular collagenous stroma. The intralobular connective tissue and the terminal ductules are sensitive to hormones. Because of hormonal fluctuations during the normal menstrual cycle, there is premenstrual swelling of breasts and their detumescence after menstruation. The ducts and the interlobular connective tissue and the fat tissue do not respond to hormonal stimulation once they have reached full development at puberty.

The differentiation of breasts into a functional mammary gland occurs only during pregnancy and postpartum lactation. At that time, the terminal ductules undergo hyperplasia and form acini. Acini are lined by secretory vacuolated cuboidal cells. The lumen of ducts and acini of secreting breasts contain milk that is produced under the influence of prolactin. After pregnancy, the acini regress. After menopause and especially with advancing age, the lobules undergo involution and the interlobular connective tissue becomes more prominent.

The male breast consist only of ducts and contains no acini. Nevertheless, male breasts can respond to female sex hormones, swell, and enlarge. This is called **gynecomastia**. The enlarged breast consists of dilated ducts lined by hyperplastic multilayered epithelium. The stroma consists of loosely arranged fibroblasts. It appears edematous and resembles the intralobular stroma of the female breast.

OVERVIEW OF PATHOLOGY

The most important lesions of breast are the tumors. Other conditions, such as inflammatory lesions and fibrocystic change, are described because they must be distinguished from tumors, which they might resemble clinically.

Inflammatory Lesions

Acute mastitis is typically found in lactating breast and is related to staphylococcal or streptococcal infection. Bacteria invade the breast through the ducts, causing suppurative inflammation that spreads from the ducts into the adjacent fibroadipose tissue. Similar acute mastitis can develop, albeit less commonly, in nonlactating infected breasts (Fig. 14.1). This infection may spread throughout the ductal system and evolve into abscesses.

Chronic mastitis may accompany other breast diseases, but its clinical significance usually is limited. It accompanies *mammary duct ectasia*, a disease of unknown etiology marked by dilatation of ducts filled with inspissated breast secretions (Fig. 14.2). The walls of these dilated ducts are filled with chronic inflammatory cells. There may be periductal inflammation that is characterized by infiltrates of plasma cells. This accounts for the other name for this disease, *plasma cell mastitis*.

Reactive lesions caused by foreign material and trauma are not uncommon in the breast. *Silicone implants* may leak, and the material from such implants may cause a foreign body giant cell reaction (Fig. 14.3) and nonspecific chronic inflammation. *Fat necrosis* accompanied by chronic inflammation may be secondary to trauma, but often occurs without any obvious causes. The necrotic fat cells are taken up by macrophages that have foamy cytoplasm (Fig. 14.4). Such lesions also contain giant cells, lymphocytes, and fibroblasts and may undergo calcification.

Fibrocystic Change

Fibrocystic changes affects approximately 10% of women of reproductive age. The breasts feel beady and are tender on palpation. The changes are usually diffuse and bilateral, and they fluctuate in size during the menstrual cycle.

Fibrocystic changes present histologically in several forms, which usually involve a combination of three basic tissue responses: *epithelial proliferation*; *fibrosis*, and *cyst formation* (Diagram 14.2). The proliferation of epithelial cells results in **adenosis**, which is sometimes accompanied by prominent fibrosis and is thus called **sclerosing adenosis**. Adenosis is benign and should not be considered preneoplastic, although in the sclerosing form it may be occasionally confused with carcinoma. In other cases, **fibrosis** predominates and the epithelial proliferative changes are less apparent. Obstructed ducts form **cysts** lined by flattened epithelium. Ductal epithelium may occasionally transform into cuboidal eosinophilic cells, resembling sweat glands. This change is called *apocrine metaplasia*.

The form of fibrocystic change comprising adenosis, fibrosis, and cysts is called **simple**, to distinguish it from **proliferative fibrocystic disease** proliferative, which is characterized by intraductal proliferation. The **intraductal proliferation** may occlude small ducts in a cribriform pattern (Fig. 14.5) or form small papillae (**intraductal papillomatosis**) that project into the lumen of dilated ducts. The proliferative intraductal lesions that show signs of atypia, known as **atypical ductal hyperplasia,** represent one step further to neoplasia. The lobular units can also proliferate and expand, giving rise to atypical lobular hyperplasia. These are considered premalignant and warrant close clinical observation. Such lesions are recognized primarily by cytological atypia, i.e., the atypical appearance of their nuclei and specific architectural patterns of proliferation.

Gynecomastia

Gynecomastia is hormonally induced enlargement of male breasts. Histologically, the tissue consists of hyperplastic elongated and/or dilated ducts surrounded by connective tissue (Fig. 14.6).

Benign Tumors

Benign tumors of breast that are of clinical significance are fibroadenoma, intraductal papilloma, and phyllodes tumor. It should be noted, however, that phyllodes tumor also occurs in a malignant form.

Fibroadenoma is the most common tumor of the breast. It occurs predominantly in young women, and presents as a well circumscribed, firm, and mobile mass, 1 to 10 cm in diameter.

Histologically, fibroadenomas are composed of epithelial and stromal cells. In the *pericanalicular form,* the epithelial and myoepithelial cells form round to elongated ducts, surrounded by loose fibroblastic stroma (Fig. 14.7). *Intracanalicular fibroadenomas* contain elongated ducts that are also lined by cuboidal epithelial and myoepithelial cells. The ducts appear distorted and are compressed by stroma, taking on

many bizarre forms (e.g., "giraffe neck like").

Phyllodes tumor, also called *giant fibroadenoma*, has the basic histological features of fibroadenoma. However, the tumors tend to grow faster and may reach larger proportions within a relatively short period. On cut section, the tumor tissue may "open like a book" with each leaf composed of loose cellular stroma admixed with epithelial and myoepithelial cells (Fig. 14.8). Most phyllodes tumors are benign. However, about 30% are locally invasive and 15% have distant metastases. The malignant phyllodes tumors are true sarcomas, i.e., they have a malignant stromal component. Histologically, their stroma is highly cellular and dense, and it shows pronounced mitotic activity.

Intraductal papillomas are benign tumors that occur in women of reproductive age, slightly older than those who have fibroadenomas and younger than those with carcinomas. The tumors occur in larger ducts, typically causing nipple discharge or bleeding. Therefore, most intraductal papillomas are discovered early and are relatively small—less than 1 cm at the time of surgery. Histologically, the tumors are composed of fibrovascular papillae lined with hyperplastic cuboidal epithelium (Fig. 14.9) and an underlying myoepithelial layer. The papillae may show complex branching and fill the entire ductal lumen. The tumors are benign and do not invade the wall of the ducts from which they arose.

Carcinoma of the Breast

Carcinoma of the breast is one of the most common malignancies; it accounts for approximately 20% of all cancer related death in women. One in nine of all American women is at risk for developing breast cancer in her lifetime.

Breast carcinomas originate from the epithelial cells lining the ducts or lobules, and are thus divided into **ductal,** which account for 90–95%, and **lobular,** which account for 5–10% of all malignant breast tumors. Either of these two forms can be localized to the anatomical structure of its origin, i.e., *intraductal or intralobular*, or can be invasive. Invasive ductal carcinoma can be further classified into several types, the most important being *infiltrating duct carcinomas, medullary carcinoma, mucinous carcinoma,* and *Paget disease* (Diagram 14.3).

Ductal Carcinoma

Intraductal carcinoma accounts for 5% of all breast carcinomas. The malignant cells grow inside the small and medium-sized ducts but do not invade the wall of the ducts (Fig. 14.10). The ducts may be filled completely with cells that form solid sheets or line narrow lumina in a cribriform pattern. In some tumors, the central area is necrotic. This tumor is called *comedo carcinoma* since the necrotic material can be expressed from the ducts like the sebum from comedos ("blackheads") of the skin. The tumor cells may spread into the lobule ("cancerization of the lobule"), still without any signs of invasion of connective tissue stroma. If untreated, all intraductal carcinomas become invasive and spread into adjacent tissue (Fig. 14.11). Invasion can also follow intralobular spread of tumor cells. Intraductal papillary carcinomas also may become invasive (Fig. 14.12).

Infiltrating ductal carcinoma accounts for 65–70% of all breast cancers. It is also called *scirrhous* carcinoma because it evokes a strong desmoplastic reaction and contains large amounts of fibrous connective tissue stroma. On gross examination, invasive duct carcinoma is firm on palpation and gritty on sectioning. Histologically, it consists of glands or solid nests enclosed within strands of connective tissue (Fig. 14.13).

Paget disease of the breast is a ductal carcinoma that spreads through the lactiferous ducts and invades the epidermis of the nipple (Fig. 14.14). In the epidermis, these cells displace keratinocytes and are most prominent along the basal membrane. However, they may permeate the entire thickness of the epidermis. These cells contain and secrete mucus and can ulcerate normal skin.

Medullary carcinoma is relatively rare, accounting for only 1–2% of all breast carcinomas. However, it has a better prognosis than other forms of breast cancer and therefore deserves special recognition. On gross examination, medullary carcinoma presents as a well circumscribed mass. The tumor is soft because it is composed of tumor cells that are closely apposed one to another without intervening stroma (Fig. 14.15). Nests of tumor cells are often surrounded by infiltrates of lymphocytes.

Mucinous carcinoma, also called colloid or gelatinous carcinoma, accounts for less than 1% of breast cancers. It too has a better prognosis than the infiltrating ductal carcinoma. On gross examination, the tumor appears bulky, soft, and jelly-like. Histologically, this adenocarcinoma produces large amounts of mucin, which is found in the lumen of neoplastic glands and around them (Fig. 14.16).

Lobular Carcinoma

Lobular carcinoma accounts for 5–10% of breast cancer. If detected in the preinvasive form confined to the terminal ductules, such *lobular carcinoma in situ* has an excellent prognosis. The *infiltrating lobular carcinoma* has the same prognosis as the infiltrating ductal carcinomas.

Lobular carcinoma in situ consists of uniform small cells that have round nuclei and a moderate amount of eosinophilic cytoplasm. The cells form solid sheets that appear to distend the terminal lobule (Fig. 14.17). **Infiltrating lobular carcinoma** often forms concentric layers of single cell strands around the intralobular foci (Fig. 14.18). As the tumor cells invade further, they invoke a strong desmoplastic reaction and are typically arranged into single cell strands ("Indian files") surrounded by dense collagen.

Carcinoma of the male breast is 100 times less common than carcinoma of the female breast. Histologically, most tumors in the male are scirrhous infiltrating duct carcinomas characterized by dense connective tissue (desmoplastic) reaction.

NOTES

PLATE 14.1. NON–NEOPLASTIC LESIONS

Figure 14.1. Acute mastitis. The duct contains inspissated milk and inflammatory cells. Inflammation extends into the adjacent connective tissue.

Figure 14.3. Silicone induced foreign body reaction. A. The encysted foreign material has a honeycomb appearance. **B.** The material is taken up by multinucleated foreign body giant cells, which are surrounded by fibrous tissue.

Figure 14.2. Mammary duct ectasia. A. The small duct is distended with inspissated material and its wall is infiltrated with chronic inflammatory cells. **B.** The connective tissue surrounding the ducts contains lymphocytes and plasma cells.

Figure 14.4. Fat necrosis. The fat tissue is replaced by fibrous tissue infiltrated with macrophages, lymphocytes, and giant cells.

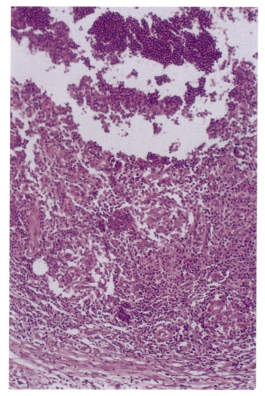

Figure 14.1

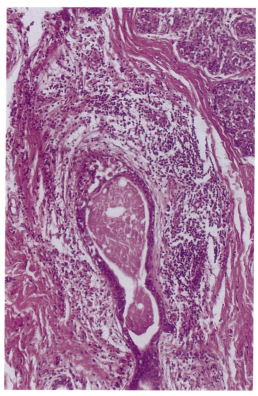

Figure 14.2A

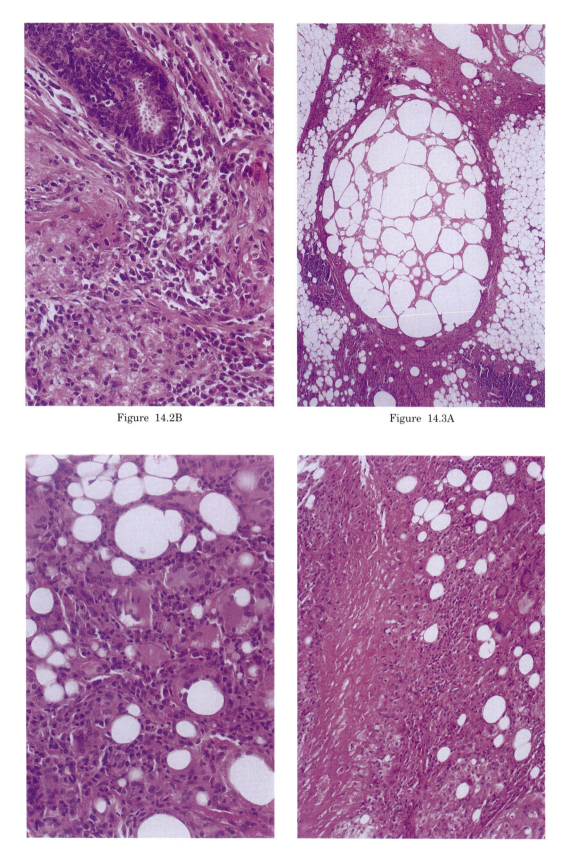

Figure 14.2B

Figure 14.3A

Figure 14.3B

Figure 14.4

PLATE 14.2. FIBROCYSTIC CHANGE

Figure 14.5.   Fibrocystic change. A. The normal lobular structure of the breast is lost, and the border between intralobular and dense interlobular connective tissue is obscured. The ducts appear dilated. **B.** Sclerosing adenosis. The proliferated ducts are surrounded by dense connective tissue. **C.** Intraductal hyperplasia leads to formation of small papillary protrusions. **D.** Atypical lobular hyperplasia is characterized by formation of solid nests of cells inside the terminal ducts.

Diagram 14.2.   Fibrocystic change. A. The normal lobule consists of hormone-sensitive epithelial and stromal cells, whereas the interlobular stroma is composed of dense hormone-nonresponsive collagenous tissue. During each menstrual cycle, the lobule enlarges because of epithelial cell proliferation and hydration of the intralobular stroma. This enlargement is reversible, however. **B.** Hormonally induced proliferation of ductular cells leads to adenosis. **C.** Replacement of the hormone-sensitive intralobular stroma by dense intralobular stroma leads to fibrosis. Such breasts cannot respond to cyclic hormonal changes, and appear firm because of increased amounts of collagen. **D.** Cystic dilatation of ductules occurs because of obstruction and severance of proliferative ductules from the main duct by dense connective tissue that has replaced the loose intralobular stroma.

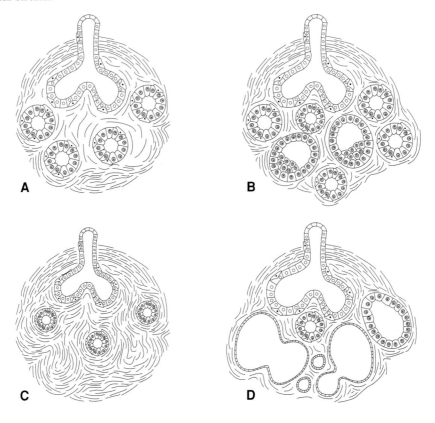

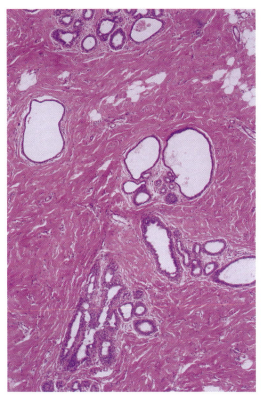

Figure 14.5A

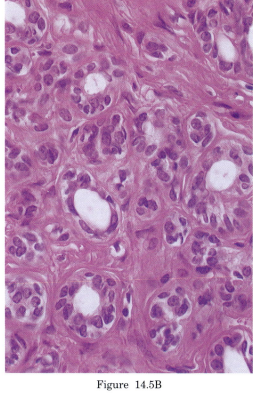

Figure 14.5B

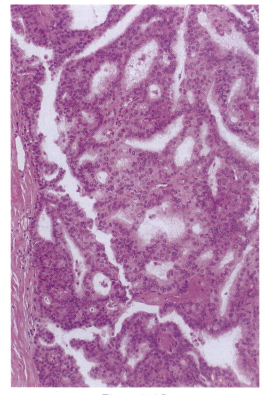

Figure 14.5C

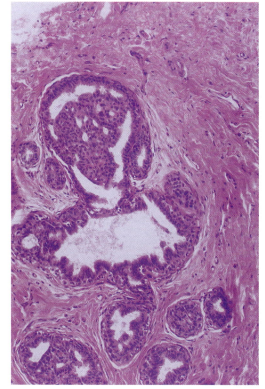

Figure 14.5D

PLATE 14.3. GYNECOMASTIA AND BENIGN TUMORS

Figure 14.6.   Gynecomastia. The male breast consists of elongated ducts surrounded by connective tissue.

Figure 14.8.   Phyllodes tumor. A. Most phyllodes tumors are benign and are composed of connective tissue folds lined by cuboidal epithelium. **B.** Malignant phyllodes tumor has dense stroma surrounding small glands.

Figure 14.7.   Fibroadenoma. A. Pericanalicular form is composed of ducts surrounded by loose fibroblastic stroma. **B.** The intracanalicular form consists of elongated ducts compressed with fibroblastic stroma.

Figure 14.9.   Intraductal papilloma. The tumor is composed of papillae that have fibrovascular cores and are lined by cuboidal cells.

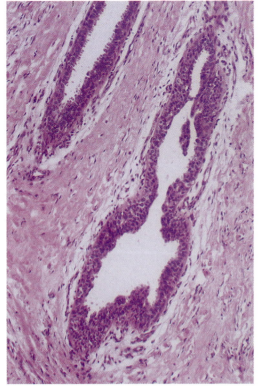

Figure 14.6

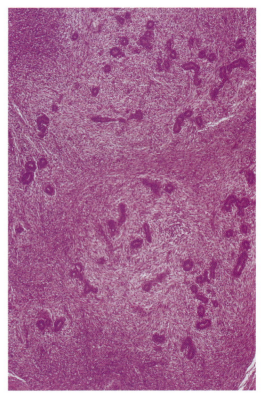

Figure 14.7A

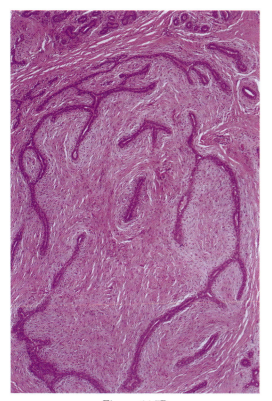

Figure 14.7B

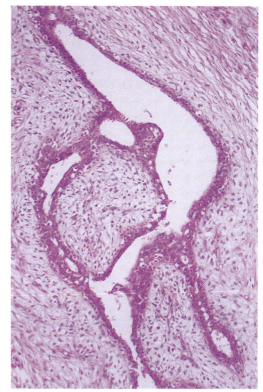

Figure 14.8A

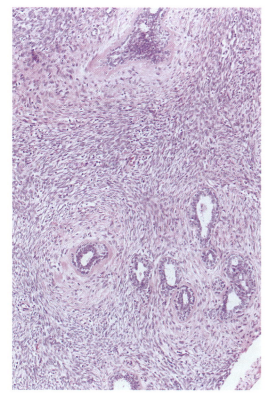

Figure 14.8B

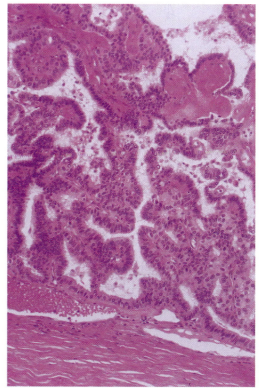

Figure 14.9

PLATE 14.4. INTRADUCTAL CARCINOMAS

Figure 14.10.   Intraductal carcinoma. A. The ducts contain tumor cells that show central necrosis ("comedo carcinoma"). **B.** Cribriform pattern of intraductal carcinoma.

Figure 14.11.   Intraductal and invasive carcinoma. Intralobular spread of ductal cancer distends markedly the terminal ducts and is accompanied by focal early invasion (arrows).

Figure 14.12.   Papillary carcinoma. The tumor is still papillary, but its growth is not limited to the lumen of ducts only.

Diagram 14.3.   Carcinoma of breast. A. Intraductal carcinoma. **B.** Infiltrating duct carcinoma. **C.** Mucinous carcinoma. **D.** Medullary carcinoma. **E.** Lobular carcinoma in situ. **F.** Invasive lobular carcinoma.

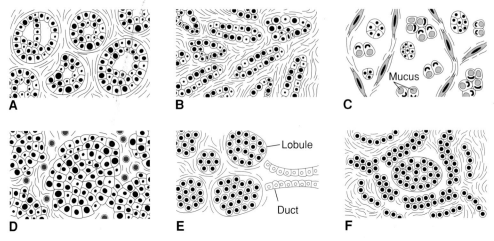

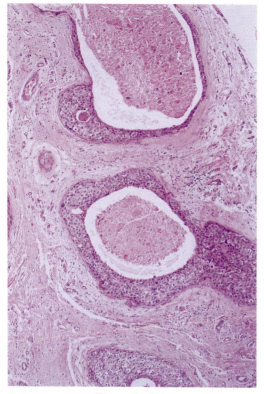

Figure 14.10A

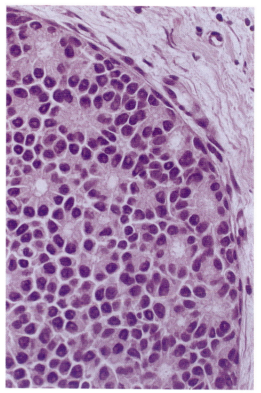

Figure 14.10B

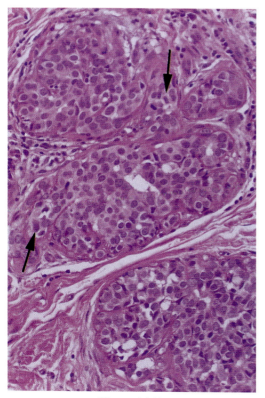

Figure 14.11

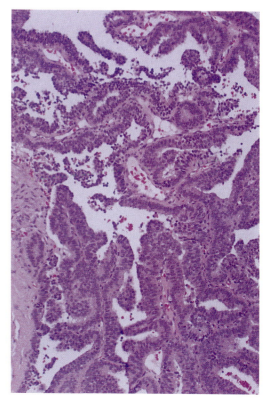

Figure 14.12

PLATE 14.5. INFILTRATING DUCT CARCINOMA

Figure 14.13.   Infiltrating duct carcinoma is a desmoplastic adenocarcinoma. A. Radial growth of tumors into the stroma and fat tissue. **B.** Infiltrating ducts are surrounded by loose and dense connective tissue. **C.** Tumor cells form solid strands. **D, E, F.** Higher-magnification views of invasive tumor cells surrounded by connective tissue.

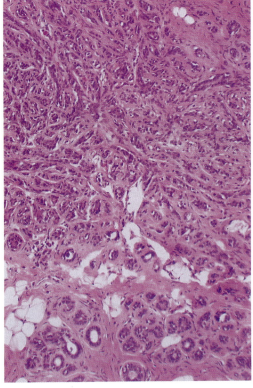

Figure 14.13A

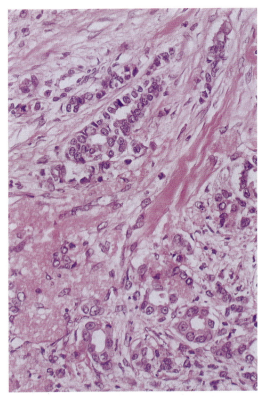

Figure 14.13B

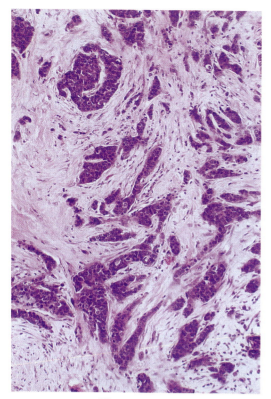

Figure 14.13C

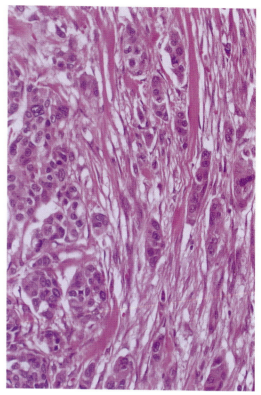

Figure 14.13D

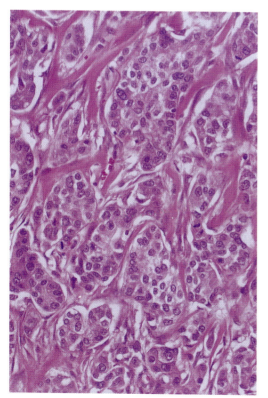

Figure 14.13E

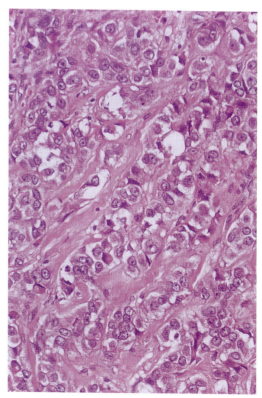

Figure 14.13F

PLATE 14.6. VARIANTS OF BREAST CARCINOMA

Figure 14.14.   Paget disease. Tumor cells invade the epidermis, forming compact nests.

Figure 14.15.   Medullary carcinoma. The tumor is composed of solid masses of cells without intervening stroma. Infiltrates of lymphocytes are often present.

Figure 14.16.   Mucinous adenocarcinoma. The neoplastic glands are surrounded by copious mucus.

Figure 14.18.   Invasive lobular carcinoma. Single cell strands are surrounded by dense stroma.

Figure 14.17.   Lobular carcinoma in situ. The terminal ductules are dilated and are filled with tumor cells. The tumor cells have uniformly round nuclei.

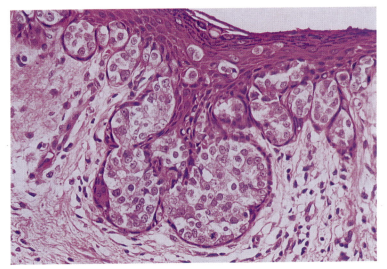

Figure 14.14

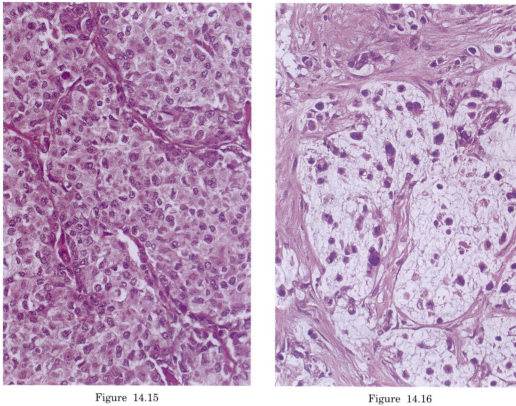

Figure 14.15

Figure 14.16

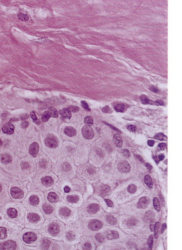

Figure 14.17

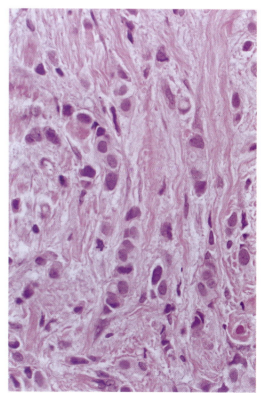

Figure 14.18

NOTES

CHAPTER 15

Endocrine Glands

NORMAL HISTOLOGY

The endocrine system includes cells that are grouped into organs with specific endocrine function, such as the pituitary, thyroid, parathyroids, and adrenals; cells that form distinct components of organs that have endocrine as well as other functions, such as ovary, testis, or the pancreas; single cells scattered throughout the gastrointestinal and parts of the respiratory tract; and parts of the central nervous system, most notably hypothalamic nuclei (Diagram 15.1). This chapter deals only with the pathological changes in the pituitary, thyroid, parathyroid, and adrenal glands.

The pituitary is a small bean-shaped endocrine gland located at the base of the brain in the sella turcica. It consists of an anterior lobe (*adenohypophysis*) and a posterior lobe (*neurohypophysis*). The anterior pituitary consists of five cell types: somatotropic, lactotropic, thyrotropic, corticotropic, and gonadotropic. Each is named after the hormone it secretes and can be identified by immunohistochemistry, using the appropriate antibodies. Almost 20% of anterior pituitary cells do not belong to any of these groups. These cells do not stain with antibodies to known pituitary hormones and comprise nondifferentiated stem cells, support cells, functionally exhausted cells, and cells whose function has not been fully elucidated. By light microscopy, the pituitary cells are recognized by the staining of their cytoplasm as acidophilic, basophilic, or chromophobic. The posterior pituitary is composed of neural cells that represent the cytoplasmic extensions of hypothalamic nuclei.

The thyroid is a large endocrine gland located in the anterior neck. It is composed of follicles that contain colloid rich in thyroglobulin. The epithelium of follicles is composed of cuboidal thyroxin-secreting cells interspersed with calcitonin secreting C cells. Follicular cells cannot be distinguished from C cells on light microscopy unless special immunohistochemical techniques are used and the tissue sections are stained with antibodies to calcitonin or thyroxin.

Parathyroid glands are small endocrine glands located on the neck behind the thyroid. There are four parathyroid glands. These glands are composed of three types of cells arranged into solid nests. These cells are known as chief cells, water-clear cells, and oxyphilic cells. The connective tissue stroma between these cells consists of fibroblasts and prominent fat cells.

Adrenal glands are paired endocrine glands located on the upper pole of the kidneys. Each gland is composed of cortex and medulla. The cortex consists of three layers: zona glomerulosa that secretes mineralocorticoids, such as aldosterone; zona fasciculata that secretes glucocorticoids, such as cortisol; and zona reticularis that secretes sex hormones, i.e., androgens and estrogens. The medulla is composed of cells that secrete epinephrine and norepinephrine.

OVERVIEW OF PATHOLOGY

The most important diseases of the endocrine systems present as one of the following:

- Hypofunction
- Hyperfunction

Hypofunction can be caused by various diseases that cause destruction of endocrine cells, such as immune or infectious diseases. Hyperfunction is most often caused by tumors of endocrine glands or various diseases that lead to hyperstimulation and overproduction of hormones.

Pituitary Tumors

Pituitary tumors almost invariably originate from the anterior lobe. The vast majority of tumors (96%) are benign *adenomas*. Many small benign tumors measure only a

Diagram 15.1. Endocrine glands. The hypothalamic releasing factors act on the pituitary to produce tropic hormones that act on the thyroid, adrenal cortex, and gonads. The hormones produced by effector endocrine glands act through negative feedback to inhibit the hypothalamus or the pituitary.

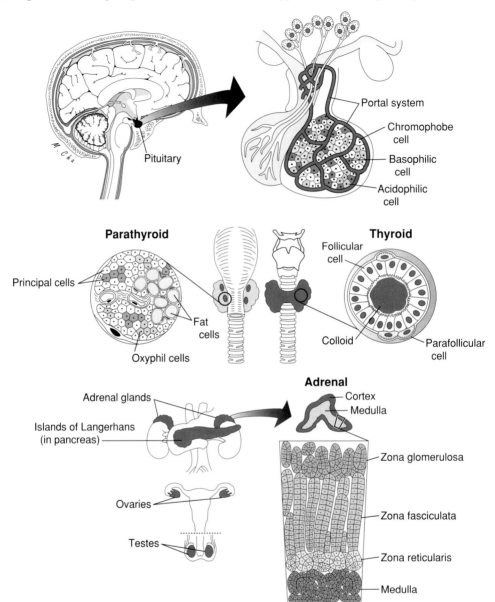

few millimeters in diameter and are called *microadenomas*. *Carcinomas* are very rare. Histologically, these tumors can be classified as acidophilic, basophilic, or chromophobic (Fig. 15.1). However, it is better to classify the tumors on the basis of the hormones that they produce (Table 15.1).

Somatotropic adenomas account for 25% of tumors. These tumors secretes growth hormone. In children, such tumors produce gigantism; in adults, such tumors produce acromegaly.

Prolactinoma (lactotropic adenoma) is the most common functioning pituitary tumor, accounting for 30% of all lesions. Many lactotrophic adenomas are very small (mi-

Table 15.1
Classification of Pituitary Adenomas

Type of Adenoma	Prevalence (%)	Hormone Secreted	Clinical Manifestations
Prolactinoma	30	Prolactin	*Women:* amenorrhea, galactorrhea, infertility *Men:* decreased libido, impotence
Somatotropic	20	Growth hormone	Acromegaly, gigantism (children)
Corticotropic	15	ACTH	Cushing disease
Gonadotropic	15	FSH/LH	Menstrual irregularities
Thyrotropic	1	TSH	Hyperthyroidism
Multihormonal	10	Two or more adenohypophyseal hormones (GH, with prolactin is the most common combination)	Depends on type of hormone secreted
Nonfunctioning	25	None	Localized symptoms: headache, visual disturbances, dysfunction of cranial nerves, hypopituitarism

croadenomas) and barely visible to the unaided eye. They secrete prolactin. In females, prolactinoma causes the amenorrhea-galactorrhea syndrome. In males, prolactinoma may be asymptomatic or cause impotence and a loss of libido.

Corticotropic adenoma accounts for 10% of pituitary tumors. It secretes adrenocorticotropic hormone (ACTH) and causes Cushing disease, marked by hypersecretion of glucocorticoids and sex hormones from the zona fasciculata and reticularis of the adrenal cortex.

Thyrotropic adenomas, which secrete thyroid-stimulating hormone (TSH), cause hyperthyroidism. *Gonadotropic* adenomas are rare tumors, which secrete follicle-stimulating hormone (FSH), luteinizing hormone (LH), or both. These tumors cause disturbances in sexual function.

Nonsecretory adenomas ("null cell adenomas") account for one-fourth of all pituitary tumors. These tumors do not produce hormonal hypersecretion but rather cause hypopituitarism due to the compression of the normal gland. *Pituitary carcinomas* are rare; they invade into the base of the skull and brain.

Hypopituitarism

Hypopituitarism may develop acutely or slowly, depending on the nature of the pituitary insult. The most important causes of hypopituitarism are listed in Table 15.2.

Acute hypopituitarism is typically due to a vascular incident resulting in infarction

15.2
Causes of Hypopituitarism

Acute
Postpartum necrosis (Sheehan syndrome)
Head trauma
Neurosurgery
Chronic
Tumors
 • Pituitary adenoma
 • Craniopharyngioma
 • Glioma, meningioma
 • Histiocytosis
Inflammation
 • Sarcoidosis
 • Encephalitis
 • Meningitis
Congenital
 • Pituitary dwarfism
 • Hypogonadism

of the pituitary. At least 90% of the gland must be destroyed for symptoms to appear. The best example of this form of injury is *Sheehan syndrome,* or postpartum pituitary necrosis. Disseminated intravascular coagulation that complicates postpartum shock also may result in pituitary infarction and destruction (Fig. 15.2).

Chronic hypopituitarism may develop as a consequence of compression of the pituitary or the hypothalamus by a tumor or inflammatory lesion. Among the tumors prominently featured are nonfunctioning pituitary adenomas, histiocytosis-X (Fig. 15.3), meningiomas, and gliomas of the hypothalamus.

Craniopharyngiomas, benign tumors derived from the epithelium of the Rathke pouch, also may produce hypopituitarism.

The Rathke pouch is the primordium of the adenohypophysis and originates as an outpouching of the fetal nasopharynx. The tumor is composed of squamous epithelium, which is arranged into nests with central keratinization. Some craniopharyngiomas form epithelial nests reminiscent of oral dentigerous epithelium and resemble ameloblastomas (Fig. 15.4).

Chronic inflammation of the pituitary or the meninges that cover the sella and the hypothalamus may also destroy the pituitary or the hypothalamus and cause hypopituitarism. Tuberculosis, which once was common, is rare today, but fungal infections, viral and bacterial meningitis, and encephalitis and sarcoidosis are still important (Fig. 15.5).

THYROID GLAND

Goiter

Goiter is a term for any enlargement of the thyroid, but in practice it is used for multinodular hyperplasia of the thyroid. In most instances there is no thyroid hyperfunction or hypofunction, and it is therefore called *nontoxic or euthyroid goiter*. It may occur *sporadically* or in an *endemic* form in iodine-deficient areas.

Diffuse multinodular goiter consists of nodules of thyroid follicles that vary in size and shape. Some follicles are distended by colloid and are lined by flattened epithelium, whereas others are small and lined by cuboidal epithelium (Fig. 15.6). Connective tissue encapsulates groups of follicles and extends between them. Secondary changes such as hemorrhage and calcification are common but clinically insignificant. Thyroidectomy is usually performed for cosmetic reasons and only rarely to relieve symptoms of compression.

Thyroiditis

Thyroiditis occurs in several forms (Diagram 15.2). It usually is a chronic inflammation that is usually immune-mediated. The disease often is associated with systemic autoimmune disorders. Isolated infectious thyroiditis caused by bacteria or other pathogens is extremely rare in immunocompetent persons but may occur in generalized sepsis and AIDS patients.

Graves disease is an autoimmune disorder caused by antibodies to the TSH receptor on follicular cells. It typically presents with hyperthyroidism, thyroid enlargement, and exophthalmus. It may be associated with other autoimmune phenomena.

Histologically, the enlarged thyroid is composed of follicles that are lined by tall cuboidal epithelium (Fig. 15.7). The colloid adjacent to the follicular cells appears vacuolated and "scalloped" because of its rapid turnover. The thyroid also contains infiltrates of lymphocytes, usually arranged into follicles with germinal centers.

Hashimoto thyroiditis is an autoimmune disease of unknown etiology. The disease is characterized by the appearance of circulating antibodies to thyroglobulin, but it seems that these antibodies are more a reaction to thyroid injury and extravasation of thyroglobulin from damaged follicles than a cause of inflammation. In early stages, the thyroid may be enlarged and hyperfunctioning. In later stages, there is destruction of the parenchyma and hypothyroidism. Histologically, the thyroid is densely infiltrated with lymphocytes (Fig. 15.8). There is destruction of thyroid follicles, with replacement by lymphocytes and fibrous tissue. The remaining follicles undergo oncocytic transformation. Oncocytes, also called Hürthle cells, are recognized by their eosinophilic granular cytoplasm. As proven by electron microscopy, this granularity is due to the accumulation of mitochondria.

Riedel thyroiditis is a chronic fibrosing process in which dense fibrous tissue replaces the damaged thyroid follicles (Fig. 15.9). There are no antithyroid antibodies in this disease, and it is probably not autoimmune in nature. Association with other fibromatoses suggests that it might be a multisystemic disorder involving the marked proliferation of fibroblasts and inappropriate deposition of collagen.

DeQuervain (subacute) thyroiditis, also known as *giant cell* or *granulomatous thyroiditis*, is characterized by a sudden painful enlargement of the thyroid. It is presumed to be of viral origin. Follicles damaged by infection rupture and extrude thyroglobulin, which elicits a foreign body giant cell reaction (Fig. 15.10).

Neoplasms

Most thyroid tumors originate from follicular cells, but they may also evolve from C cells, albeit less often (Diagram 15.3). Primary tumors may be benign or malignant. Occasionally, the thyroid is involved by lymphoma and extremely rarely by metastatic neoplasms.

Follicular adenoma is the most common benign tumor. It typically presents as a solitary nodule that may take up radioactive iodine ("*hot nodule*") but more often does not ("*cold nodule*"). These tumors infrequently cause hormonal symptoms and even more rarely present as "a toxic nodule."

Histologically, adenomas are composed of follicles that contain colloid and are lined by cells that resemble normal thyroid cells (Fig. 15.11). Follicular adenomas are well encapsulated, which distinguishes them from well differentiated follicular carcinomas. In contrast to multinodular goiter, follicular adenomas are solitary lesions. Several histological subtypes are known, such as Hürthle cell adenoma and embryonal adenoma, but such subtyping is of no clinical significance.

Papillary carcinoma is the most common thyroid malignancy. Most tumors are diagnosed as small solitary nodules that do not concentrate iodine (cold nodule). At the time of surgery, many tumors have already metastasized to the contiguous lymph nodes. However, most still have an excellent prognosis. Papillary carcinomas are hormonally inactive.

On gross examination, the tumor presents as a small whitish nodule that may contain cystic cavities. Histologically, the tumor is composed of cuboidal cells arranged into papillae (Fig. 15.12), which project into the cavity spaces and may contain calcifications (*psammoma bodies*). The nuclei of tumor cells appear clear and are described as like "ground glass" or the eyes of the cartoon character, Orphan Annie. Many nuclei show a cleft or a linear fold. All papillary tumors are considered malignant, and there are no papillary adenomas.

Follicular carcinoma accounts for 20% of thyroid malignant tumors. The tumor has a less favorable prognosis and tends to metastasize to distant sites, most notably lung and bones.

Histologically, these tumors are composed of well differentiated cells that form colloid filed follicles. Poorly differentiated tumor cells may be arranged in solid sheets and groups devoid of colloid (Fig. 15.13). Nuclear and histological features are not entirely reliable signs of malignancy in assessing follicular neoplasms, and many well differentiated follicular carcinomas cannot be distinguished from benign follicular adenomas. The only definitive sign of malignancy in such cases is the extension of the tumor beyond the capsule, evidenced by the invasion of lymphatics and blood vessels and spread of tumor outside the thyroid or distant metastases.

Medullary carcinoma of the thyroid is a tumor composed of calcitonin-secreting C cells. Tumors may occur sporadically or in families affected by multiple endocrine adenomatosis syndrome (MEA-II).

Histologically, medullary carcinoma is composed of small cells with round or oval nuclei that are arranged into solid groups, nests, or cords, reminiscent of carcinoids and other neuroendocrine tumors (Fig. 15.14). The stroma is hyalinized and consists of collagen and amyloid. Special stains for amyloid and immunohistochemical stains for calcitonin are useful for diagnosis of neoplasms without the typical histological features.

Anaplastic carcinoma is a rare but deadly form of thyroid cancer. It occurs mostly in older persons and is slightly more common in women than in men. It has a dismal prognosis, and most patients die during the first 2 years. Histologically, the tumor is composed of undifferentiated cells that may be very small or very large and grow without any distinct pattern (Fig. 15.15). The tumor cells invade into the surrounding tissues of the neck and tend to metastasize widely.

PARATHYROID GLANDS

Parathyroid diseases (Diagram 15.4) present as hypoparathyroidism or hyperparathyroidism.

Hypoparathyroidism may be congenital, due to gland aplasia as seen in *DiGeorge syndrome* (congenital aplasia of the parathyroids and thymus). In adults, it is most often iatrogenic, due to accidental removal of parathyroids during neck surgery for thyroid disease or laryngeal cancer.

Hyperparathyroidism is caused by a solitary parathyroid adenoma in 80% of cases; the remaining cases are secondary to *parathyroid hyperplasia*. The hyperplasia may be *primary* (idiopathic) or *secondary,* due to metabolic or renal diseases that affect calcium and phosphate homeostasis.

Parathyroid adenoma is a benign tumor composed of parathyroid cells. It is usually hormonally active and typically involves only one gland. The remaining three glands are usually normal. An average tumor measures 1–2 cm in diameter. Adenomas secrete parathyroid hormone and clinically present with hypercalcemia, bone resorption, and hypercalciuria. Histologically, they either are composed of all three cell types or one type predominates (Fig. 15.16). The histological composition of tumors does not correlate with their functional activity. Tumors may be sharply demarcated from the normal gland, which may be compressed into a peripheral rim. Between 1% and 3% of solitary parathyroid nodules are true carcinomas, which are difficult to distinguish from adenomas on the basis of their histological features (Fig. 15.17). A high mitotic rate is often the only clue, and the presence of metastases is the only reliable sign of the malignancy of such tumors.

Parathyroid hyperplasia has histological features similar to those of parathyroid adenoma (Fig. 15.18). Neoplastic parathyroids can be distinguished from hyperplastic parathyroids only after all four glands have been examined: adenomas are typically solitary, whereas in hyperplasia, all four glands are enlarged. Hyperplastic glands differ from normal parathyroids in that the hyperplastic glands are generally enlarged and contain fewer stromal fat cells than normal parathyroids do.

ADRENAL GLANDS

The diseases affecting the adrenals present as *adrenal cortical insufficiency, adrenal cortical hyperfunction (hypercorticism),* or *adrenal medullary hyperfunction* (Diagram 15.5).

Adrenal cortical insufficiency is a rare disease that could be caused by many pathogenetic mechanisms, most of which lead to a destruction of the adrenals (Table 15.3). Acute destruction of adrenal glands may occur in shock and is a typical feature of the *Waterhouse-Friderichsen syndrome.* This syndrome typically occurs during meningococcal sepsis and is characterized by petechial skin hemorrhages and bilateral adrenal hemorrhage (Fig. 15.19). Necrosis of both glands results in acute adrenal insufficiency.

Chronic adrenal cortical insufficiency was previously a common complication of **tuberculosis** (Fig. 15.20). **Autoimmune adrenalitis** with destruction of cortical cells has supplanted tuberculosis as the most important inflammatory cause of adult adrenal insufficiency in modern times (Fig. 15.21). It may occur in an isolated form or as a component of the multiglandular autoimmune syndrome involving the gonads, pituitary, and thyroid (*Schmidt syndrome*).

Adrenal insufficiency may occur in sarcoidosis, amyloidosis (Fig. 15.22), and hemochromatosis. Bilateral metastases of breast or lung carcinoma also may destroy the adrenals. Regardless of the cause, bilateral destruction of the adrenal cortex results in Addison disease.

Adrenal Cortical Hyperfunction

Adrenal cortical hyperfunction may be due to hyperstimulation by ACTH or due to pri-

Table 15.3
Causes of Adrenal Insufficiency

Congenital
Acquired
1. Autoimmune adrenalitis
   • Schmidt syndrome (autoimmune multiglandular failure)
2. Infections
   • Tuberculosis
   • Histoplasmosis
3. Circulatory disorders
   • Thromboembolism
   • DIC and shock
   • Waterhouse-Friderichsen syndrome
4. Tumors
   • Metastatic carcinoma to adrenals
   • Lymphoma
5. Other causes
   • Amyloidosis
   • Hemochromatosis
   • Sarcoidosis
   • Idiopathic

mary adrenal disease such as adrenal cortical hyperplasia or functioning neoplasms.

Three distinct clinical syndromes are recognized, which depend on the predominant hormones secreted. Hyperfunction or tumors of zona glomerulosa cause hyperaldosteronism (*Conn syndrome*); zona fasciculata lesions result in *Cushing syndrome*; and zona reticularis disease causes the *adrenogenital syndrome*. Although these syndromes are clinically distinct and biochemically defined, the underlying pathology is not distinctive enough to make a definitive diagnosis of each syndrome on morphological grounds.

Adrenal cortical hyperplasia may be diffuse or nodular (Fig. 15.23). In diffuse hyperplasia, the cortex as a whole or one of the three zones is diffusely thickened. The cells are usually rich in lipids, which are essential for the synthesis of steroid hormones. Lipid-rich cells have clear cytoplasm; those depleted of lipids have eosinophilic cytoplasm.

Adrenal cortical adenoma is a benign tumor composed of well differentiated adrenal cortical cells that resemble the normal or hyperplastic cortex (Fig. 15.24). The nuclei of such cells are usually uniform and round, although some pleomorphism is seen occasionally.

Adrenal cortical carcinoma is a malignant tumor originating from any of the three cortical zones. The tumor cells show varying degrees of nuclear and cytoplasm pleomorphism (Fig. 15.25). Mitoses may be prominent. However, there are no reliable histological criteria of malignancy, and the definitive diagnosis is made only if the tumor is obviously invasive and/or has metastasized Functionally, malignant tumors may be hormonally active or inactive.

Adrenal Medullary Tumors

The most important tumors of the adrenal medulla are: pheochromocytoma, neuro-blastoma, ganglioneuroblastoma, and ganglioglioma (Diagram 15.6). Like the normal adrenal medullary cells, all of these tumors are derivatives of cells that have emigrated from the fetal neural crest.

Pheochromocytoma is a tumor composed of well differentiated adrenal medullary cells. Like the normal medullary cells, the tumor secretes catecholamines, although usually in reverse proportions, i.e., more norepinephrine than epinephrine.

Histologically, the tumor is composed of large polygonal cells that have round nuclei and clear or finely granular cytoplasm (Fig. 15.26). By electron microscopy, the tumor cells contain membrane-bound granules with excentric densities typical of secretory catecholamine granules. Immunohistochemically, such cells have neuroendocrine cells features and react with antibodies to chromogranin, synaptophysin, and related polypeptides that are found in the neuroendocrine cytoplasmic granules.

Neuroblastoma is a malignant tumor of infancy and childhood. Most tumors originate from the neuroblasts of the adrenal medulla. These neuroblasts are migratory cells that emerge from the embryonic neural tube to give rise to neural crest and structures derived from the neural crest. In the fetal adrenal, these neuroblasts form the medulla. In autonomic ganglia, these cells differentiate into ganglion cells. The tumors originating from the undifferentiated embryonic neuroblast are composed of cells that retain their embryonic phenotype (Fig. 15.27). If the tumor cells retain some ability to differentiate into neural elements, such tumors are called **ganglioneuroblastoma** (Fig. 15.28). If the neuroblasts differentiate completely into ganglion cells, the tumor is a benign **ganglioneuroma** (Fig. 15.29). It is of interest to note that some neuroblastomas may "heal spontaneously" by differentiating into benign ganglioneuromas.

PLATE 15.1. PITUITARY ADENOMA

Figure 15.1. **Pituitary adenoma.** It should be noted that the pituitary tumors cannot be classified into cell-specific varieties without immunohistochemistry. **A.** Acidophilic adenoma. This tumor is composed of eosinophilic cells. Growth hormone was demonstrated in tumor cells by immunohistochemistry and, therefore, it was classified as a somatotropic adenoma. **B.** Basophilic adenoma. Tumor cells were found to be immunoreactive with antibodies to ACTH; thus, the tumor was classified as corticotropic adenoma. **C.** Chromophobe adenoma. The cells of this tumor have scant cytoplasm that is neither eosinophilic nor basophilic. By immunochemistry, this tumor contained prolactin and was classified as prolactinoma. **D.** Microadenoma. This small tumor, embedded within a normal pituitary, was an incidental microscopic finding.

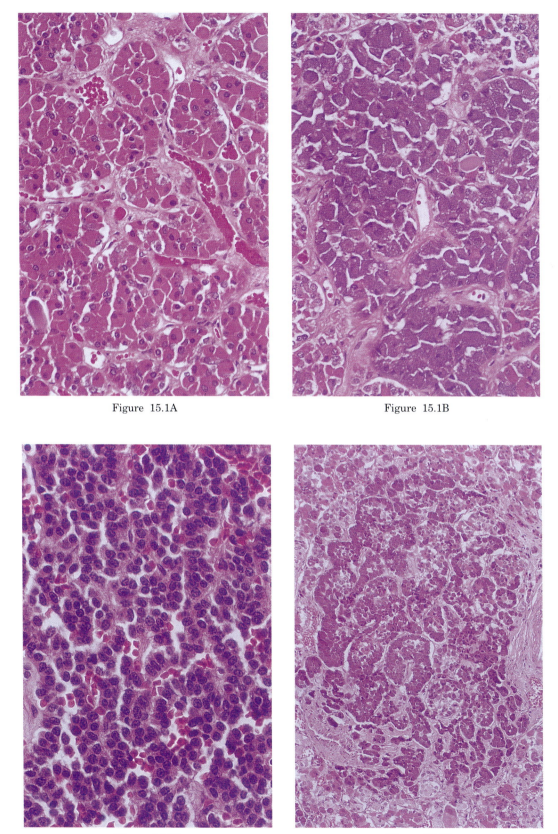

Figure 15.1A

Figure 15.1B

Figure 15.1C

Figure 15.1D

PLATE 15.2. DISEASES CAUSING HYPOPITUITARISM

Figure 15.2. **Pituitary necrosis.** The necrosis of the anterior pituitary was caused by an infarction.

Figure 15.4. **Craniopharyngioma.** The tumor is composed of clear and opaque keratinizing cells arranged in nests. The tumor cells at the periphery of nests appear palisaded.

Figure 15.3. **Histiocytosis-X.** The pituitary is infiltrated with Langerhans histiocytes and lymphocytes.

Figure 15.5. **Sarcoidosis of the pituitary.** The gland contains noncaseating granulomas.

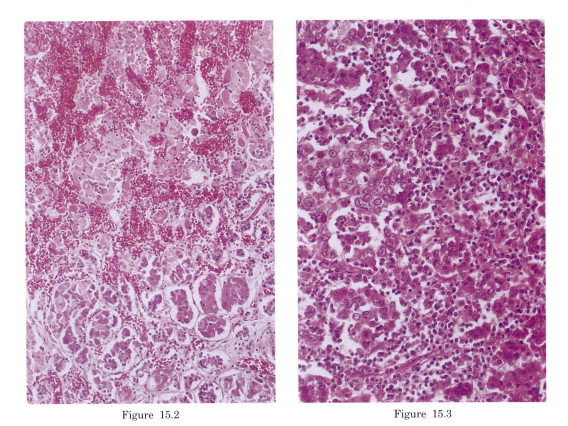

Figure 15.2

Figure 15.3

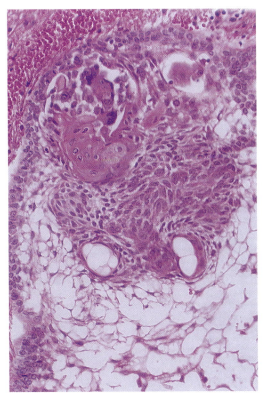

Figure 15.4

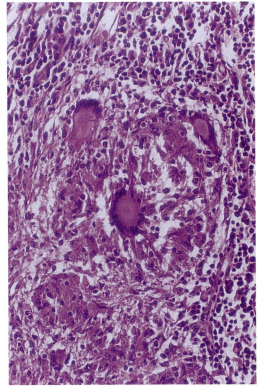

Figure 15.5

PLATE 15.3. NON–NEOPLASTIC THYROID DISEASES

Figure 15.6. Nodular goiter. A. The follicles vary in size and shape and contain varying amounts of colloid. The larger follicles seem to compress the small ones. **B.** Secondary changes include fibrosis, hemorrhage, and calcification. This photograph shows broad areas of fibrosis between the nodules composed of follicles that vary in size and shape.

Figure 15.7. Graves disease. A. The follicles are lined by tall cuboidal cells. The colloid appears rarefied and "scalloped." The intestinal spaces contain lymphocytes. **B.** Hyperplastic epithelium of the follicles project into the lumen in the form of papillary in foldings.

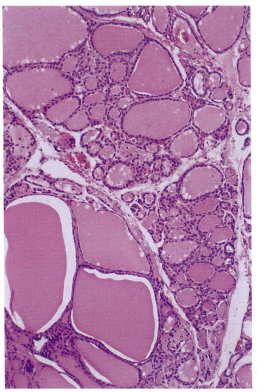

Figure 15.6A

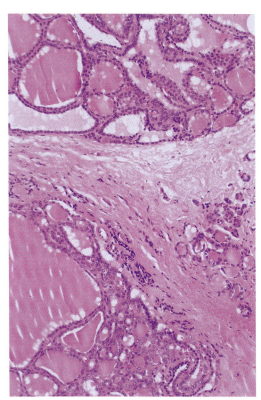

Figure 15.6B

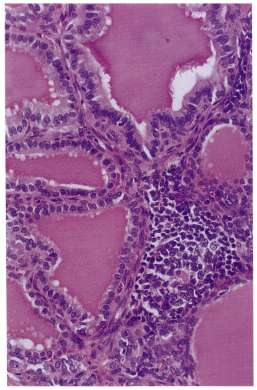

Figure 15.7A

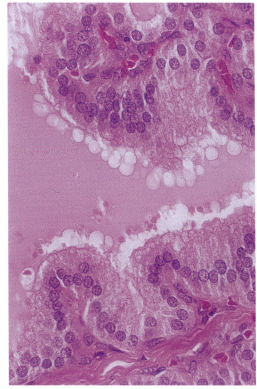

Figure 15.7B

PLATE 15.4. THYROIDITIS

Figure 15.8. Hashimoto thyroiditis. A. A marked stromal lymphocytic infiltrate replaces partially the follicles. The remaining follicles are lined by Hürthle cells that have an eosinophilic cytoplasm. **B.** In burnt-out Hashimoto thyroiditis, the thyroid shows atrophy of follicles, interstitial fibrosis, and a few residual chronic inflammatory cells.

Figure 15.9. Riedel thyroiditis. Fibrous tissue has replaced most of the thyroid. Only a few atropic follicles remain.

Figure 15.10. DeQuervain thyroiditis. Multinucleated giant cells and lymphocytes infiltrate the thyroid.

Diagram 15.2. Thyroiditis. A. Graves disease. Follicles are lined by cells that show signs of hyperfunction, and the stroma contains lymphoid follicles. **B.** Hashimoto thyroiditis. The thyroid is diffusely infiltrated with lymphocytes. A part of the thyroid is destroyed, and many follicles are lined by Hürthle cells. **C.** de Quervain thyroiditis. The rupture of follicles is associated with an inflammatory response that includes macrophages and giant cells. **D.** Riedel struma. The thyroid follicles have been replaced by fibrous tissue.

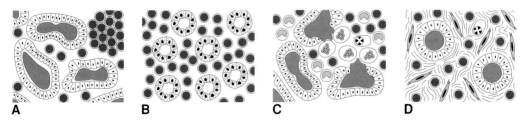

A   **B**   **C**   **D**

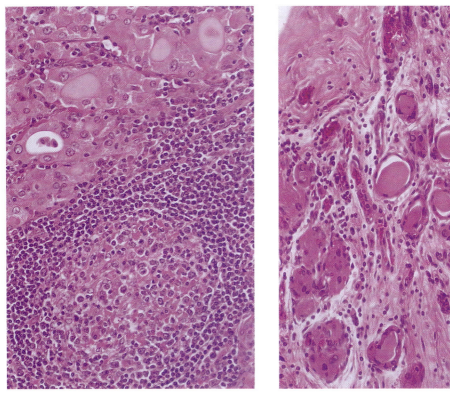

Figure 15.8A

Figure 15.8B

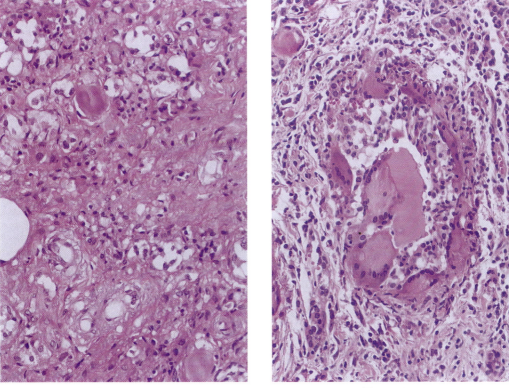

Figure 15.9

Figure 15.10

PLATE 15.5. THYROID TUMORS

Figure 15.11. Follicular (Hürthle cell) adenoma of the thyroid. Hürthle cell adenoma is composed of cuboidal cells that have eosinophilic cytoplasm. These so-called Hürthle cells form solid sheets, and only focally are they arranged into follicles devoid of colloid.

Figure 15.13. Follicular carcinoma of the thyroid. A. Tumor cells are arranged into irregular follicles and solid nests. **B.** Invasion is the only reliable criterion for distinguishing follicular carcinoma from follicular adenoma. Here the tumor is seen invading into the blood vessels and adjacent parenchyma.

Figure 15.12. Papillary carcinoma of the thyroid. A. Well circumscribed tumor in the thyroid. The tumor consists of numerous papillae. **B. Inset** shows a papilla. It has a central vascular core and is lined by tumor cells, the nuclei of which appear clear ("ground glass" or "Orphan Annie" nuclei).

Figure 15.14. Medullary carcinoma of the thyroid. The tumor is composed of small cells with clear cytoplasm. The cells grow in solid nests with a prominent stroma. The stroma appears hyalinized and contains collagen and amyloid.

Figure 15.15. Anaplastic carcinoma of the thyroid. The tumor is composed of large, undifferentiated cells that grow without any distinct pattern. There is marked nuclear pleomorphism and high mitotic activity.

Diagram 15.3. Thyroid tumors originate from follicular or C cells. A. Follicular adenoma and carcinoma. **B.** Papillary carcinoma. **C.** Anaplastic carcinoma. **D.** Medullary carcinoma.

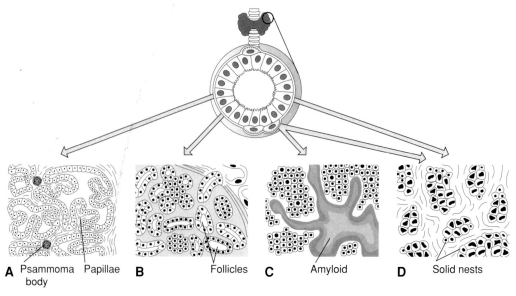

A Psammoma body Papillae **B** Follicles **C** Amyloid **D** Solid nests

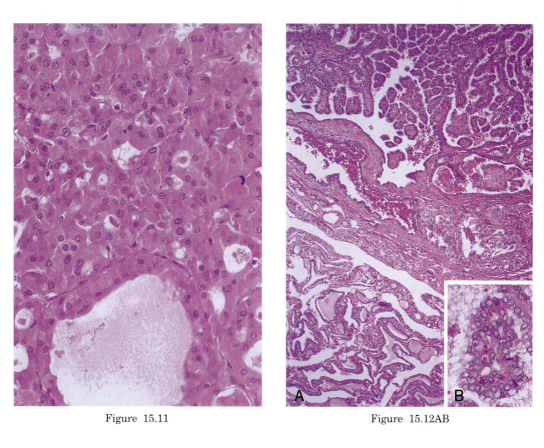

Figure 15.11

Figure 15.12AB

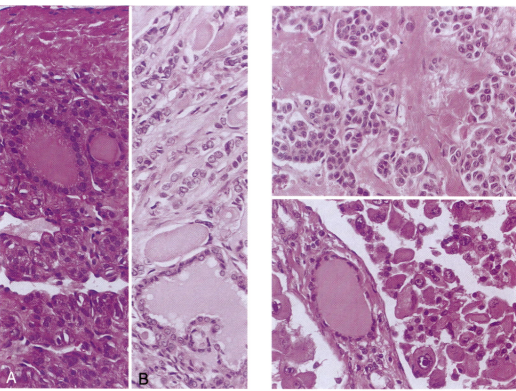

Figure 15.13AB

Figure 15.14, 15

PLATE 15.6. PARATHYROID LESIONS

Figure 15.16.   Parathyroid adenoma. A. The tumor is composed of a solid mass of uniform cells compressing the normal parathyroid, which consists of similar cells (lower part). **B.** Tumor composed of chief cells and oxyphilic cells.

Figure 15.17.   Parathyroid carcinoma. Histologically, these malignant tumors may resemble adenomas. Invasion and metastases are the only definitive proof that a tumor is malignant.

Figure 15.18.   Parathyroid hyperplasia. Histologically, hyperplastic parathyroids are indistinguishable from adenomas. This gland consists of several hyperplastic nodules.

Diagram 15.4.   Parathyroid diseases. A. Adenoma. **B.** Primary hyperplasia. **C.** Secondary hyperplasia. **D.** Carcinoma. Adenoma leads to an enlargement of one gland, whereas all others are of normal size. In hyperplasia, all four glands are symmetrically enlarged. Carcinomas are invasive tumors of irregular size and indistinct borders.

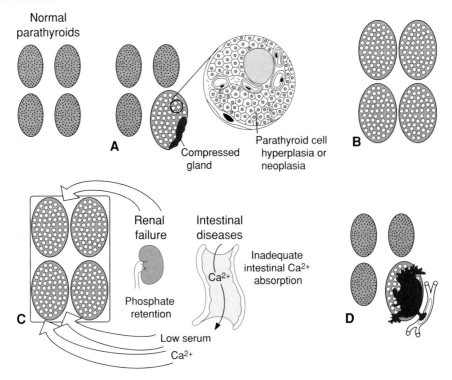

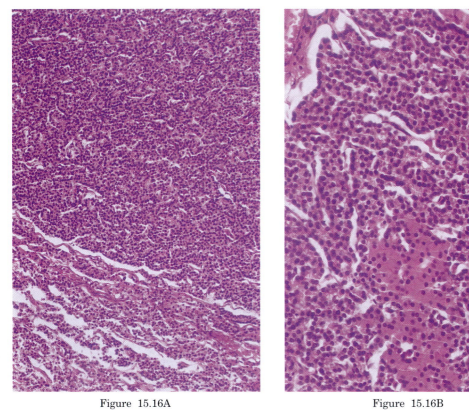

Figure 15.16A

Figure 15.16B

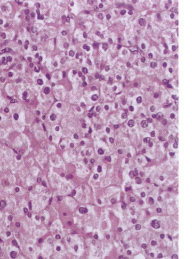

Figure 15.17

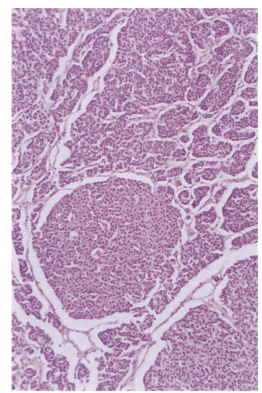

Figure 15.18

PLATE 15.7. ADRENAL LESIONS

Figure 15.19. Waterhouse-Friderichsen syndrome. The adrenal gland has been destroyed by hemorrhage.

Figure 15.21. Autoimmune adrenalitis. The gland is infiltrated with lymphocytes and plasma cells.

Figure 15.20. Tuberculosis of the adrenal. The cortex has been partially destroyed by granulomas.

Figure 15.22. Amyloidosis of adrenal. The cords of adrenal cells are compressed by deposits of amyloid. The wall of blood vessels is also infiltrated with amyloid.

Diagram 15.5. Adrenal cortical diseases. Adrenal insufficiency, illustrated in the upper row, follows adrenal destruction by immunological or infectious diseases and tumors. Adrenal cortical hyperplasia, illustrated in the second row, may be either diffuse or nodular. Adrenal tumors, illustrated in the third row, may be benign or malignant. Adenomas are distinct adrenal cortical nodules. Adrenal cortical carcinomas form irregular masses obliterating the normal adrenal and invading the adjacent tissues.

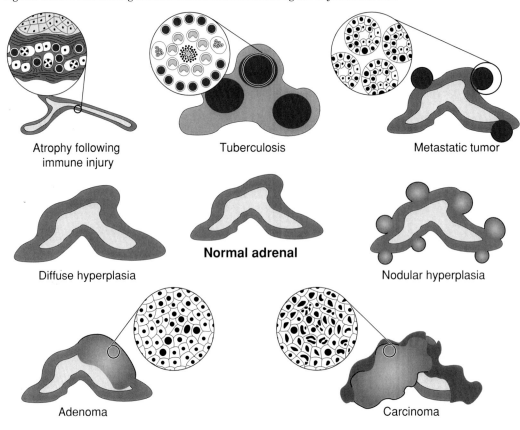

Atrophy following immune injury

Tuberculosis

Metastatic tumor

Diffuse hyperplasia

Normal adrenal

Nodular hyperplasia

Adenoma

Carcinoma

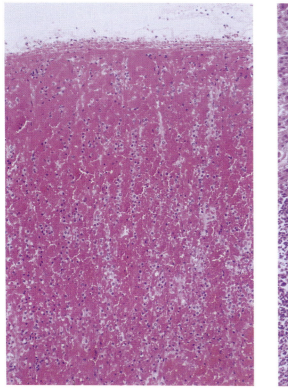

Figure 15.19

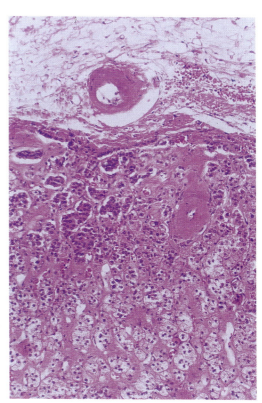

Figure 15.20

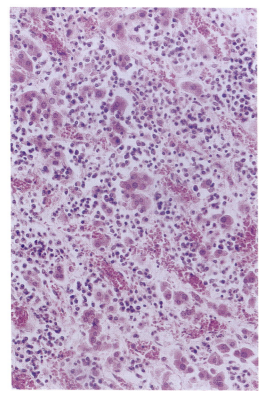

Figure 15.21

Figure 15.22

PLATE 15.8. ADRENAL CORTICAL HYPERFUNCTION

Figure 15.23.   Adrenal cortical hyperplasia. The hyperplastic cells are arranged into small nodules.

Figure 15.24.   Adrenal cortical adenoma. A. The adrenal contains a discrete nodule. **B.** The tumor is composed of eosinophilic cells resembling adrenal cortical cells depleted of lipids.

Figure 15.25.   Adrenal cortical carcinoma. The tumor consists of anaplastic cells that vary in size and shape. There is prominent nuclear pleomorphism. Mitotic figures are prominent.

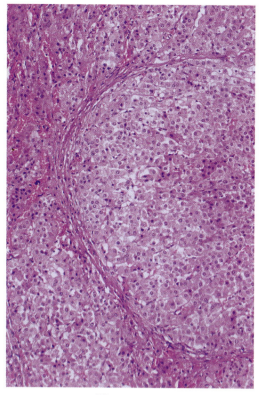

Figure 15.23

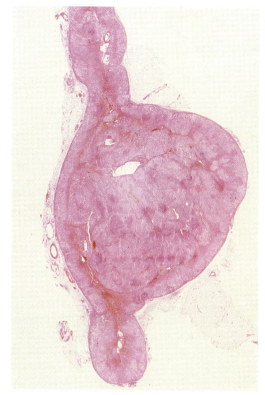

Figure 15.24A

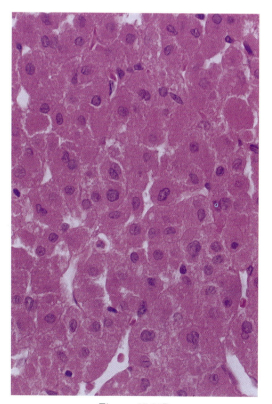

Figure 15.24B

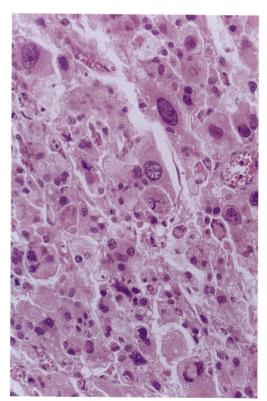

Figure 15.25

PLATE 15.9. ADRENAL MEDULLA

Figure 15.26. Pheochromocytoma. The tumor cells have round nuclei and well developed cytoplasm. These cells are arranged into nests surrounded by connective tissue septa rich in small blood vessels.

Figure 15.28. Ganglioneuroblastoma. The tumor consists of neuroblasts that occasionally form neural rosettes and neural tissue. This "neuropil" resembles brain tissue and is composed of myelinated and unmyelinated nerves. It appears as loose eosinophilic material and may contain ganglion cells.

Figure 15.27. Neuroblastoma. The tumor is composed of sheets of small blue cells.

Figure 15.29. Ganglioneuroma. The tumor is composed of mature ganglion cells, myelinated and unmyelinated nerves, and fibrous tissue.

Diagram 15.6. Embryogenesis and tumors of adrenal medulla. The neuroblasts derived from the neural tube form the neural crest, which gives rise to peripheral ganglia and the adrenal medulla. The tumors may be composed of undifferentiated neuroblasts (neuroblastoma), a mixture of neuroblasts and ganglion cells (ganglioneuroblastoma), or only mature neural tissue (ganglioneuroma). Pheochromocytomas are composed of neoplastic cells corresponding to mature adrenal medullary cells.

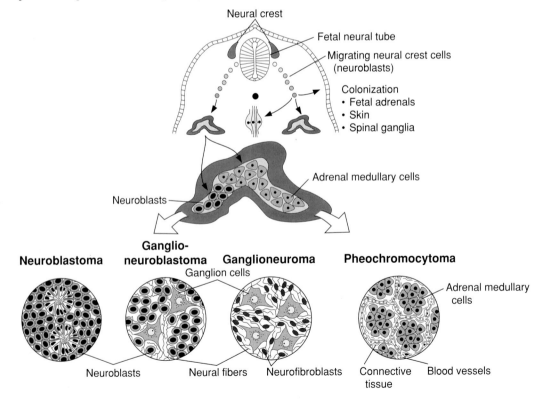

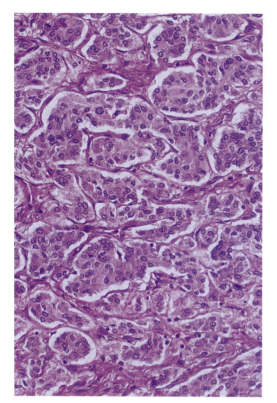

Figure 15.26

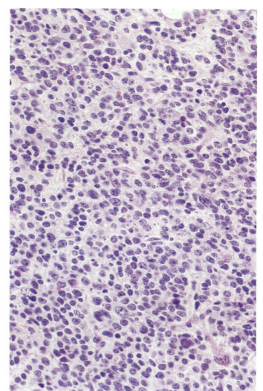

Figure 15.27

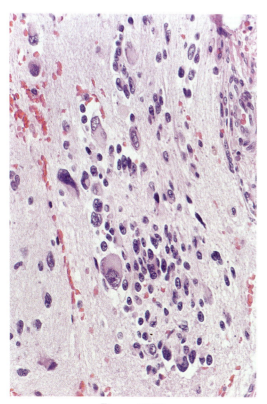

Figure 15.28

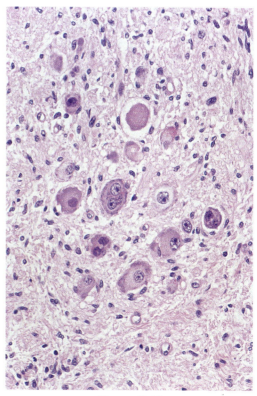

Figure 15.29

NOTES

CHAPTER 16

Skin

NORMAL SKIN

The skin consists of three layers: epidermis, dermis, and subcutaneous tissue (Diagram 16.1 and Fig. 16.1).

The epidermis, the outer layer of the skin, is composed of four cell types: *keratinocytes,* which form the vast majority of cells and produce keratin; *melanocytes*, the pigment-producing cells; *Langerhans cells*, the phagocytic cells involved in the uptake and processing of antigens; and *Merkel cells*, the neuroendocrine cells of unknown function.

The keratinocytes are arranged into several layers: the *basal* layer, composed of dividing cells; the *spinous* layer, composed of polygonal cells interconnected with one another by prominent intercellular bridges; the *granular* layer, composed of somewhat flattened cells rich in bluish cytoplasmic keratohyaline granules; and finally, the *keratinized* surface layer, composed of anucleated keratin squames. This layering of epidermis reflects the gradual maturation of keratinocytes, which move from the basal layer to the surface, over a period of about 30 days. It is important to note that the mitoses occur only in the basal layer, that the normal skin (in contrast to the mucosal squamous epithelium) contains a granular layer, and that the squames of the keratin layer do not contain nuclei. Nucleated keratin layer is an abnormality called *parakeratosis.*

Melanocytes and Merkel cells are restricted to the basal layer. Langerhans cells occur in all layers at random. These three cell types have a clear cytoplasm and can be recognized with certainty only with special stains or by electron microscopy.

The epidermis is separated from the dermis by a basement membrane, the principal component of the *epidermodermal junction.* The dermis is composed of loose connective tissue and small blood vessels, and it contains the *hair follicles.* The superficial zone forms *dermal papillae,* whereas the deeper dermis is composed of dense connective tissue. It merges imperceptibly with the *subcutaneous tissue* that consists predominantly of fat tissue. The dermis also contains the *sweat glands,* which have their own ducts, and *sebaceous glands,* which are attached to hair follicles.

OVERVIEW OF PATHOLOGY

The response of the skin to injury may take several forms, which roughly reflect various aspects of inflammation, circulatory disturbances, cell injury and necrosis, regeneration and repair, or tumor formation. The most important skin diseases include:

- Idiopathic diseases, which often have a genetic component
- Diseases caused by chemical and physical irritants in the environment (exogenous injury)
- Infectious diseases
- Immunological diseases
- Neoplasms

These pathological processes result in distinct lesions visible by the naked eye, which all have their histological equivalents. The most important terms of dermatopathology are summarized in Table 16.1 and illustrated in Diagram 16.2.

Idiopathic Skin Diseases

Many skin diseases are poorly understood and develop without a well defined cause. This heterogeneous group includes diseases that are inherited as Mendelian traits; diseases that are often familial but that do not show a distinct inheritance pattern, such as psoriasis; and diseases that show a predilection for patients of a certain sex and age. For example, lichen planus occurs more often in women than in men, affecting mostly persons in the 30 to 60 age group. Pityriasis rosea is most prevalent in persons between the ages of 20 and 30 years. Some of these idiopathic diseases are possibly caused by

Table 16.1
Common Skin Lesions

Skin Lesion	Microscopic Findings	Disease (Examples)
Erythema	Dilated, congested vessels	Acute inflammation
Macule	Focal hyperpigmentation of epidermis	Freckle
Patch	Edema and inflammation of dermis	Rubella
Wheal	Dermal edema and mild inflammation	Poison ivy skin lesion
Papule	Dermal inflammation and acanthosis	Atopic dermatitis
Plaque	Epidermal thickening	Psoriasis
Nodule	Infiltrate of inflammatory or tumor cells	Nevus
Tumor	Tumor cell infiltrates	Benign and malignant skin tumors
Papilloma	Acanthosis and papillomatosis	Wart
Cyst	Epithelium-lined cavity	Epidermal inclusion cyst
Vesicle	Edema and inflammation and/or necrosis	Herpesvirus (early lesion)
Bulla	Edema and/or cell necrosis inflammation	Burns
		Bullous drug reaction
Pustule	Suppurative inflammation	Impetigo
Ulcer	Epidermal defect	Syphilitic chancre
Crust	Wound or defect filled with clotted plasma	Healing scratched chickenpox lesion

immunological mechanisms. For example, atopic dermatitis of children responds well to steroid ointments. Despite these facts suggesting an immune pathogenesis, the cause of atopic dermatitis and many similar diseases has not been proven.

Idiopathic skin diseases of the skin present clinically with diverse symptoms that correspond to various pathological lesions. These heterogeneous lesions result from various pathogenetic mechanisms affecting the epidermis, the basal membrane of the epidermodermal junction, the dermal connective tissue, the dermal and subcutaneous blood vessels, or the entire skin. Four paradigms of idiopathic skin diseases have been chosen to illustrate both the heterogeneity of diseases in this category and skin reactions to various pathogenetic mechanisms.

Ichthyosis is a term applied to several congenital disorders of keratinization, all of which result in thickening of the epidermis in the form of fish scales. Common to all these disorders, which typically become clinically apparent early in life, is massive thickening of the stratum corneum and excessive accumulation of keratin scales on the surface (Fig. 16.1).

Psoriasis is a chronic disease marked by the formation of erythematous or whitish scaly papules and plaques. Lesions appear symmetrically on the body surface and pre-

dominantly affect the extensor dorsal surfaces of the extremities, especially those that are easily traumatized (e.g., elbows). The face and the scalp are often involved, and the nails are affected in 50% of cases. Some evidence of psoriasis can be found in 1–2% of all persons but the severe, generalized form of the disease is less common. The classic psoriatic plaques have a typical histological appearance that includes:

- Thickening of the epidermis predominantly due to elongation of the epidermal rete ridges and parakeratosis of the surface layer (Fig. 16.2).
- Elongation of the papillae and edema of the reticular dermis. These papillae contain dilated small blood vessels that have the features of venules rather than capillaries, a process known as "venulization of capillaries." The epidermis overlying the papillae is thin and lacks the granular layer. If the plaques are removed by scraping, punctate bleeding will occur from the venules in the exposed papillae ("Auspitz sign").
- Inflammatory cells in the dermal papillae and in the epidermis. Leukocytes may even form small aggregates in the keratin layer ("abscess of Monroe").

It is thought that psoriasis represents a disorder of epidermal cell proliferation and maturation and abnormal microcirculation of blood in the reticular dermis. The changes in the structure of dermal blood vessels facilitates the exit of inflammatory cells, which add an inflammatory aspect to this disease and account for its chronicity.

Epidermolysis bullosa is a term used to denote several hereditary disorders, all of which are characterized by formation of blisters on minor trauma. The bullae are subepidermal (Fig. 16.3). This probably reflects a defect in the attachment of the basal layer to the basement membrane at the epidermodermal junction.

Scleroderma is a chronic disease of dermal connective tissue. It may present as part of *systemic sclerosis*, a disease affecting many internal organs characterized by hidebound skin or local skin patches known as *morphea*. The basic defect underlying the numerous manifestations of the systemic disease is poorly understood, and even the biochemical changes in the connective tissue are still obscure. These patients have autoantibodies to various nuclear compo-

Diagram 16.1. The normal skin comprises three layers: epidermis, dermis, and subcutaneous tissue. The basal layer, spinous layer, granular layer, and keratinized layer of the epidermis are composed of keratinocytes. Melanocytes, Langerhans cells, and Merkel neuroendocrine cells also are found in the epidermis. The basement membrane separates the epidermis from the dermis. In the dermis, which is primarily composed of connective tissue, there are blood vessels, hair follicles, sebaceous glands, and sweat glands.

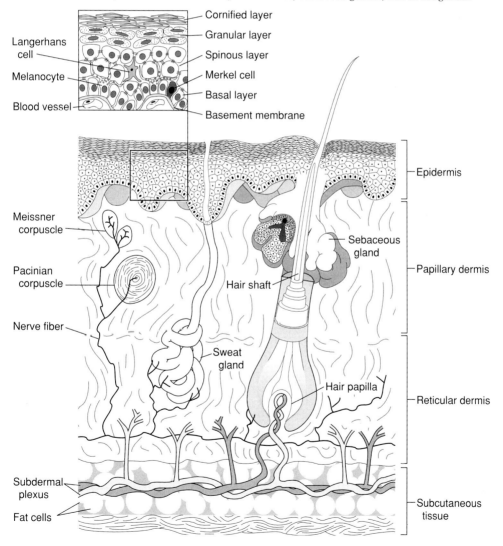

nents (antinuclear antibodies, or ANAs), usually to centromere and topoisomerase I. It is thought, therefore, that scleroderma might be an autoimmune disorder. Nevertheless, it is difficult to relate pathogenetically the various autoimmune phenomena with the increased amounts of collagen in various tissues, and the reason for collagen deposition remains unknown.

The histological changes in the skin are characteristic (Fig. 16.4). These include a marked increase in the amount of dermal collagen, typically arranged into dense bundles replacing the normal components of the dermis. Only a few atrophic sweat glands and hair follicles remain embedded in the dense hyalinized collagen. The overlying epidermis shows signs of atrophy. The collagen fibers also extend into the subcutaneous fat, obliterating the borders between the dermis and the subcutis.

Exogenous Injury

The skin is the outer surface of the body, and its primary function is to protect the body from external injuries. Accordingly, the skin is most susceptible to exogenous insults, such as mechanical trauma; thermal injury—excessive heat (burns) or cold (frostbites); ultraviolet, infrared, x-ray, or corpuscular radiation; chemical injury following exposure to strong acids or alkali, heavy metals, and various drugs; and insect bites and foreign bodies.

Wounds are lesions marked by a defect in surface epithelium caused by sharp objects, such as a knife; blunt objects, such as a club; or missiles, such as bullets. The defect of epidermis (*ulcer*) is first filled with plasma that coagulates, producing a scab. Further healing of the wound is mediated by dermal granulation tissue (Fig. 16.5), which leads to scar formation. Epidermis regenerates from the margin of the wound, thus covering the defect and restoring the integrity of the damaged skin.

Wound healing occasionally results in hypertrophic scars, which are called **keloids**. Such scars contain broad, irregularly interwoven bundles of collagen fibers (Fig. 16.6).

Sunlight injury is caused by a wide spectrum of rays, from ultraviolet to infrared rays. Acute injury is predominantly due to infrared (thermal) rays that scorch the skin and cause a sequence of erythema, edema, and blistering (Fig. 16.7). Longer exposure induces hyperpigmentation ("suntanning"), which protects the underlying dermis from the adverse effects of sun rays. The protection is not absolute, however, and persons exposed to sun for prolonged periods of time show typical degenerative alterations of dermal elastic fibers and collagen (*solar degeneration*). The dermis in such cases is filled with amorphous, granular, faintly basophilic material resembling fragmented elastic fibers (Fig. 16.8).

Actinic keratosis. Prolonged exposure to sunlight produces changes in the epidermis known as *actinic* or *solar keratosis*. Actinic keratosis occurs in two forms: a *hypertrophic*, more common form, and an *atrophic form*. Usually, there is disorganization of the epidermal layers (Fig. 16.9). Irregularly shaped cells with hyperchromatic nuclei may be seen in all layers of the epidermis, which indicates that this is a premalignant condition and that it may progress to invasive cancer. The dermis usually contains chronic inflammatory cells and shows solar degeneration.

Infectious Diseases

Infections of the skin may be caused by a variety of pathogens, including bacteria, viruses, fungi, protozoa, and parasites. Depending on the pathogen, the diseases may be acute or chronic, localized or diffuse. Furthermore, the pathological changes vary, reflecting on one hand the propensity of various microbes to invade various structures of the skin, and on the other hand their ability to invoke various forms of inflammation (Diagrams 16.3 and 16.4).

Viral infections. Some viruses, such as chickenpox, are epidermotropic and invade the epidermis, whereas others, such as measles, are dermotropic and affect dermis. Chickenpox or herpes virus produce vesicles (Fig. 16.10) that may heal without scarring or transform into pustules, which ulcerate and transform into scabs, leading to shallow scar formation. Smallpox causes similar lesions, but the necrosis affects deeper layers of the skin and usually causes scarring. Measles are marked by an acute, short-lived rash and pathological changes limited to dermis without any epidermal lesions.

Molluscum contagiosum and human papilloma virus (HPV) produce typical histological changes. The cells forming the papules of molluscum contagiosum contain prominent aggregates of viral particles (Fig. 16.11). Warts caused by HPV appear as papillomas with hyperkeratosis (Fig. 16.12).

Bacterial infections. *Pyogenic bacteria,* such as *Streptococcus* and *Staphylococcus,* cause pus-containing lesions.

Impetigo is a purulent inflammation limited to the epidermis (Fig. 16.13).

Folliculitis is accumulation of pus in the hair follicle (Fig. 16.14).

Confluent folliculitis results in an abscess involving more than one hair follicle that is called a *carbuncle.* Suppurative infection extending into the deeper dermis and subcutis is called *cellulitis.*

Mycobacterium tuberculosis and *M. leprae* produce granulomatous dermal lesions (Fig. 16.15). Syphilis causes perivascular inflammation of the dermis with overlying maculopapular lesions of the epidermis known as *condyloma latum*. Histologically, condyloma lata show nonspecific inflammation and perivascular accumulation of plasma cells.

Rickettsiae tend to invade the endothelium of small blood vessels of the dermis and, by disrupting the blood vessels, cause skin petechiae. Petechiae are prominent in typhus and Rocky Mountain spotted fever.

Protozoa, like *Leishmania,* invade the dermis and are taken up by macrophages, which form dermal infiltrates. This results in formation of papules and plaques that tend to ulcerate.

Fungi of the *Dermatophyton* species invade the keratin scales and do not penetrate deeper into the skin. *Blastomyces dermatitidis* and other more invasive fungi, especially those in the tropics, tend to produce deep dermatomycoses or even subcutaneous tumor-like lesions called "mycetomas." Histologically, such dermal lesions show suppuration or granuloma formation (Fig. 16.16).

Insects such as fleas or mosquitoes feed on human blood. Insect bites cause acute inflammation in the dermis. Other insects, such as *Sarcoptes scabiei*, the cause of scabies, tend to attach to the skin or to bury themselves in the superficial layers of the skin, causing chronic inflammation.

Immunological Diseases

Skin is exposed to numerous exogenous substances, many of which may act as antigens and elicit a localized or systemic immune reaction. Systemic immune disorders, such as systemic lupus erythematosus, may also produce skin lesions. Allergy to food or drugs may also produce skin lesions.

Pathogenetically, the immune reactions are divided into four categories; the members of each type of immune reaction can cause skin lesions (Diagram 16.5).

Type I immune reaction, or *atopic reaction,* is mediated by immunoglobulin E (IgE) and mast cells. Allergens from the environment react with the specific IgE, which in turn binds to the mast cells, thus triggering a release of histamine, serotonin, and other vasoactive substances. This increases the permeability of blood dermal blood vessels, causing edema of the dermis and the overlying epidermis (called spongiosis). Clinically, type I reactions present as *wheals (hives)* or localized skin edema. Atopic dermatitis, childhood eczema, and acute swelling of skin in anaphylactic reaction following bee-sting or drug allergy are all caused by type I immune reactions (Fig. 16.17).

Type II immune reaction, or *cytotoxic cell* reaction, is mediated by antibodies that bind to cell membranes and cause cell necrosis by activating complement or by cytotoxic lymphocytes. The prototype of type II immune reaction in the skin is **pemphigus vulgaris**. In this disease of unknown origin, antibodies to keratinocytes bind to epidermal cells, disrupting the intercellular adhesion sites. Separation of epidermal cells from one another results in a widening of intercellular spaces filled with the fluid. Coalescence of the fluid-filled spaces leads to the formation of intraepidermal vesicles and bullae (Fig. 16.18). Antibodies bound to the cell surface of keratinocytes (usually IgG) can be demonstrated by immunofluorescence microscopy.

Type III immune reaction, or *circulating immune complex–mediated reaction,* is due to the deposition of antigen antibody complexes and complement in tissues. This immune reaction accounts for the skin lesions in **systemic lupus erythematosus** (Fig. 16.19). Immune deposits along the epidermodermal junction, which may appear fibrinoid on light microscopy, cause lique-faction degeneration of the basal layer of the epidermis and edema of the dermis. Activated complement products are chemotactic and attract chronic inflammatory cells, which are most prominent around the dermal vessels. The epidermis is usually atrophic and shows hyperkeratosis and keratin plugs in the follicular skin. Immune complexes can be demonstrated by immunofluorescent microscopy as granular deposits along the epidermodermal junction.

Type IV immune reaction, or cell-mediated reaction, includes participation of T lymphocytes. This reaction occurs in *contact dermatitis* or the *so-called graft-versus-host reaction* after bone marrow transplantation. In **contact dermatitis,** the sensitized T lymphocytes invade the dermis and epidermis and cause edema of the dermis or spongiosis of the epidermis. These changes are histologically nonspecific. Sarcoidosis, another cell-mediated disease, is marked by formation of granulomas.

Neoplasms

Neoplasms of the skin are among the most common tumors of humans. The most important are:

- Epithelial cell tumors
- Melanocytic tumors
- Dermal stromal tumors

Tumors of the epithelial cells. The most important epithelial cell tumors presented in Diagram 16.6 are:

- Benign neoplasms (e.g., seborrheic keratosis)
- Invasive tumors of low malignancy (e.g., basal cell carcinoma)
- Preinvasive carcinoma in situ of the epidermis, which if untreated will progress to invasive carcinoma (e.g., Bowen disease)
- Invasive carcinoma (e.g., squamous cell carcinoma)

Seborrheic keratosis, also called *basaloid cell papilloma* or *senile wart,* is an exophytic benign tumor (Fig. 16.20). There are several histological types of seborrheic keratosis, all of which show three common features: thickening of the epidermis (acanthosis), papillomatosis, and hyperkeratosis. The thickened epidermis consists of either squamous or basaloid cells, which abruptly

undergo keratinization and form prominent "keratotic plugs". These are located between the epithelial papillae and on cross sectioning appear as concentric keratin pearls. Seborrheic keratosis presents clinically in form of pigmented warts in the elderly. It is a benign lesion and it does not evolve into carcinoma, even if left untreated.

Basal cell carcinoma, also known as *basal cell epithelioma,* is an invasive tumor of low-grade malignancy. The tumor is derived from epidermal basal cells that invade the dermis, forming nests and islands. Typically, these nests are composed of small blue cells (Fig. 16.21). Tumor cells may appear palisaded at the periphery, i.e., have their elongated nuclei lined-up like a picket fence ("palisade") and parallel to each other. Clinically, basal cell epitheliomas present as slightly elevated waxy papules, often with central ulceration ("rodent ulcer"). Treatment includes wide excision of the tumor and surrounding skin. Even if left untreated, basal cell epitheliomas do not metastasize.

Bowen disease, or *carcinoma in situ,* of the epidermis is a preinvasive form of squamous cell carcinoma. Clinically, it presents as scaly patches on sun-exposed skin. Histologically, it is characterized by thickening of the irregularly structured epidermis (acanthosis), hyperkeratosis and parakeratosis, and elongation of rete ridges, which usually appear plump and widened or flattened and effaced (Fig. 16.22). The maturation of the epidermis is in complete disarray. Cells with large and hyperchromatic nuclei can be found throughout the epidermis except the basal layer, which is relatively preserved. Mitoses are not limited to the basal layer. Single-cell keratinization occurs at random and can be seen even in the suprabasal parts of spongiose layer. Thickened keratin and parakeratin layers may invaginate deep into the lesion and thus appear as keratin pearls on cross-section. The basement membrane of the epidermis is intact, however, and tumor cell invasion into the dermis, which usually shows signs of chronic inflammation, is not seen.

Squamous cell carcinoma is an invasive malignant tumor of the epidermis. It may be preceded by actinic keratosis or

Bowen disease or arise de novo without obvious precursor lesions. Squamous cell carcinoma may occur on any part of the body, but these tumors generally are more common in the skin exposed to the sun. The lesions appear as plaques or ulcers with indurated margins. Histologically, the tumor is composed of strands of epithelial cells that often show atypical, pleomorphic, and hyperchromatic nuclei (Fig. 16.23). Aberrant keratinization and formation of keratin pearls may be seen in better differentiated tumors, whereas the undifferentiated tumors consist of nondescript cells, spindle-shaped cells, or bizarre cells showing no resemblance to normal epidermal cells. These malignant tumors invade the underlying tissues and give rise to local lymph node and distant metastases.

Pigmentary Lesions. Melanocytes, the pigment-producing cells of the skin, form several pigmentary lesions outlined in Diagram 16.7: freckles, lentigo, nevus, and melanoma.

Freckles (*ephelides*) are pigmentary spots (macules) of the skin composed of morphologically normal melanocytes that tend to overreact to sunlight. Exposed to sunlight, freckles become darker because the melanocytes produce more melanin, injecting it into the adjacent keratinocytes and thus darkening the skin spot.

Lentigo is a benign pigmentary lesion representing a local hyperplasia of melanocytes and hyperpigmentation of neighboring keratinocytes. This is usually associated with elongation and thinning of epidermal rete ridges, which thus increase the total surface occupied by the pigmentary cells in one area (Fig. 16.24). In contrast to freckles, lentigo does not darken upon exposure to sunlight.

Nevocellular (melanocytic) nevus, or *mole,* is a benign hamartoma composed of melanocytes. They can be *congenital* or *acquired.* Congenital nevi are found in 1% of newborns. Acquired nevi appear later, usually at puberty. These nevi gradually involute in old age. Depending on the location of melanocytes, nevocellular nevi are classified as *dermal* if the nevus cells are in the dermis, *junctional* if the cells are at the dermoepidermal junction, or *compound* if the nevus cells are both in the dermis and at the dermoepidermal junction (Fig. 16.25).

Malignant melanomas are malignant neoplasms of melanocytes (Fig. 16.26). In contrast to lentigo or nevi, melanoma cells have large, irregular nuclei and prominent nucleoli. The tumor cells occupy initially the dermoepidermal junction. During the horizontal phase of growth, the tumor cells spread along the epidermodermal junction. These lesions are called *superficial spreading melanomas.* Thus, horizontal spread is followed by a vertical growth phase during which the cells invade the dermis, giving rise to *nodular melanoma.* Malignant melanomas that have spread deeper into the dermis are prone to metastasis.

Dermal and Subcutaneous Tumors. Dermal tumors may originate from normal components of the dermis, such as fibroblasts, blood vessels, or adnexal glands; or from cells that have immigrated into the skin, such as lymphocytes and mast cells. The most important benign dermal tumors are listed in Table 16.2. Malignant equivalents of these tumors occur as well but are less common.

Dermatofibroma and related tumors originating from fibroblasts such as *atypical fibroxanthoma* and *dermatofibrosarcoma protuberans* are common dermal and subcutaneous lesions. They present as small dermal nodules that are mostly well circumscribed. Histologically, dermatofibromas are composed of intertwined and anastomosing bundles of fibroblasts surrounded by dense collagen (Fig. 16.27). Larger dermatofibromas extend imperceptibly into the subcutaneous tissue, but the tumors usually are separated from the epidermis by a thin zone of normal loose connective tissue.

Adnexal gland tumors are usually benign tumors composed of cells equivalent to those in normal apocrine and eccrine sweat glands or sebaceous glands. These tumors occur under several names, such as *syringomas* and *eccrine poromas.* The tumor cells are typically arranged into well circumscribed lobules and consist of ducts and acini (Fig. 16.28).

Dermal tumors composed of blood-borne cells are most often *lymphomas,* which are

Table 16.2
Benign Tumors of the Dermis and Subcutaneous Tissue

Neoplasm	Origin or Type of Differentiation	Typical Location
Dermatofibroma	Fibroblast	Extremities, but also elsewhere
Blue nevus	Melanocyte	Ubiquitous
Neurofibroma	Neurofibroblast multiple in neuro	Ubiquitous, may be
Schwannoma	Schwann cell	Fibromatosis
Hemangioma	Angioblast, congenital	Ubiquitous, usually
Trichoepithelioma	Hair shaft	Face, may be mutliple
Pilomatrixoma	Hair shaft	Ubiquitous, mainly in children
Calcifying epithelioma of Malherbe	Hair shaft	Face, upper extremity
Syringoma	Eccrine sweat gland	Lower eyelid, often multiple, chest
Syringocystadenoma papilliferum	Eccrine sweat gland	Scalp
Eccrine poroma	Eccrine sweat gland	Soles of feet and palms
Eccrine spiradenoma	Eccrine sweat gland	Ubiquitous, tender or painful
Cylindroma	Apocrine sweat glands	Scalp, may be multiple ("turban tumor")
Hidradenoma papilliferum	Apocrine sweat glands	Only in females—vulva
Nevus sebaceus	Sebaceous glands	Face, scalp; congenital, may be associated with tuberous sclerosis
Sebaceous adenoma	Sebaceous glands	Face and scale, very rare

discussed in the chapter on hematopathology (Chapter 7). T-cell lymphomas have a pronounced dermatotropism and may present with skin lesions typical of *mycosis fungoides*. *Histiocytosis-X* is characterized by dermal infiltrates of malignant Langerhans cells. In *juvenile xanthogranuloma*, the dermis is infiltrated with lipid-laden macrophages (Fig. 16.29). These cells often coalesce into multinucleated Touton giant cells.

Urticaria pigmentosa is a term used to describe several skin diseases caused by dermal infiltrates of mast cells. Urticaria pigmentosa usually occurs in children presenting with multiple lesions that disappear spontaneously by puberty. The more serious form of urticaria pigmentosa has its onset in young adults and may be associated with systemic symptoms. Malignant mastocytosis is rare. Histologically, urticaria pigmentosa is characterized by dermal infiltrates of mast cells. Mast cells have round to bean-shaped nuclei and a moderate amount of pink or slightly bluish (amphophilic) cytoplasm (Fig. 16.30). Overall, these cells resemble histiocytes, and it may be necessary to perform special stains or electron microscopic studies to prove that the cells are mast cells rather than some other inflammatory cells. Mast cell granules react with metachromatic stains such as crystal violet or methyl violet, rendering the dye red-violet in contrast to all other cells, which stain blue.

NOTES

PLATE 16.1. IDIOPATHIC SKIN DISEASES

Figure 16.1. Ichthyosis. This congenital skin disease is marked by extensive keratinization. Note the thick superficial keratinized layer.

Figure 16.2. Psoriasis. The skin lesion shows elongation of the rete ridges and surface parakeratosis that contribute to the thickening of the skin. Note also the elongation of the dermal papillae, which contain dilated blood vessels and scattered chronic inflammatory cells.

Figure 16.3. Epidermolysis bullosa. This congenital defect in the attachment of the basal layer to the basement membrane of the epidermodermal junction results in a subepidermal bulla.

Figure 16.4. Scleroderma. The dermis contains an increased amount of dense collagen, and the epidermis is atrophic.

Diagram 16.2. Principal skin lesions. A. Macule is a flat, focal, colored skin lesion. **B.** Papule is a slightly raised lesion. Larger papules are called plaques. **C.** Nodule is a solid slightly elevated lesion. Larger nodules are called tumors. **D.** Papilloma is an elevated exophytic epidermal outgrowth. **E.** Cyst is a cavity filled with fluid or some other material, such as sebum or keratin. **F.** Vesicle is a fluid-filled, raised lesion. Larger vesicles are called bullae. **G.** Pustule is a vesicle filled with pus. **H.** Crust is dried-out clotted blood or inflammatory exudate covering a skin defect. **I.** Ulcer is a defect of epidermis.

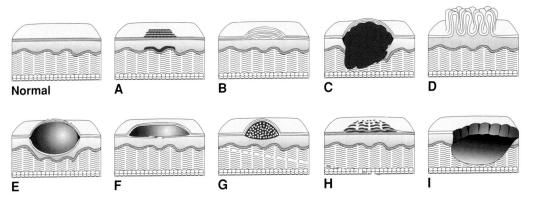

Normal   A   B   C   D

E   F   G   H   I

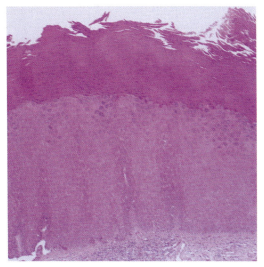

Figure 16.1

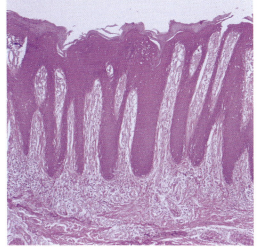

Figure 16.2

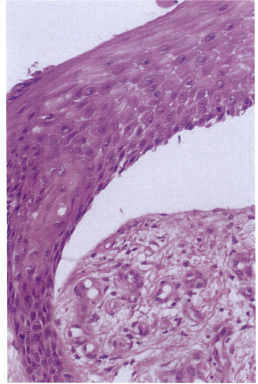

Figure 16.3

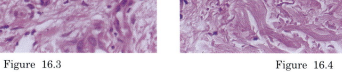

Figure 16.4

PLATE 16.2. LESIONS CAUSED BY EXOGENOUS PHYSICAL INJURY

Figure 16.5. **Ulcer.** The epidermis is missing, and the defect is filled with granulation tissue.

Figure 16.6. **Keloid.** In this hypertrophic scar, the dermis contains broad bands of collagen.

Figure 16.7. **Vesicle caused by sunburn.** Note acantholysis and accumulation of fluid within the epidermis.

Figure 16.8. **Solar degeneration of the dermis.** Fragmented coiled bluish material, corresponding to altered elastic fibers, is seen to replace the normal collagen in the dermis.

Figure 16.9. **Actinic keratosis.** The hypertrophic form of actinic keratosis shows thickening of the epidermis and hyperkeratosis. The epidermis lacks normal layers and shows no evidence of maturation. The cells appear hyperchromatic and have a high nuclear/cytoplasmic ratio.

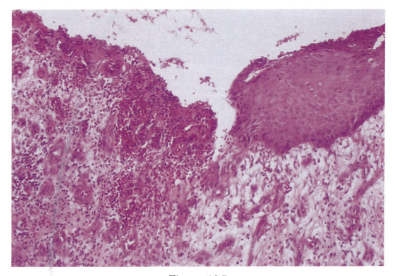

Figure 16.5

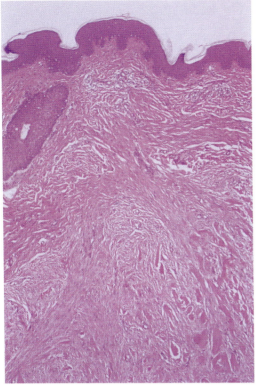

Figure 16.6

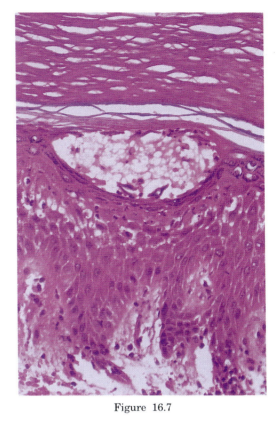

Figure 16.7

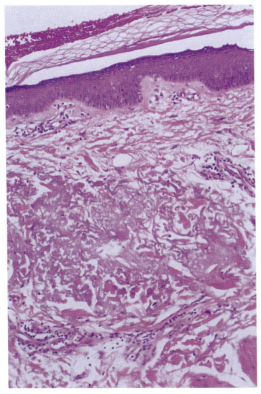

Figure 16.8

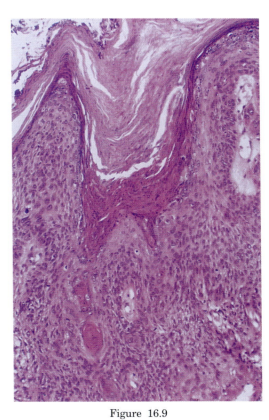

Figure 16.9

PLATE 16.3. INFECTIOUS DISEASES (VIRAL)

Figure 16.10.   Herpesvirus vesicle. A. The intraepidermal vesicle resulted from dissociation of epidermal cells (acantholysis) followed by the influx of fluid. **B.** The virus produces the typical nuclear changes—ground-glass appearance of nuclear matrix and multinucleated cells.

Figure 16.11.   Molluscum contagiosum. The epidermal cells contain viral inclusions that are either red or bluish.

Figure 16.12.   Common wart. The lesion looks like a hyperkeratotic squamous papilloma. It shows acanthosis (thickening of epidermis), papillomatosis (prominent dermal papillae), and prominence of the granular layer.

Diagram 16.3.   Infectious diseases. Viral diseases may present as acute red macules (rubella), blister (varicella), or chronic papules or nodules (molluscum contagiosum) and papilloma (warts caused by papilloma virus).

Skin Infections
Viral

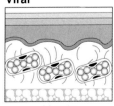
Macule

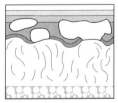
Blister

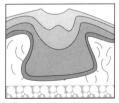
Papule of molluscum contagiosum

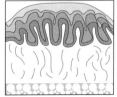
Wart

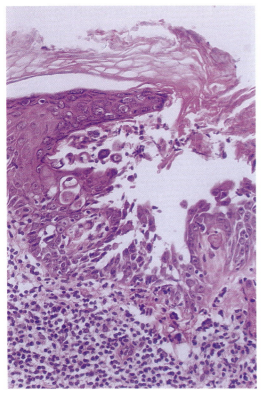

Figure 16.10A

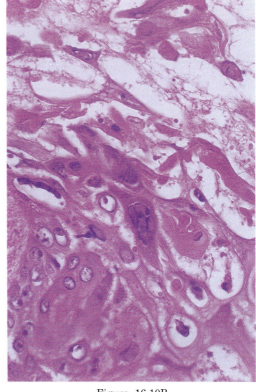

Figure 16.10B

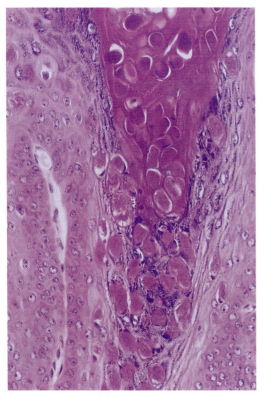

Figure 16.11

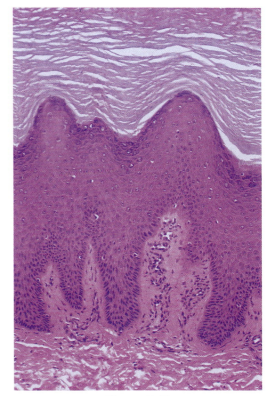

Figure 16.12

PLATE 16.4. INFECTIOUS DISEASES (BACTERIAL AND FUNGAL)

Figure 16.13. Impetigo. This superficial skin infection is characterized by subcorneal intraepidermal pustules.

Figure 16.14. Folliculitis. The pus fills the hair follicle and extends into the adjacent structures, forming a dermal abscess.

Figure 16.15. Leprosy. In tuberculoid leprosy, the epidermis contains confluent granulomas composed of epithelioid macrophages, giant cells, and a few lymphocytes.

Figure 16.16. Blastomycosis. The round yeasts in the dermis are surrounded by neutrophils, macrophages, and giant cells.

Diagram 16.4. Infectious diseases. Bacterial diseases may present as superficial pustules (impetigo caused by *Streptococcus*), as folliculitis or carbuncle involving the hair follicles (caused by *Staphylococcus* or *Streptococcus*), or as dermal granulomas (tuberculosis or leprosy). Fungal infection may be limited to the superficial keratinized layer, but may be also marked by deep seated abscesses and granulomas. Rickettsiae invade the dermal blood vessels and cause petechial hemorrhages and macules. Protozoa such as *Leishmania* are intracellular parasites that live in dermal macrophages, and thus cause dermal mononuclear infiltrates or granuloma-like lesions.

Skin Infections

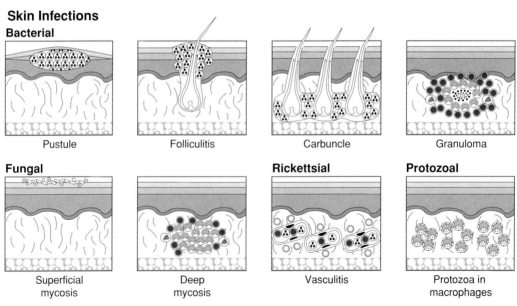

Bacterial

Pustule | Folliculitis | Carbuncle | Granuloma

Fungal | **Rickettsial** | **Protozoal**

Superficial mycosis | Deep mycosis | Vasculitis | Protozoa in macrophages

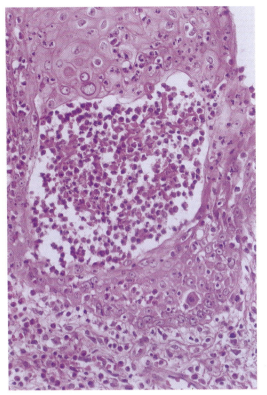

Figure 16.13

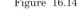

Figure 16.14

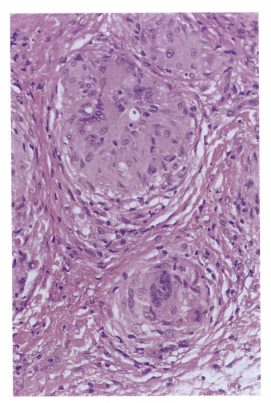

Figure 16.15

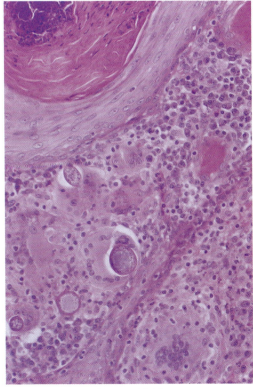

Figure 16.16

PLATE 16.5.   IMMUNOLOGICAL DISEASES

Figure 16.17.   Wheals. Type I allergic reaction caused massive edema of the dermis and subepidermal bulla. The dermis shows a mononuclear cell infiltrate.

Figure 16.18.   Pemphigus vulgaris. This immune-mediated disease is marked by the formation of suprabasal intraepidermal vesicles.

Figure 16.19.   Lupus erythematosus. A. In systemic lupus erythematosus, the dermoepidermal junction is indistinct and there is liquefaction degeneration of the basal layer. **B. (Inset)** By immunofluorescence microscopy, one can demonstrate deposits of antibodies along the epidermodermal junction. **C.** In discoid lupus, the dermis shows lymphocytic infiltrates, especially around the blood vessels and hair follicles.

Diagram 16.5.   Immune diseases. A. Type I immune reaction is marked by edema of epidermis and dermis (wheals). The dermis contains infiltrates of mast cells, which are the primary mediators of this reaction. The surface of mast cells is studded with IgE, which reacts with the antigen and thus triggers the release of histamine from mast cell granules. IgE is produced locally by plasma cells. Eosinophils interact with mast cells and are also present in the dermis. **B.** Type II immune reaction is mediated by antibodies to antigens expressed on tissue components. These include the cell surface of keratinocytes (pemphigus vulgaris) or basal layer (bullous pemphigoid). This causes dissociation of epidermal cells and formation of vesicles and bullae, which may be intraepidermal or subepidermal. **C.** Type III immune reaction is characterized by deposits of immune complexes at the epidermodermal junction, typical of lupus erythematosus. These immune complexes activate complement and thus damage the epidermal cells (liquefaction degeneration of basal cell layer). The dermis contains inflammatory cells, especially around the blood vessels. These are mostly lymphocytes, macrophages, and plasma cells. **D.** Type IV immune reaction is mediated by T lymphocytes and macrophages. In graft-versus-host reaction, these mononuclear cells invade the epidermis from the dermis, causing cell injury and edema. Sarcoidosis, another type IV reaction, is marked by the formation of dermal granulomas composed of macrophages, lymphocytes, and giant cells.

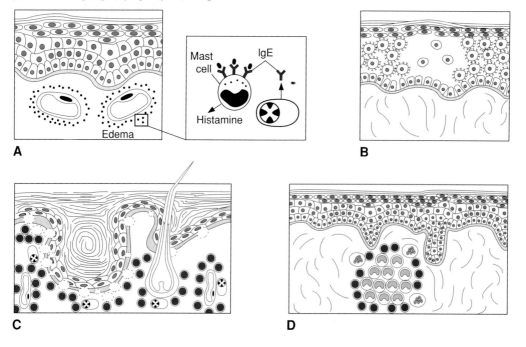

A

B

C

D

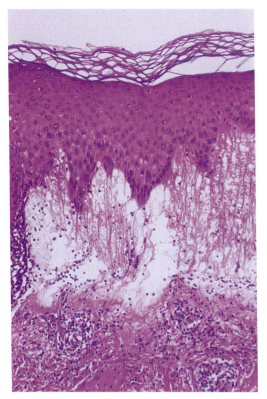

Figure 16.17

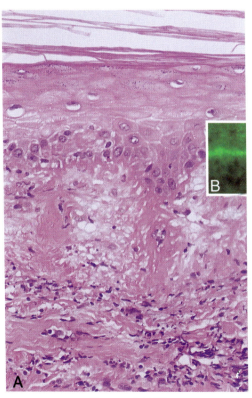

Figure 16.19AB

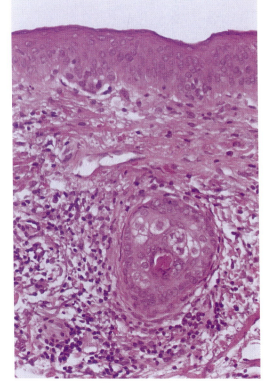

Figure 16.18

Figure 16.19C

PLATE 16.6. NEOPLASMS (EPITHELIAL)

Figure 16.20. Seborrheic keratosis. The lesion is an exophytic papilloma lined by thickened epithelium showing surface keratinization.

Figure 16.22. Bowen disease. The epidermis shows irregular layering, dyskeratotic cells, and mitotic figures outside of the basal layer. The basement membrane appears intact.

Figure 16.21. Basal cell epithelioma. Tongues of bluish cells, resembling those in the basal cell layer, extend from the surface epithelium into the dermis.

Figure 16.23. Squamous cell carcinoma. Invasive tumor composed of cells resembling normal epithelium and focal keratinization.

Diagram 16.6. Tumors of epithelial cells. A. Exophytic lesions typically found in seborrheic keratosis consist of acanthosis, papillomatosis, and hyperkeratosis. **B.** Basal cell carcinoma is a locally invasive tumor extending into the epidermis in the form of tongues of cells resembling those in the normal basal layer. **C.** Bowen disease is a preinvasive carcinoma in situ limited to the epidermis. The epidermis is thickened or disorganized and does not show the usually layering or maturation. There is hyperkeratosis, and the rete ridges are effaced. **D.** Squamous cell carcinoma is an invasive malignant tumor that also may have indurated and elevated margins. The malignant keratinocytes may mature into keratinous layers, which form concentric layers ("keratin pearls"). The tumors may extend into deeper layers of the skin, and it may metastasize through lymphatic or hematogenous spread.

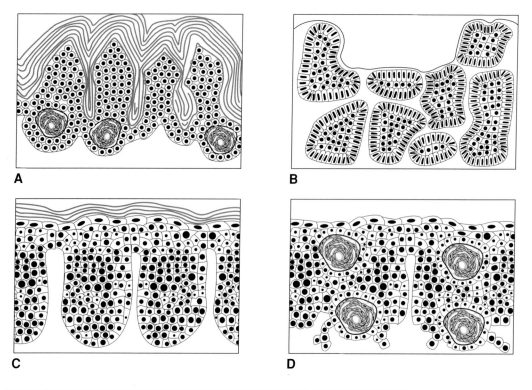

A

B

C

D

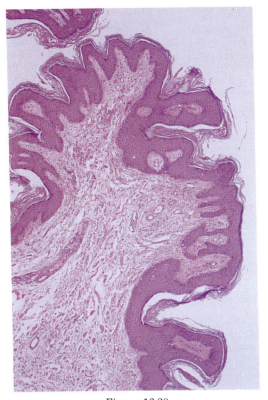

Figure 16.20

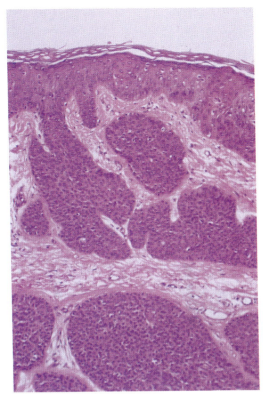

Figure 16.21

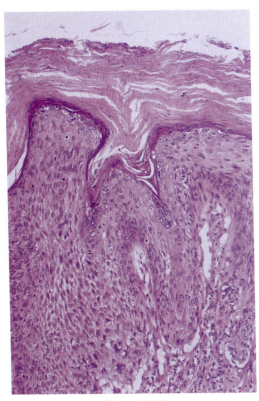

Figure 16.22

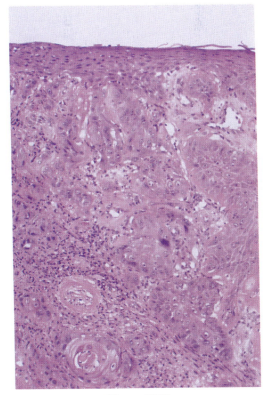

Figure 16.23

PLATE 16.7. PIGMENTED LESIONS

Figure 16.24. Lentigo. The epidermis shows elongation of rete ridges. The basal layer contains numerous melanocytes.

Figure 16.25. Nevus. Compound nevus has a junctional and a dermal component. The nevus cells form sharply demarcated nests.

Figure 16.26. Melanoma. A. Superficial spreading melanoma. Malignant melanocytes are restricted to the epidermis. **B.** Nodular melanoma. Tumor cells invade the dermis. The dermis contains melanin-laden macrophages (melanophages) and lymphocytes.

Diagram 16.7. Pigmented lesions. A. Freckle shows increased pigmentation of basal layer but a normal number of melanocytes. **B.** Lentigo is marked by an increased number of pigmented cells in the basal layer over the elongated rete ridges. **C.** Nevus is characterized by an increased number of nevus cells in the dermis (*dermal nevus*), at the epidermodermal junction (*junctional nevus*), or in both the dermis and the epidermis (*compound nevus*). Dysplastic nevus is a compound nevus composed of atypical melanocytes that replace the basal layer of the epidermis. **D.** Malignant melanoma. Level I tumor is limited to the epidermis. Level II tumors are composed of cells that have penetrated into the upper papillary dermis. These lesions do not measure more than 0.75 mm in thickness. Level III tumors are composed of cells that widen the papillary dermis and impinge on the reticular dermis and are 0.76 mm thick. Level IV tumors invade into the reticular dermis and are more than 2.6 mm thick.

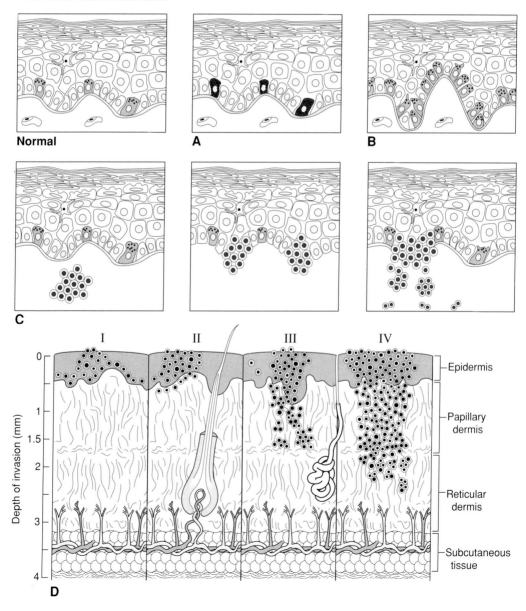

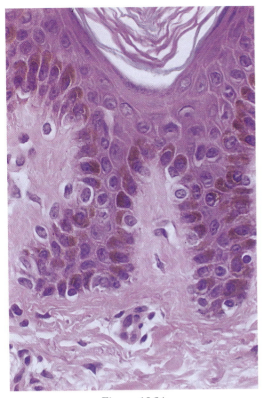

Figure 16.24

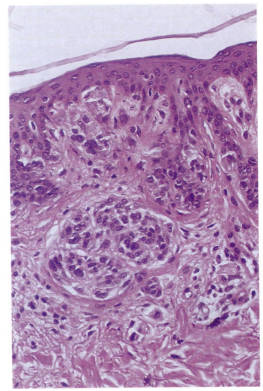

Figure 16.25

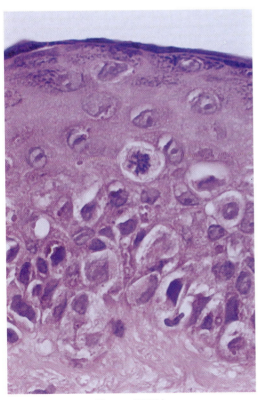

Figure 16.26A

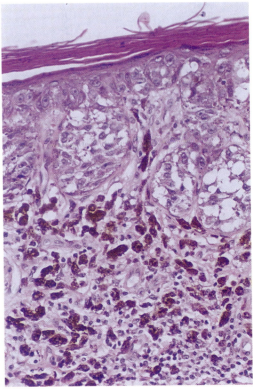

Figure 16.26B

PLATE 16.8. DERMAL TUMORS

Figure 16.27. Dermatofibroma. The tumor is composed of fibroblasts arranged into bundles. The interstitial spaces contain abundant collagen.

Figure 16.28. Sweat gland adenoma. The tumor is located in the dermis and consists of ducts and acini.

Figure 16.29. Juvenile xanthogranuloma. The dermis is infiltrated with macrophages (histiocytes), many of which are multinucleated.

Figure 16.30. Urticaria pigmentosa. The dermis is infiltrated with mast cells that have bean-shaped nuclei and amphophilic cytoplasm.

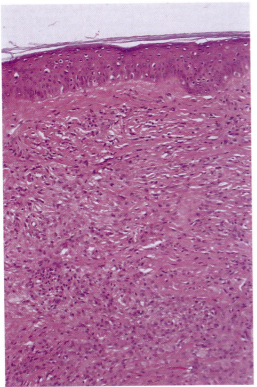

Figure 16.27

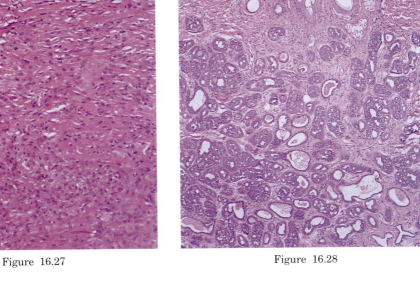

Figure 16.28

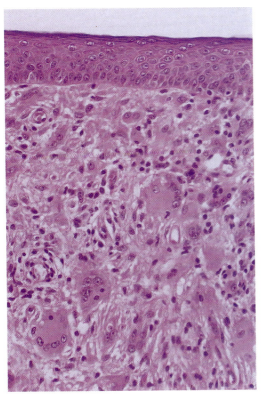

Figure 16.29

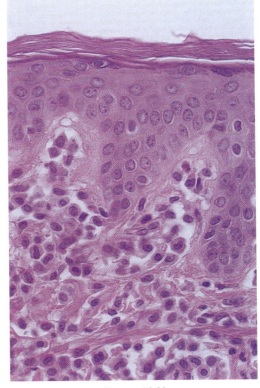

Figure 16.30

NOTES

CHAPTER 17

Bones and Joints

NORMAL HISTOLOGY

The bones are the main support structures of the body. Their primary functions are to provide a mechanical framework and protection to other organs, and to enable the movement of body parts and locomotion. The bones have also metabolic functions, serving as the primary storage site for calcium and phosphorus, and they provide the microenvironment for hematopoiesis.

All bones are composed of bone cells and matrix arranged into functional units called *osteons*. The articular surfaces of the bones are covered with *cartilage*, which is composed of chondrocytes and extracellular matrix. The lateral surfaces of the long bones are covered with the *periosteum*, composed of fibroblasts and collagenous extracellular matrix (Diagram 17.1).

The *osteon* is delimited from adjacent units by cement lines. The osteon receives its blood supply through centrally located vessels in the so-called haversian canal. The haversian canal is surrounded by concentric lamellar bone with lamellar bone lacunar spaces containing mature bone cells, the osteocytes. The medullary surface of cortical bone and the bone trabeculae of the spongiosa are lined with bone-forming *osteoblasts* and bone-resorbing *osteoclasts*. Multinucleated osteoclasts actively participate in the removal and restructuring of bone. The mononuclear osteoblasts participate in the formation of new bone, which entails the synthesis of an organic matrix called *osteoid*. Osteoid undergoes *calcification,* which marks its transformation into bone.

Osteoblasts and osteoclasts also participate in endochondral ossification, which typically occurs in the growth plate of long bones. In contrast to intramembranous ossification, in which the bone trabeculae are formed in a background of embryonic fibrous tissue, endochondral ossification is based on the transformation of a provisional cartilaginous matrix into bone. The newly formed bone appears under polarized light as *woven*. As the bone matures, it transforms into *lamellar bone*. The woven bone contains more bone cells and is composed of haphazardly arranged collagen fibers as opposed to lamellar bone, which has fewer cells and an orderly matrix composed of collagen fibers aligned into parallel bundles. The woven bone is found only in growing bones and under pathological conditions. Histological evidence of woven bone in adults is therefore always abnormal.

The joints are specialized junctions between the bones. There are different types of joints, which can be classified into two major groups: joints that are movable (*synovial* or *diarthrodial* joints) and those that allow very little movement (*synarthrosis*). Most of the clinically significant diseases affect the synovial joints, but the synarthroses joining the vertebrae are often pathologically altered as well.

Synovial joints serve to oppose the terminal positions of the long bones of extremities and the phalanges. The joint is held together by a fibrous capsule that encloses a space filled with a few drops of joint fluid (Diagram 17.1). Inside, the joint space is lined by a synovial membrane that is continuous with the periosteum of the adjacent bones. The articular surface of bones is covered with hyaline cartilage.

Developmental Disorders

Many genetic diseases directly affect the development of bones (Diagram 17.2). These diseases may:

- Retard or impede the normal growth of bones as in *achondroplasia*, a disease affecting the epiphyseal growth plate
- Adversely affect the matrix formation, as in *osteogenesis imperfecta*
- Result in abnormally structured bone, as in *osteopetrosis*

Bone development is also affected secondarily in many systemic inborn defects of metabolism, especially in the *mucopolysaccharidoses* (e.g., Morquio syndrome, Hurler syndrome), which typically produce skeletal deformities ("gargoylism"). Congenital *hypopituitarism* or deficiency of thyroid function (*congenital hypothyroidism*) cause

dwarfism because growth hormone and the thyroid hormone are essential for normal bone growth).

Achondroplasia is an autosomal dominant Mendelian defect of endochondral ossification. The growth of long bones, which

Diagram 17.1. Anatomy and histology of a typical long bone. The shaft is called the *diaphysis*. The part of the bone between the growth plate and articular cartilage is called the *epiphysis*. The terminal parts of the diaphysis and the adjacent growth plate are called *metaphysis*. The central part of the shaft is occupied by the medulla, and the outside is covered with periosteum. The compact cortical bone is composed of osteons, and the medullary spongiosa is composed of trabeculae. The joint is held together by a fibrous capsule. The inside of the joint is lined by synovial membrane.

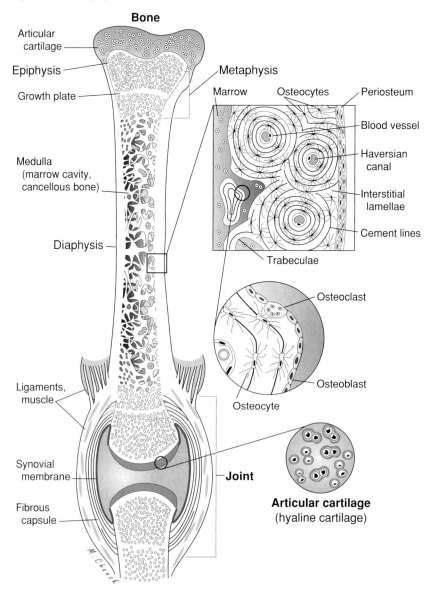

Bone

Articular cartilage
Epiphysis
Growth plate
Medulla (marrow cavity, cancellous bone)
Diaphysis
Ligaments, muscle
Synovial membrane
Fibrous capsule

Metaphysis
Marrow
Osteocytes
Periosteum
Blood vessel
Haversian canal
Interstitial lamellae
Cement lines
Trabeculae
Osteoclast
Osteoblast
Osteocyte
Joint

Articular cartilage (hyaline cartilage)

elongate through endochondral ossification, is stunted, resulting in a typical form of dwarfism marked by short arms and legs and normal body size. Histologically, achondroplastic long bones have an abnormal epiphyseal growth plate. The growth plate is thin. Within it, the cartilaginous cells do not form the typical columns and do not provide the matrix for provisional calcification, which is essential for normal bone growth. Calcification of the cartilage matrix appears to be irregularly distributed and is most prominent at the demarcation line between the bone marrow and the rest of the cartilage (Fig. 17.1). Osteoclasts, which normally remodel the provisionally calcified matrix, do not remove the calcified demarcation line. In essence, this calcified cartilage serves as a barrier that limits the axial growth of long bones.

Osteogenesis imperfecta is a term encompassing several genetic inborn errors of collagen metabolism. Without collagen type I, the basic component of osteoid, bone matrix, cannot form. The bones are brittle and prone to fracture. Short stature, bone deformities, and pathological fractures are typical in severe cases. Histologically, the bone trabeculae are thin and irregularly shaped (Fig. 17.2). Microfractures heal by irregular callus formation marked by excessive osteoid that is probably deficient in collagen type I.

Osteopetrosis is a genetic defect in bone formation. The basic flaw is probably related to the inability of osteoclasts to remove and remodel the calcified bone trabeculae. The bones of extremities remain short and compact. On radiographs, bones appear extremely radiodense ("marble bone disease").

Thick cortical and spongiose bone expands into the marrow, compressing and ultimately replacing the hematopoietic cells. This causes bone marrow failure and aplastic anemia. Histologically, the bones have thick trabeculae and narrow marrow spaces (Fig. 17.3).

Fibrous dysplasia is a term for localized tumor-like bone lesions probably related to abnormal development. These lesions may be monostotic or polyostotic, and are typically located within the cancellous bones (spongiosa) of the ribs, long bones of the lower extremities, or the jaws. In the polyostotic form, more than 50% of cases present with involvement of facial bones. Both the monostotic and the polyostotic lesions are histologically composed of spindle-shaped fibroblastic cells and irregular trabeculae of osteoid and woven bone. The trabeculae are not lined with osteoblasts, but appear to arise from direct osseous metaplasia of the fibroblastic stroma (Fig. 17.4).

Metabolic Bone Disorders

Metabolic disorders affecting bones are of two kinds: *idiopathic*, as in the cases of osteitis deformans (Paget disease) and osteoporosis of old age, or *secondary* to an identifiable cause or disease (Diagrams 17.3, 17.4, and 17.5). These disorders include:

- Excess or deficiency of hormones (e.g., growth hormone, parathyroid, thyroid, estrogenic, and androgenic hormones)
- Nutritional deficiency (e.g., deficiency of vitamins D and C, protein malnutrition, or lack of calcium)
- Diseases of another organ systems (e.g., end-stage disease of the kidneys)

Osteoporosis is a metabolic bone disease marked by a loss of total bone mass ("osteopenia"). Osteoporosis may be primary *(idiopathic)* or secondary, which is related to another metabolic disorder, such as Cushing syndrome, intestinal malabsorption syndromes, or hypogonadism.

Histologically, the bones show thinning of cortical and trabecular bone (Fig. 17.5) but are normally mineralized. Trabeculae of the spongiosa are thin and reduced in number. Microfractures are common and are characterized by the formation of spindle-shaped microcalluses in various stages of healing.

Osteomalacia is a metabolic disturbance of osteoid mineralization related to a deficiency of abnormal metabolic activation of vitamin D. Affected bones are composed of unmineralized matrix, which renders them soft and prone to deformities or fractures.

Osteomalacia presents histologically with an excess of unmineralized osteoid (Fig. 17.6). The bone trabeculae are of normal width but rimmed with unmineralized osteoid. In slides stained with hematoxylin and eosin, this border appears as a bluish seam. Special stains for calcium show the core of the trabeculae to be calcified, whereas the osteoid is not. Osteoblastic activity may be increased, contributing to the irregular shape of the trabeculae.

Vitamin D deficiency in growing infants and children results in **rickets**. The hallmark of rickets is abnormal endochondral ossification, as outlined in Diagram 17.4.

Histologically, the epiphyseal growth plates of rachitic bones appear disorganized and widened laterally (Fig. 17.7). The osteoid is abundant but shows very little mineralization. The cartilage cells are not arranged in columns that undergo regular calcification; rather, they form irregular nests that show only spotty calcification. Rachitic bones contain fewer blood vessels than normal growing bones do.

Hyperparathyroidism is associated with distinct bone lesions (Diagram 17.5). *Primary* hyperparathyroidism, owing to parathyroid gland adenoma or parathyroid hyperplasia, and *secondary* hyperparathyroidism, caused by chronic renal failure, produce similar bone changes (Fig. 17.8). Depending on the duration of hyperparathyroidism, the lesions show demineralization of bone, increased numbers of osteoclastic cells, or fibrosis of the bone marrow.

The osteoclasts form lacunae within the trabeculae as well as in the compact cortical bone, which they invade from the subperiosteal and endosteal side. The cortical bone appears ragged. Microfractures occur and are accompanied by rupture of blood vessels and bleeding into the affected area. Hemosiderin generated from extravasated blood is taken up by macrophages, imparting a brownish-red color to these lesions—hence the name *brown tumors of hyperparathyroidism*. Brown tumors of hyperparathyroidism consist of osteoclasts, fibroblasts, hemosiderin-laden macrophages, and scattered osteoblasts, and they are histologically indistinguishable from giant cell tumors of the bones.

Osteitis deformans (Paget disease) is a common bone disorder of unknown etiology characterized by an imbalance of bone formation and bone resorption. Approximately 10% of all people over 65 have some evidence of Paget disease. It occurs in a less common *monostotic* form predominantly involving tibia, femur, or calvaria and the

pelvic bones; and a *polyostotic* form that accounts for 85% of cases. Predominant sites of involvement are the vertebrae and pelvic bones. Other parts of the skeleton are affected unpredictably. Clinically, Paget disease presents with deformities, bone pain, and fractures. Approximately 1–2% of all patients with Paget disease develop osteosarcoma.

In either form, the disease begins as an *osteolytic* process. This is followed by a *mixed osteolytic and osteoblastic phase* that terminates in an *osteosclerotic phase* (Fig. 17.9). The osteolytic lesions are dominated by large, multinucleated osteoclasts. New bone is laid down by osteoblasts, which are typically lined up along broad rims of osteoid. Paget lesions are typically hypervascular. The osteosclerotic bone of the final stage is composed of broad, irregularly shaped trabeculae with a mosaic pattern imparted by broad calcified seams and wide borders of unmineralized osteoid. The bone marrow space is fibrotic. Secondary changes, such as fractures and hemorrhages, are common.

Infectious Bone Diseases

Osteomyelitis can be caused by a variety of microorganisms. Clinically, it may present as a primary infection or as secondary superinfections of fractures of bones. Among the bone infections unrelated to trauma or surgery, the most important are those that result from the hematogenous spread of pyogenic bacteria such as *Staphylococcus aureus. Salmonella* is a common cause of osteomyelitis in patients with sickle cell anemia. *Mycobacterium tuberculosis* was a significant cause of chronic osteomyelitis in the past but occurs less frequently today.

Osteomyelitis shares many histological features of acute or chronic inflammation in other organs (Fig. 17.10). Depending on duration of infection, the inflamed bone will show various reactive changes, including new bone formation, increased osteoblastic reactivity, and endosteal and periosteal fibrosis.

Fractures

Fractures of bones are the most frequently encountered bone lesions in orthopedic practice. Simple sterile fractures that do not require surgical intervention heal spontaneously upon immobilization over several weeks. Healing occurs in several phases (Diagram 17.6), which follow one another sequentially and include:

- Destruction of normal bone
- Hemorrhage into the site of fracture
- Clot formation
- Ingrowth of granulation tissue
- Removal of cell debris and old bone fragments
- Callus formation
- Remodeling of the callus
- Permanent bone formation

Following the disruption of intact bone, the site of fracture is flooded by extravasated blood. Fibrin clots form, enmeshing the disrupted tissue fragments and providing the scaffolding for the ingrowth of granulation tissue. The newly formed blood vessels in this granulation tissue (called "procallus") allow the influx of macrophages and the removal of cellular detritus (Fig. 17.11). The connective tissue cells of the procallus lay down collagen and other cell matrix components. Newly formed cartilage and bone appear within the granulation tissue, which is at this point called *callus*. With time, the granulation tissue regresses as the need for the clean-up is superseded by the need for structural reinforcement of the callus. The callus becomes firmer as the inflammatory cells are replaced by fibroblasts, chondrocytes, and osteoblasts. Foci of endochondral and intramembranous ossification result in the formation of bone trabeculae, which are partly composed of osteoid and partly of woven bone. These provisional trabeculae undergo remodeling through the action of osteoclasts, and are replaced by lamellar bone. The remodeling phase may last months and even years.

Neoplasms

Primary tumors of bone can originate from the hematopoietic bone marrow, bone-forming cells, cartilage cells, and nonspecific stromal and vascular cells. If one eliminates the hematopoietic neoplasms, which account for approximately 40% of bone tumors, the remaining primary neoplasms are derived mostly from bone-forming cells (osteoblasts), cartilage cells, fibroblasts, and undifferentiated mesenchymal cells. Secondary bone tumors, i.e., metastases from other sites, are actually the most common malignancies of bones and outnumber the primary tumors 10 to 1.

Each individual type of bone tumor usually has the following:

- Characteristic radiological features
- Distinct peak age incidence
- Specific predilection for anatomical site
- Typical histological features

In view of the above facts, it is imperative that the definitive pathological diagnosis of bone tumors be made only after the clinical and radiological data have been correlated with the gross and microscopic findings.

Typical anatomical sites of the most important bone tumors are shown in Diagram 17.7. Selected important facts about bone tumors are summarized in Table 17.1.

Table 17.1
Bone Tumors

Tumor	Age	Location	Histology	Clinical Behavior
Osteoma	40–50	Skull and facial bones	Mature lamellar bone	Benign
Osteoid osteoma	10–20	Diaphysis of long bones and short bones	Osteoid, osteoblasts	Benign
Osteosarcoma	10–25	Metaphysis of long bones	Osteoblasts osteoid, bone	Malignant
Chondroma	10–40	Hands, feet, ribs	Cartilage	Benign
Chondrosarcoma	30–60	Axial skeleton, metaphysis of long bones	Immature cartilage	Malignant
Ewing sarcoma	5–25	Diaphysis of long bone	Small undifferentiated cells	Malignant
Giant cell tumor	20–40	Metaphysis and epiphysis of long bones (around knee)	Giant cell and spindle mononuclear cells	Benign, may recur and be malignant
Metastases	50–90	Any place	Variable; most often adenocarcinoma	Malignant

Chondromas are cartilaginous nodules located in the medullary cavity; they are also called *enchondromas* because of their location and are composed of mature cartilage cells without atypia (Fig. 17.12). Solitary enchondromas are innocuous. Multiple enchondromas typical of *Ollier* or *Maffucci syndrome* tend to give rise to chondrosarcomas in almost 50% of cases and should be watched carefully.

Osteoid osteoma is a benign tumor, usually 1 cm or less in diameter, composed of osteoid. Histologically, the osteoid is lined by osteoblasts and surrounded by fibrous tissue (Fig. 17.13). The tumor is encased by dense bone and appears as a well circumscribed, punched-out lesion with dense margins on radiograph. Tumors composed of mature compact bone are called **osteomas** (Fig. 17.14).

Giant cell tumors are mostly benign but locally aggressive tumors that tend to recur if not removed completely. Giant cell tumors are composed of mononuclear and fibroblast-like cells admixed with giant multinucleated giant cells resembling osteoclasts (Fig. 17.15). In about 10% of cases, the tumors are composed of highly atypical fibroblastic cells and are, thus, classified as sarcomas.

Osteosarcoma is a malignant mesenchymal tumor composed of bone-forming cells. Osteosarcomas occur in several histological variants, all of which contain, however, the diagnostic foci of osteoid or woven bone directly produced by tumor cells (Fig. 17.16). Tumor cell populations can vary and could include spindle-shaped cells (resembling fibroblasts or osteoblasts), small undifferentiated cells, or large multinucleated giant cells. Histological subclassification of osteosarcomas has no clinical significance.

Chondrosarcomas are malignant tumors of cartilaginous cells. Two-thirds of tumors originate de novo, usually in bones of the trunk (pelvis, vertebrae, and ribs) and adjacent proximal ends of long bones of the extremities. These are called *primary chondrosarcomas*. The remaining tumors are considered *secondary chondrosarcomas*, evolving from pre-existing chondromas.

In contrast to osteosarcomas, which are all highly malignant, chondrosarcoma may be of low, intermediate, or high grade. The well differentiated chondrosarcomas resemble normal cartilage. The signs of malignancy include nuclear atypia, enlarged nuclei, and multinucleation (Fig. 17.17). In contrast to normal cartilage cells, each of which is located in a single lacuna, low-grade chondrosarcomas often contain more than one cell in each lacuna. High-grade tumors show marked nuclear pleomorphism. Many tumor cells appear undifferentiated, resembling fibroblasts or nonspecific mesenchymal cells.

Ewing sarcoma is an undifferentiated small cell bone tumor of undetermined origin. The tumor originates in the medullary cavity in the diaphysis of long bones, then infiltrates through the cortical bone and extends into the adjacent soft tissues. About 25% patients have multiple lesions. Tumors of identical histological appearance also may originate in soft tissues (*extraosseous Ewing sarcoma*).

Histologically, Ewing sarcoma consists of sheets of small cells. The cells have relatively uniform round nuclei, scant cytoplasm, and no distinct cell borders (Fig. 17.18). There is no intercellular stroma except at the periphery of cell islands and around the blood vessels. Areas of necrosis may be prominent. Tumor cells contain cytoplasmic glycogen that can be demonstrated with the PAS stain.

Metastases are the most common malignant tumors of bone. The most common primary tumors that metastasize to bones are: lungs, breast, prostate, kidneys, and thyroid. Histologically, the bone lesions contain tumor cells and variable amounts of fibrosis (Fig. 17.19). The surrounding bone shows signs of bone destruction ("osteolytic lesions") and/or reactive new bone formation ("osteoblastic lesions").

Joint Diseases

The diseases affecting the joints are caused by:

- Trauma—e.g., luxation
- Degeneration of cartilage—e.g., degenerative joint disease or osteoarthritis
- Infection—e.g., pyogenic arthritis
- Immunological injury—e.g., rheumatoid arthritis
- Metabolic disorders—e.g., gout

The most important of these diseases are degenerative joint disease, also known as osteoarthritis, rheumatoid arthritis, pigmented villonodular synovitis, and gout.

Osteoarthritis is a degenerative joint disease caused by wear and tear and biochemical change in the articular cartilage (Diagram 17.8).

The primary site of injury is the articular cartilage. Histologically, the cartilage shows fraying, irregular thinning, and disintegration (Fig. 17.20). The degenerated cartilage may become detached and may appear as free-floating intra-articular bodies (*"joint mice"*). The denuded articular bone surface may be covered with fibrous tissue. The underlying bone, now unprotected by the cartilage layer, is exposed to additional stress and often shows degenerative changes such as *cysts* and restructuring of the trabeculae. On the lateral sides of the joint surface, new bone appears in the form of *osteophytes*. Typically, there is no inflammation in the joint or in the periarticular connective tissue.

Rheumatoid arthritis is a systemic immune disorder of unknown etiology that affects joints (Diagram 17.9), as well as many other organs. Histologically, rheumatoid arthritis manifests itself with chronic inflammation of the synovium, i.e., chronic synovitis (Fig. 17.21). The synovial membrane is infiltrated with lymphocytes and plasma cells, which often form prominent aggregates and may be arranged into lymphoid follicles. The synovial lining cells proliferate with the underlying connective tissue cells, forming villous projections that extend into the joint cavity. These fronds are traumatized during joint movement, which results in intra-articular bleeding, further inflammation, and degenerative joint changes. Scavenger macrophages are attracted to the inflamed synovium, which transforms into granulation tissue called *pannus* that covers the joint surface. Acute inflammatory cells are not prominent in the pannus, although they are often seen in the intra-articular exudate.

The inflammatory process tends to spread to the surrounding connective tissue, which presents clinically as swelling and tenderness. The interposition of pannus between the articular surfaces limits joint movement. Ultimately, the joint is immobilized as the pannus undergoes fibrosis and healing. In joints attached to one another, this stiffening and ultimate loss of mobility results in *ankylosis*.

Rheumatoid arthritis is a systemic disease and it may cause lesions in the connective tissue components of other organs besides the joints. The hallmark of rheumatoid arthritis in subcutaneous tissues is the rheumatoid nodules (Fig. 17.22). These nodules have a central area of fibrinoid necrosis surrounded by palisading histiocytes and varying numbers of lymphocytes and plasma cells.

Pigmented villonodular synovitis is considered an idiopathic inflammatory process by some authorities and a benign neoplastic proliferation of synovial tissue by others. Clinically, it presents as painful swelling of joints, the cavity of which is obliterated by exuberant villonodular synovium.

Histologically, the synovium transforms into fronds (villi), which are densely infiltrated with hemosiderin-laden macrophages, foam cells, and occasional multinucleated giant cells. The lining synovial cells may appear hyperplastic (Fig. 17.23), but otherwise, there is no evidence that this lesion is neoplastic.

Gout is a term encompassing several metabolic disorders marked by hyperuricemia. Crystals of uric acid are deposited in the subcutaneous connective tissue, in the periosteum, and especially in the joint capsule. Arthritis is thus a common feature of gout and is the presenting symptom in most patients.

Etiologically, gout is classified as *primary* or *secondary*. The cause of primary gout is not known. Secondary gout is related to overproduction of uric acid in various diseases, such as leukemia treated with cytotoxic drugs or inadequate excretion of uric acid, as in chronic renal disease.

An excess of uric acid in circulation results in the deposition of urate crystals in the connective tissue of many organs but most prominently in joints and the subcutis. The acute arthritis is mediated by polymorphonuclear leukocytes, which are attracted to the joint by the chemotactic uric acid crystals. The attacks tend to recur, resulting in chronic arthritis. Chronic arthritis is characterized by massive tumor-like deposits of uric acid crystals. This nodular mass, surrounded by macrophages, fibroblasts, lymphocytes, and occasional giant cells, is called *tophus* (Fig. 17.24). The uric acid crystals in the tophus are birefringent under polarized light.

PLATE 17.1. DEVELOPMENTAL DISORDERS

Figure 17.1. Achondroplasia. The cartilage cells do not form columns. The zone in which cartilage cells have hypertrophied is relatively thin.

Figure 17.2. Osteogenesis imperfecta. Bone from a stillborn infant with multiple fractures. The bone consists of irregularly shaped trabeculae composed of matrix that lacks any lamellar structure. The surrounding stroma appears fibrotic. The cells included in the matrix that stains blue with hematoxylin are considered osteoblasts.

Figure 17.3. Osteopetrosis. The bone of this child shows irregularly shaped, thick trabeculae of the spongiosa composed of osteoid and calcified bone. The marrow spaces are reduced.

Figure 17.4. Fibrous dysplasia. The lesion consists of bone trabeculae surrounded by fibrous tissue. There are no obvious osteoblasts surrounding the trabeculae, which seem to arise through osseous metaplasia of fibroblastic stroma.

Diagram 17.2. Developmental disorders of the bone. A. Normal growing bone. Epiphysial cartilage cells form columns and undergo hypertrophy and form the matrix for calcification. Osteoclasts remove provisionally calcified cartilage, and osteoblasts form osteoid, which calcifies to become bone. **B.** Achondroplasia. The growth plate is marrow. The cartilage cells do not form the typical columns. Calcification at the innermost zone of cartilage is irregular. There is little osteoclastic and osteoblastic activity in the zone of endochondral ossification. Compact bone is of normal thickness. **C.** Osteogenesis imperfecta. The cortex is thin. The trabeculae in the spongiosa are thin, irregularly distributed, and surrounded by osteoblasts and fibrous tissue. There is an increase in the number of osteocytes. **D.** Osteopetrosis. The cortical and spongy bone are thickened, and the marrow spaces are reduced.

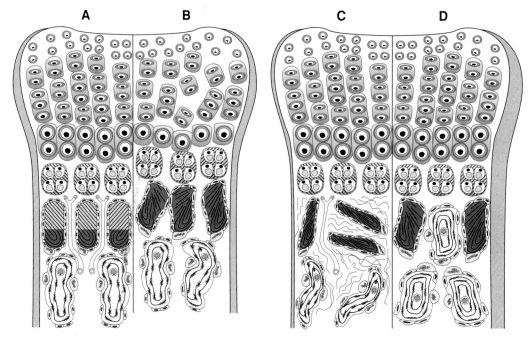

A B   C D

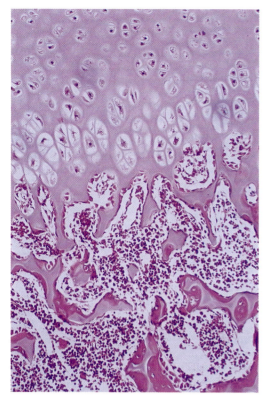

Figure 17.1

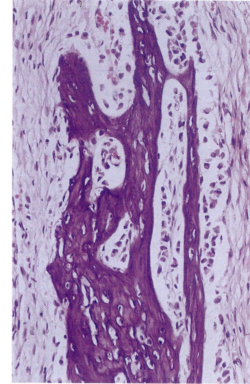

Figure 17.2

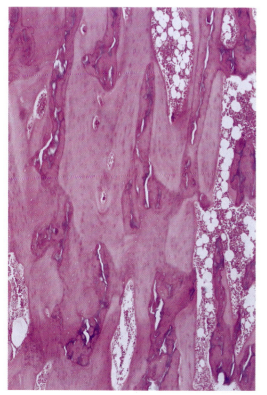

Figure 17.3

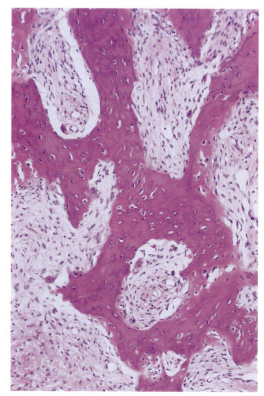

Figure 17.4

PLATE 17.2. METABOLIC DISORDERS

Figure 17.5. Osteoporosis. The trabeculae and cortical bone are thin, especially in parts of this cross-section of the femoral head.

Figure 17.6. Osteomalacia. The bone trabeculae consist predominantly of unmineralized osteoid (brownish-pink). The mineralized bone stains green.

Figure 17.7. Rickets. A. The widened growth plate contains disorganized cartilage columns and osteoid. Irregular bone trabeculae are seen in the lower part of the figure. **B.** Special stain for calcium shows that the bone consists of unmineralized matrix (red) and only minimal calcified tissue (black).

Diagram 17.3. Metabolic bone diseases. A. Normal bone. The cortex and trabeculae of spongiosa are relatively thick. Osteoblasts and osteoclasts are present on the surfaces of trabeculae and endosteal cortical bone in a ratio of 10:1. **B.** Osteoporosis. Cortex and trabeculae are thinner but well mineralized. Osteoblasts and osteoclasts are present in normal numbers. **C.** Osteomalacia. The cortical bone and trabeculae appear of normal thickness, but are composed mostly of osteoid.

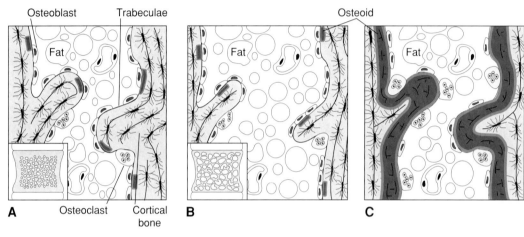

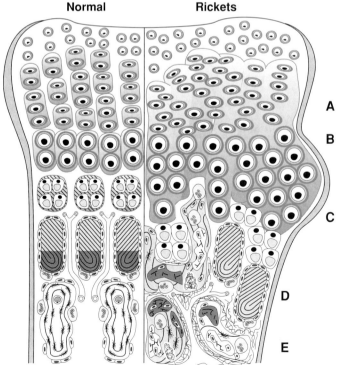

Diagram 17.4. Rickets. A. The cartilage cells do not form columns, but are arranged into irregular nests. **B.** Lateral growth of cartilage cells leads to widening of growth plate. **C.** The cartilage cells do not calcify, and the zone of provisional calcification of cartilage is not formed. **D.** Osteoid formation is not impeded. However, since the osteoclasts cannot remove the uncalcified osteoid, there is excess of osteoid, which appears to be arranged into broad plates. **E.** Bone trabeculae appears irregular, partly because of the irregularities of ossification, and partly because of deformation by mechanical forces.

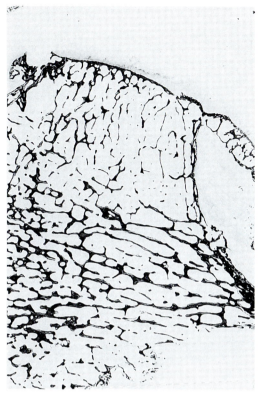

Figure 17.5

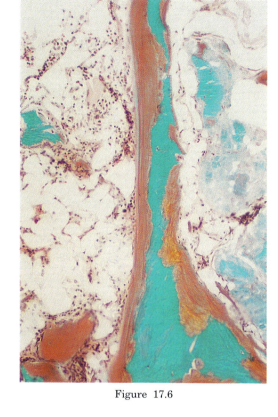

Figure 17.6

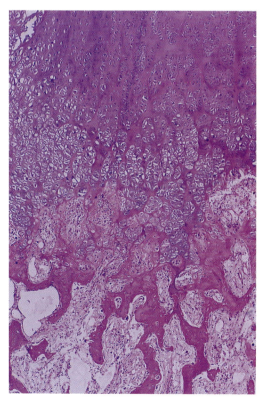

Figure 17.7A

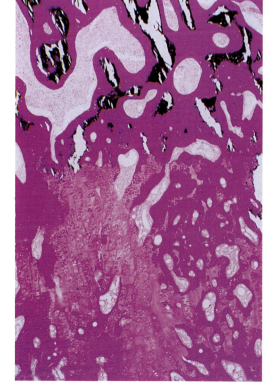

Figure 17.7B

PLATE 17.3. METABOLIC DISORDERS

Figure 17.8.   Osteitis fibrosa secondary to hyperparathyroidism. A. Demineralization of the trabeculae is associated with increased osteoclastic activity and fibrosis of the marrow. The mineralized bone is green, and the osteoid red. **B.** Brown tumor of hyperparathyroidism is composed of multinucleated osteoclasts and mononuclear cells, macrophages, and fibroblasts.

Figure 17.9.   Osteitis deformans (Paget disease). A. In early stages of the disease, osteolytic changes predominate. The bone spicules are surrounded by an increased number of osteoclasts. **B.** The late stages of Paget disease are characterized by osteosclerosis. In this slide, osteoid is red and the calcified bone green.

Diagram 17.5.   Osteitis fibrosa caused by hyperparathyroidism. A. The outer cortex is ragged, and all the bone surfaces contain an increased amount of osteoid. Osteoclasts are present in increased numbers, and the marrow shows fibrosis. **B.** Brown tumor of hyperparathyroidism. This destructive expansive bone lesion is composed of osteoclasts, macrophages, and fibroblasts.

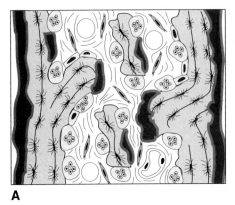

A

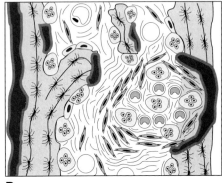

B

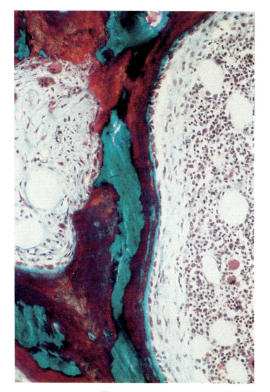

Figure 17.8A

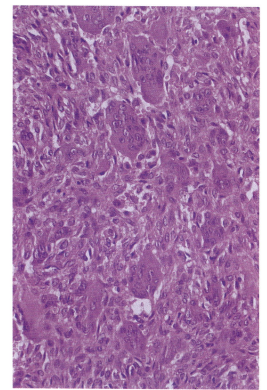

Figure 17.8B

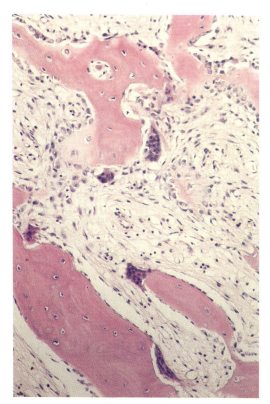

Figure 17.9A

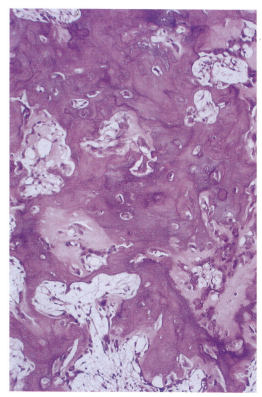

Figure 17.9B

PLATE 17.4. OSTEOMYELITIS AND FRACTURES

Figure 17.10.   Osteomyelitis. A. Acute suppurative osteomyelitis is characterized by an accumulation of neutrophils in the marrow spaces that are surrounded by thickened bone. **B.** Chronic osteomyelitis is characterized by fibrosis. Inflammatory infiltrates consist of plasma cells, lymphocytes, and macrophages.

Figure 17.11.   Healing of fracture. The healing occurs in several continuous phases. **A.** Callus consists of fibrous tissue and newly formed bone. **B.** Intramembranous ossification within a callus.

Diagram 17.6.   Healing of fracture. Left. Procallus. The area of fracture has been invaded by granulation tissue, which has replaced the extravasated blood and has removed the cell detritus that remained after injury. **Middle.** Callus. Bone spicules are formed by calcification of the trabeculae of osteoid and/or endochondral ossification. **Right.** Remodeling of the callus. The haphazardly arranged bone trabeculae are restructured, and the normal cortical and cancellous bones are reformed.

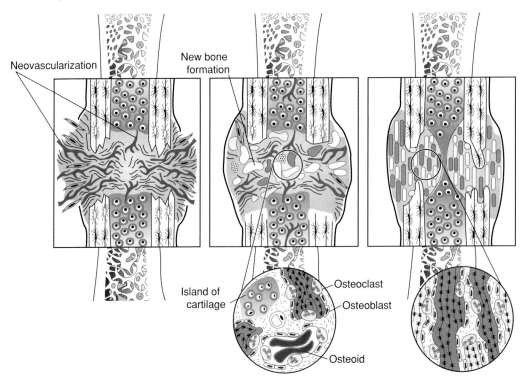

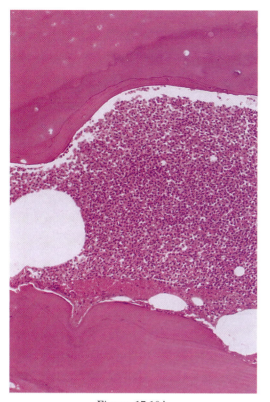

Figure 17.10A

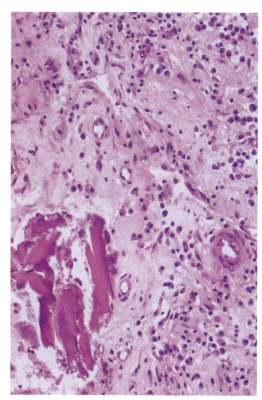

Figure 17.10B

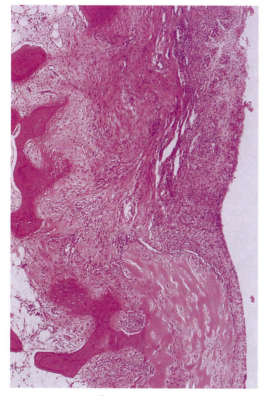

Figure 17.11A

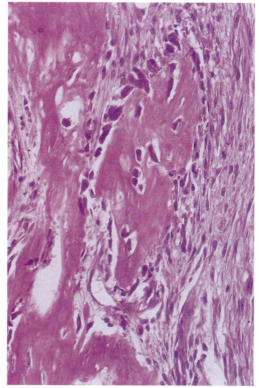

Figure 17.11B

PLATE 17.5. BENIGN BONE TUMORS

Figure 17.12. **Enchondroma.** The tumor is composed of well-differentiated chondrocytes.

Figure 17.13. **Osteoid osteoma.** The tumor is composed of anastomosing trabeculae of osteoid rimmed by osteoblasts and surrounded by fibroblastic stroma.

Figure 17.14. **Osteoma.** The tumor is composed of mature bone.

Figure 17.15. **Giant cell tumor of bone.** The tumor is composed of multinucleated giant cells resembling osteoclasts and fibroblastic mononuclear cells.

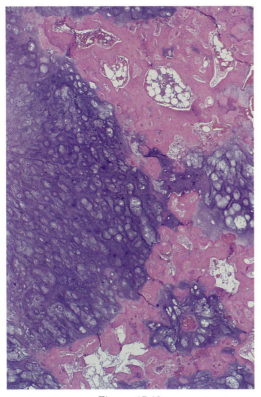

Figure 17.12

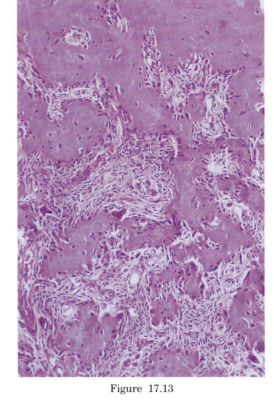

Figure 17.13

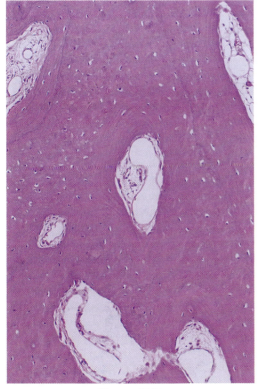

Figure 17.14

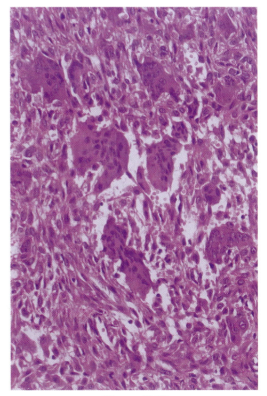

Figure 17.15

PLATE 17.6. MALIGNANT BONE TUMORS

Figure 17.16. Osteosarcoma. The tumor is composed of atypical spindle-shaped cells resembling osteoblasts and fibroblasts. The osteoid is disorganized and there is no true bone formation.

Figure 17.17. Chondrosarcoma. The tumor is composed of atypical cartilaginous cells.

Figure 17.18. Ewing sarcoma. The tumor is composed of uniform small cells with scant cytoplasm. The tumor cells occupy the medullary spaces between the trabeculae of the diaphysis.

Figure 17.19. Metastasis to the bone. This adenocarcinoma is embedded in dense connective tissue between bone trabeculae.

Diagram 17.7. Bone tumors. The most common anatomical sites of malignant bone tumors. Osteosarcomas arise in metaphysis, chondrosarcomas in the metaphysis, Ewing sarcomas in the diaphysis, and giant cell tumors in the epiphysis of long bones.

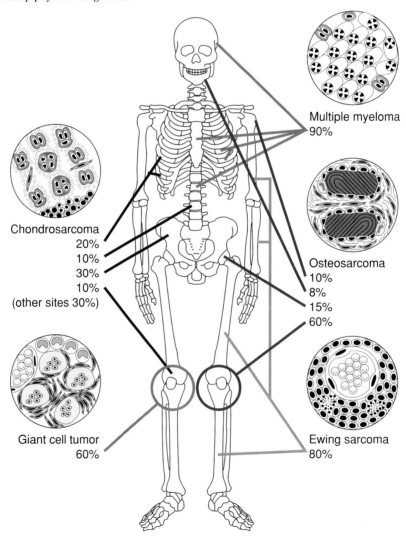

Multiple myeloma
90%

Chondrosarcoma
20%
10%
30%
10%
(other sites 30%)

Osteosarcoma
10%
8%
15%
60%

Giant cell tumor
60%

Ewing sarcoma
80%

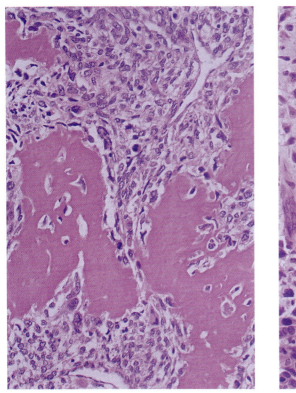

Figure 17.16

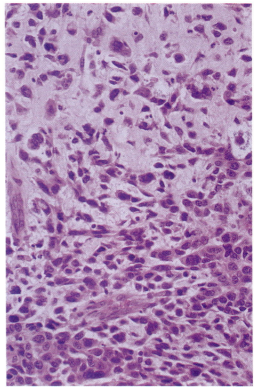

Figure 17.17

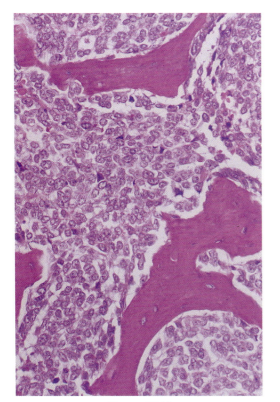

Figure 17.18

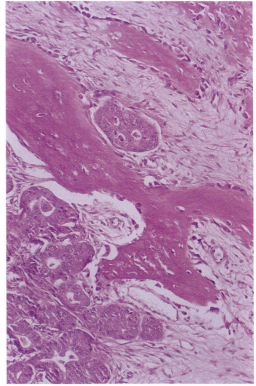

Figure 17.19

PLATE 17.7. OSTEOARTHRITIS

Figure 17.20. Osteoarthritis. A. Flaking of the cartilage. **B.** The subchondral bone appears irregular and contains cystic spaces. **C.** Sclerotic subchondral bone. **D.** Osteophytes (upper part of the figure) are formed on the lateral side of the joint. (Courtesy of Dr. Roger Smith, Cincinnati.)

Diagram 17.8. Osteoarthritis. Degenerative changes of the articular cartilage are accompanied by destructive and reactive changes in the adjacent bone. **A.** Erosion of the cartilage surface. **B.** Detached fragment of intraarticular cartilage ("joint mice"). **C.** Osteosclerosis. **D.** Cystic changes in the bone. **E.** Osteophyte.

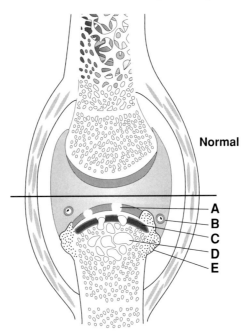

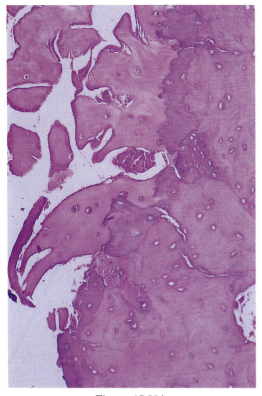

Figure 17.20A

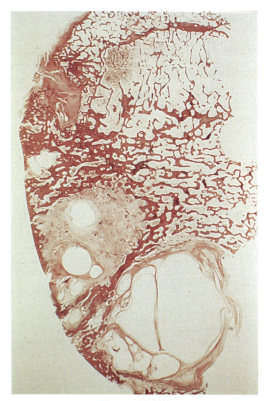

Figure 17.20B

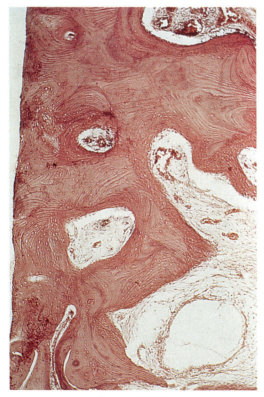

Figure 17.20C

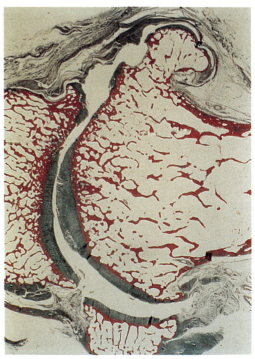

Figure 17.20D

PLATE 17.8. RHEUMATOID ARTHRITIS

Figure 17.21.   Rheumatoid arthritis. A. Villous protrusions of synovial membrane project into the joint cavity. **B.** The synovium is infiltrated with chronic inflammatory cells that form aggregates. **C.** At higher magnification, it is possible to see that the infiltrate consists of lymphocytes and plasma cells.

Figure 17.22.   Rheumatoid nodule from subcutaneous tissue. Central area of fibrinoid necrosis is surrounded by palisaded histiocytes.

Diagram 17.9.   Rheumatoid arthritis. Inflammation of the synovium leads to a destruction of the joint and finally results in ankylosis

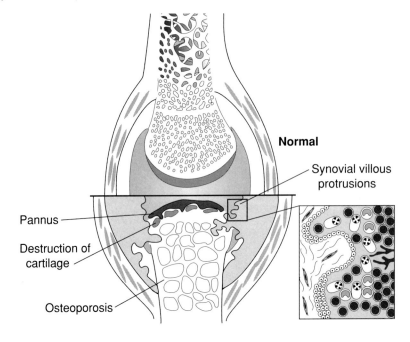

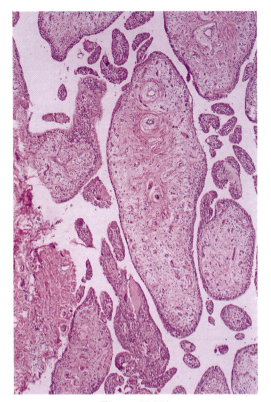

Figure 17.21A

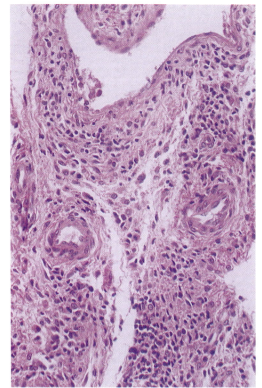

Figure 17.21B

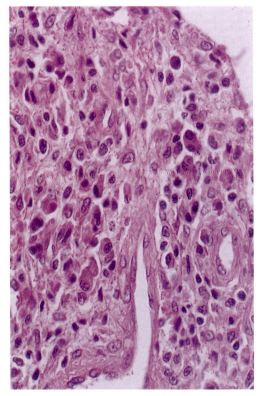

Figure 17.21C

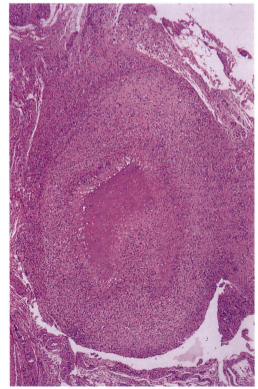

Figure 17.22

PLATE 17.9. OTHER JOINT DISEASES

Figure 17.23. Pigmented villonodular synovitis. A. Fronds of synovium densely infiltrated with inflammatory cells. **B.** At higher magnification, it is possible to identify pigment-laden macrophages and hyperplastic synovial lining cells.

Figure 17.24. Tophus. A. Uric acid accumulates in the connective tissue. **B.** Uric acid crystals are birefringent when examined under polarized light.

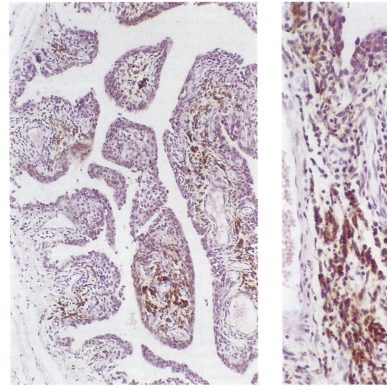

Figure 17.23A

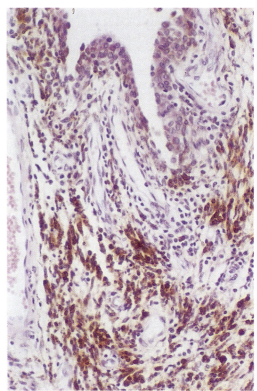

Figure 17.23B

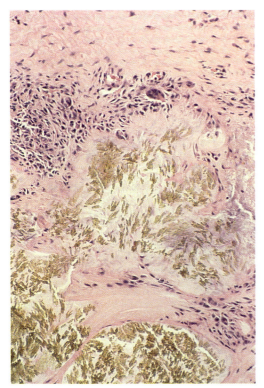

Figure 17.24A

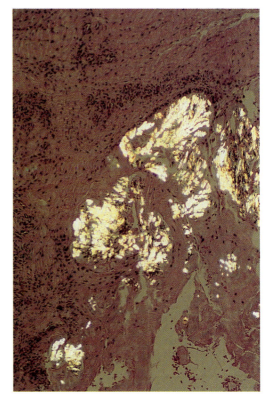

Figure 17.24B

NOTES

CHAPTER 18

Skeletal Muscles

NORMAL HISTOLOGY

Skeletal muscle is composed of striated muscle fibers and a connective tissue framework that extends into tendons on periosteum and links the muscles to the bones (Diagram 18.1). Each fascicle is enclosed by a connective tissue sheath that contains nerves and blood vessels.

Individual muscle fibers are enervated by branches of motor neuron axons. The nerve determines whether the fiber will have properties of slow-twitch (type I) or fast-twitch (type II) fibers. These fibers are comparable to red meat of chicken legs and white meat of chicken breast; in humans, however, the fibers are intermixed in a checkerboard manner. This fiber mix can be recognized by enzyme histochemistry, a technique that differentially stains type I and type II fibers. By electron microscopy, all muscle fibers have the same features. The cytoplasm consists mostly of actin, α-actinin, and myosin filaments arranged into functional units called myofibrils. Each myofibril consists of repetitive segments called sarcomeres. Within a sarcomere, one may identify the lighter I band and a denser A band, which give the muscle its striated appearance on light microscopy.

OVERVIEW OF PATHOLOGY

The most important diseases of the muscle are:

- Neurogenic muscle diseases, secondary to injury of motor neurons
- Primary myopathies, such as muscular dystrophy
- Inflammatory muscle diseases, such as polymyositis

The response of muscle to injury occurs in two predictable patterns. These can be recognized in muscle biopsy as the following two patterns:

- Neuropathic pattern
- Myopathic pattern

Neuropathic pattern is a typical consequence of denervation of the muscle (Diagram 18.2). **Myopathic pattern** is seen in primary muscle diseases such as muscular dystrophy, congenital inborn errors of metabolism, and myopathies of unknown etiology (Diagram 18.3).

It should be noted that many muscle diseases, such as myasthenia gravis, present with functional abnormalities that are not accompanied by morphological changes. In such diseases, the muscle appears normal and the muscle biopsy is of no direct diagnostic value.

Denervation Atrophy

Denervation of muscle, i.e., loss of motor neural stimuli, results in muscle atrophy that presents in a typical *neuropathic pattern* (see Diagram 18.2). Examples of denervation atrophy are muscle changes secondary to transection of the upper motor neuron and lower spinal cord motor neuron by trauma, loss of distal motor neuron in the spinal cord in poliomyelitis, and loss of upper neuron due to apoplexy.

Denervation-caused atrophy of skeletal muscles can occur in three forms: single-cell atrophy, group atrophy, and atrophy of entire fascicles. Single-cell atrophy is found under several circumstances.

Early or mild denervation atrophy is characterized by single-cell atrophy. Both type I and type II fibers may be affected at random. The atrophic fibers are angulated and compressed by adjacent normal muscle fibers (Fig. 18.1). Loss of axonal branches, as in diabetic neuropathy, results in atrophy of individual muscle fibers, which are scattered at random. Atrophy of scattered muscle fibers, usually selectively involving type II fibers, may be caused by prolonged inactivity, steroid treatment, and many nonspecific factors.

Group atrophy results from injury of small nerves or their branches. *Fascicular atrophy* reflects a more extensive denervation in which the entire muscle fascicle has lost its enervation and has undergone atrophy. In fascicular atrophy, all the muscle fibers within a motor unit are uniformly small. Such atrophy occurs in spinal motor neuron diseases. For example, it is typically found in *Werdnig-Hoffmann disease* or infantile spinal muscular atrophy.

Myopathy

Muscular dystrophies (see Diagram 18.3) are genetic disorders that present in several clinically distinct forms, such as *Duchenne* *dystrophy*, *Becker dystrophy*, and *facioscapulohumeral dystrophy*. All dystrophies show the same histological changes, which, however, vary in intensity and extent.

Duchenne muscular dystrophy is a lethal disorder involving the mutation or deletion of gene that encodes a structural protein called *dystrophin*. The disease is inherited as a recessive Mendelian sex-linked trait. The symptoms begin in childhood with involvement of pelvic and shoulder girdle muscles. The disease is progressive, and death usually occurs by the age of 25 years because of respiratory paralysis.

The histological features of muscular

Diagram 18.1.   Normal skeletal muscle.

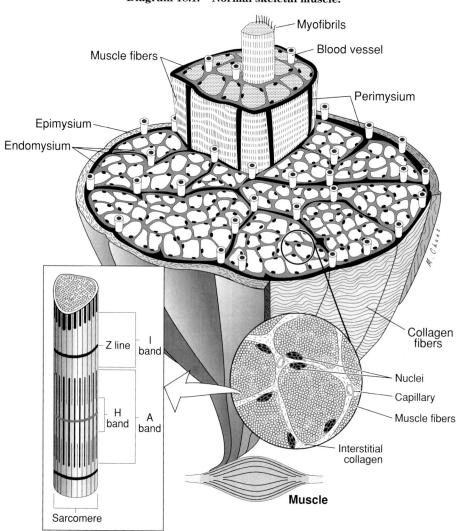

dystrophy depend on the duration of the disease. In the initial stages, there is focal muscle cell degeneration associated with hypertrophy of less affected fibers and abortive regeneration (Fig. 18.2). The degenerating muscle fibers attract scavenger cells, and the area becomes infiltrated with mononuclear macrophages. Loss of muscle fibers is accompanied by fibrosis and a replacement of destroyed muscle fibers by fat cells. Accumulation of fat cells accounts for grossly visible "pseudohypertrophy" of muscles.

Becker dystrophy is a less common and typically milder form of dystrophin gene defect. The symptoms of muscle weakness appear in adulthood. Histologically, the muscle changes are similar to those in Duchenne dystrophy but are milder (Fig. 18.3).

Limb-girdle and **facioscapulohumeral dystrophy** are milder, nonlethal muscle diseases. The muscle biopsy shows "myopathic changes" with varying degrees of muscle cell loss, atrophy, and compensatory hypertrophy.

Congenital myopathies are rare disorders that present with muscular weaknesses in infancy ("floppy baby syndrome") or childhood. Histologically, these diseases present with nonspecific changes in a myopathic pattern or show specific changes. In **glycogen storage diseases,** the fibers contain glycogen and appear clear (Fig. 18.4). **Mitochondrial myopathy** can be diagnosed only by electron microscopy (Fig. 18.5). By light microscopy, the muscle biopsy shows only nondiagnostic changes in a "myopathic pattern." *Nemaline myopathy* is characterized by fibrillar cytoplasmic bodies, "nemaline bodies" visible by light and electron microscopy (Fig. 18.6). In **myotubular myopathy,** the muscle fibers are small and have large, centrally located nuclei (Fig. 18.7).

Rhabdomyolysis

Muscle cells damaged by a variety of exogenous insults can undergo complete necrosis. Such necrosis of single muscle fibers, called rhabdomyolysis, can be induced by toxins, trauma, and even strenuous exercise. The muscle fibers lose their internal structure (Fig. 18.8) and are removed by phagocytes.

Polymyositis

Polymyositis is an autoimmune disorder of muscle that may occur in several ways:

- In an isolated form
- As a component of dermatomyositis
- As a manifestation of systemic diseases such as systemic lupus erythematosus or rheumatoid arthritis

The disease presents with proximal muscle weakness, recurrent tenderness, and episodic pain and elevated serum creatine kinase due to muscle cell destruction. Histologically, the findings vary (Fig. 18.9). One may find single-muscle degeneration and necrosis. Cell death elicits a phagocytic response. The inflammatory cell infiltrates vary and may be abundant or sparse. Degeneration and regeneration of muscle fibers are also evident but depend on the duration of the disease.

Infectious Myositis

Muscle inflammation may be caused by identifiable pathogens. *Viruses,* such as *Coxsackievirus,* cause changes indistinguishable from those of polymyositis. *Bacteria* may cause suppurative inflammation and abscesses. *Parasites* such as *Trichinella spiralis* can be readily identified, encysted in the muscle (Fig. 18 10). The cysts of the parasite may be surrounded by an acute inflammatory infiltrate, rich in eosinophils, or by fibrosis and chronic inflammatory cells. Ultimately, the remnants of the parasite may calcify.

PLATE 18.1. NEUROGENIC ATROPHY OF THE MUSCLES

Figure 18.1. Neurogenic atrophy. A. In early stages of atrophy, the fibers are smaller and angulated because of the compression by adjacent normal fibers. **B.** Inactivity leads to selective atrophy of type II muscle fibers. Type II fibers appear darker in this specimen, which was processed by enzyme histochemistry. **C.** Group atrophy seen in amyotrophic lateral sclerosis is due to loss of motor neurons innervating one area. **D.** Fascicular atrophy, as seen in Werdnig-Hoffmann disease. This spinal atrophy affects anterior spinal cord neurons and causes atrophy of entire fascicles of denervated muscles. The adjacent muscle fibers appear normal.

Diagram 18.2. Denervation of muscle due to nerve injury with subsequent reinnervation. A. The normal muscle is composed of a mixture of type I and type II fibers. **B.** Transection of nerve causes atrophy of denervated muscle cells. **C.** Reinnervation leads to fiber type grouping because the nerve sprouts reach muscle fibers in groups and thus make them all of the same type—either fast or slow.

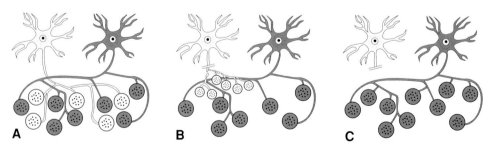

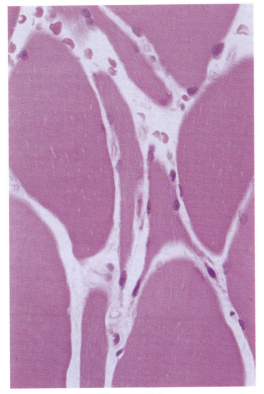

Figure 18.1A

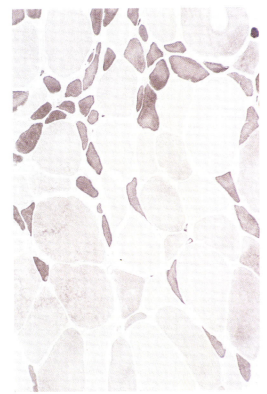

Figure 18.1B

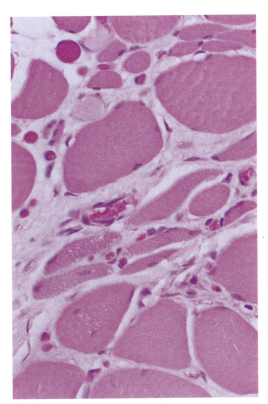

Figure 18.1C

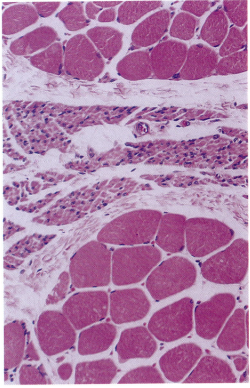

Figure 18.1D

PLATE 18.2. MUSCULAR DYSTROPHY

Figure 18.2.   Duchenne muscular dystrophy. A. The early changes include muscle cell degeneration, accompanied by phagocytic cell infiltration of the muscle and compensatory hypertrophy of preserved fibers. **B.** Endomysial fibrosis is prominent in advanced disease. **C.** Pseudohypertrophy of late stages of the disease is due to fat cells replacing the muscle fibers.

Figure 18.3.   Becker dystrophy. The disease cannot be histologically distinguished from Duchenne dystrophy except that Becker dystrophy is milder. The muscle biopsy of a teenager shown here reveals marked variation in size and shape of muscle fibers combined with interstitial fibrosis, i.e., a myopathic pattern.

Diagram 18.3.   Myopathic pattern of muscle injury. A. Normal muscle. **B.** Duchenne muscular dystrophy. **C.** Polymyositis.

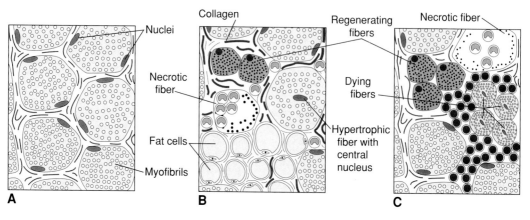

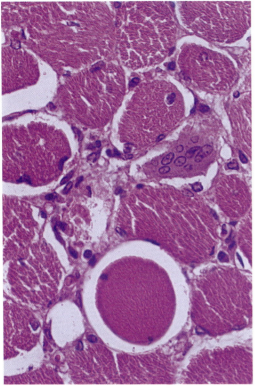

Figure 18.2A

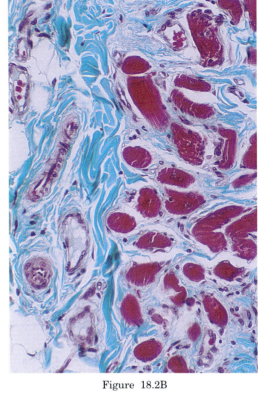

Figure 18.2B

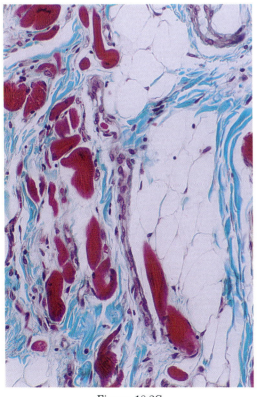

Figure 18.2C

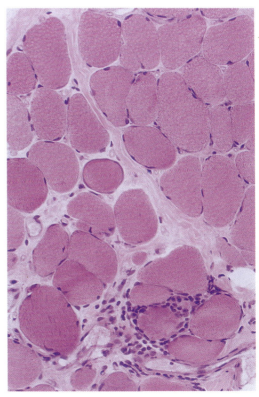

Figure 18.3

PLATE 18.3. MYOPATHY

Figure 18.4.   Glycogen storage disease. The muscle fibers appear clear because they contain large amounts of glycogen.

Figure 18.5.   Mitochondrial myopathy. Electron microscopy shows mitrochondrial abnormalities and inclusions.

Figure 18.6.   Nemaline myopathy. A. The muscle cells contain cytoplasmic inclusions ("nemaline bodies") that appear dark blue on this trichrome-stained slide. **B.** Electron microscopy shows nemaline bodies composed of filaments equivalent to Z-line material.

Figure 18.7.   Myotubular myopathy. Many fibers appear small and rounded, and have centrally located nuclei.

Figure 18.8.   Rhabdomyolysis. The necrotic muscle fiber, which has a fragmented internal structure, is surrounded by normal fibers.

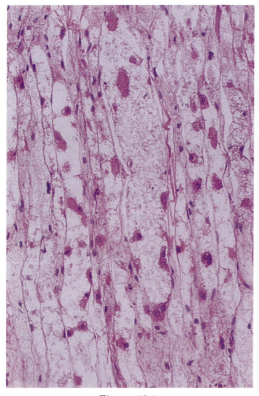

Figure 18.4

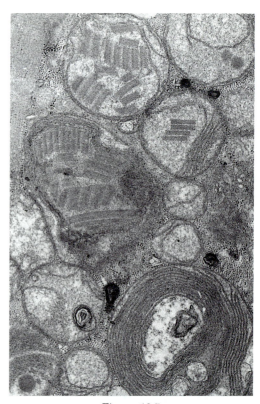

Figure 18.5

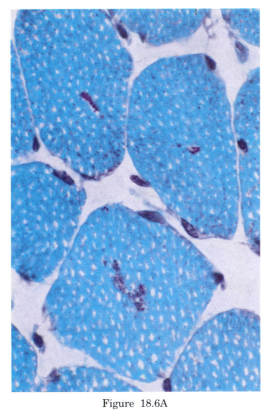

Figure 18.6A

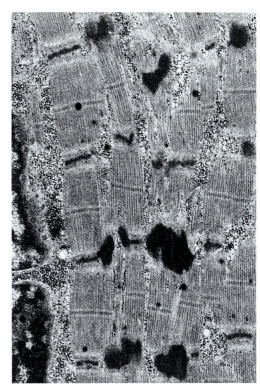

Figure 18.6B

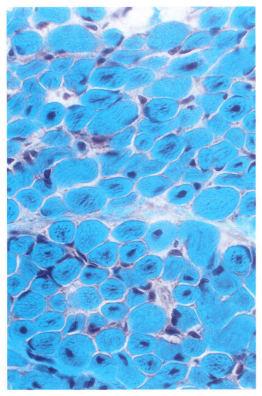

Figure 18.7

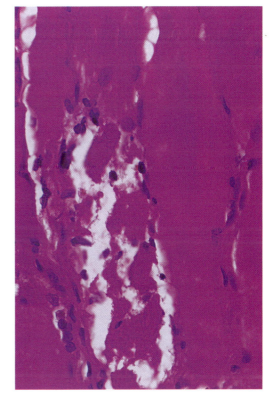

Figure 18.8

PLATE 18.4. MYOSITIS

Figure 18.9.   Polymyositis. A. Single-muscle fiber degeneration. **B.** Foci of inflammation surround necrotic muscle fibers. **C.** Extensive inflammation. The phagocytic cells replace muscle fibers, and the preserved muscle fibers show reactive changes as evidenced by central location of their nuclei. **D.** Chronic myositis. There is fibrosis and interstitial inflammation.

Figure 18.10.   Myositis caused by *Trichinella spiralis*. A. In early stages of infection, the parasite is surrounded by macrophages and degenerating muscle cells. **B.** In chronic infection, the encysted parasite is surrounded by fibrotic muscles.

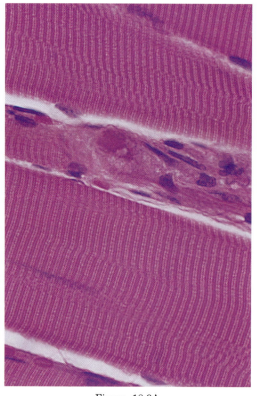

Figure 18.9A

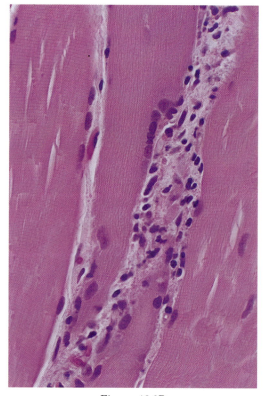

Figure 18.9B

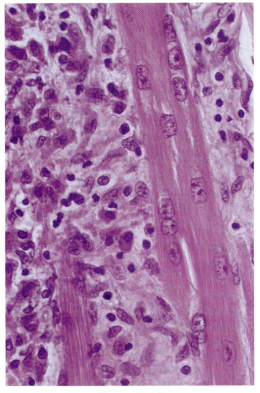

Figure 18.9C

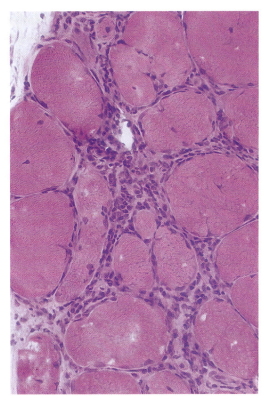

Figure 18.9D

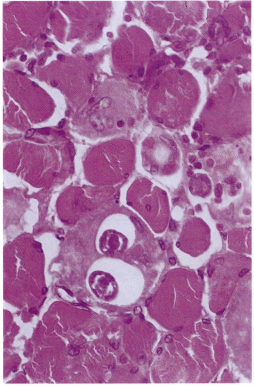

Figure 18.10A

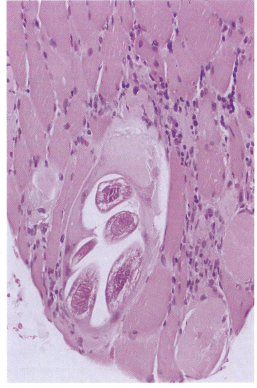

Figure 18.10B

NOTES

CHAPTER 19

Nervous System

NORMAL HISTOLOGY

The nervous system can be divided into three parts: the central nervous system (CNS), comprising the brain and spinal cord; the peripheral nervous system (PNS), which includes the peripheral nerves; and the autonomic nervous system (ANS), which includes the autonomic ganglia, paraganglia, and related nerves.

The principal cells of the nervous system are the neurons and glia cells (Diagram 19.1). The *neuron* has a body called perikaryon, from which the cytoplasm extends, forming the axon and dendrites. The cranial and the peripheral nerves are the cytoplasmic extensions of central and spinal neurons.

Glia cells are classified as astrocytes, oligodendroglia cells, microglia cells, and ependymal cells. The *astrocytes* are the most prominent glial cells, and they can be classified as protoplasmatic or fibrillar. The *oligodendroglia* cells surround the neurons in the cortex and form the myelin sheath around the axons in the white matter. The *microglia* cells are phagocytic and are the CNS equivalents of macrophages. The ependymal cells are cuboidal polarized cells lining the ventricles and the central canal of the spinal cord.

The surface of the brain is covered with *meninges,* which consist of three layers. pia, arachnoid, and dura mater. The ventricles contain *choroid plexus,* which has a papillary structure and consists of a central fibrovascular core and a cuboidal cell lining.

REACTION OF CNS CELLS TO INJURY

The principal cells of the CNS differ in their response to injury, as illustrated in Figures 19.1 to 19.5.

Neuron can be injured by anoxia, viruses, or toxic substances. Injury of the perikaryon or the axon results in cytoplasmic swelling and the degranulation of ribosomes from the rough endoplasmic reticu-

lum. This loss of RNA is seen as disappearance of cytoplasmic basophilia (bluishness), which is called *chromatolysis* (Fig. 19.1).

Neurons are a frequent site of *accumulation* of unprocessed metabolites (e.g., glycolipids) in congenital metabolic disorders such as Tay-Sachs disease or Niemann-Pick disease. *Granulovacuolar degeneration* of neurons is seen in Alzheimer disease, but can occur in other conditions as well. *Viral inclusions* are found in the cytoplasm in rabies, whereas herpesvirus and cytomegalovirus cause intranuclear inclusions. Atrophic neurons, common in the brains of old people, have less cytoplasm than normal neurons do. Hypoxic neurons have eosinophilic cytoplasm and, if the hypoxia persists ultimately, the neurons will lose their nuclei as well. Transection of axons leads to degeneration of distal segment (*Wallerian degeneration*). If the perikaryon survives, it sprouts a new axon, which will extend across the site of transection and reform the damaged nerve.

Glial cells respond to most forms of brain injury by accumulating in the lesion, or by changing their shape and function. Gliosis, i.e., an increased number of glia cells, usually includes a prominent astrocytic response (Fig. 19.2). Cytoplasmic astrocytes transform into *gemistocytes* (i.e., cells with prominent cytoplasm), whereas fibrillar astrocytes contribute to the formation of glial scars. Glial scars are soft because they consist of cytoplasmic processes of astrocytes. Firm fibrous scars do not form readily in the brain because the brain does not contain fibroblasts, except in the larger vessels.

Astrocytes also react to metabolic disorders. For example, in hepatic failure, the astrocytic nuclei become vacuolated and contain nuclear inclusions of glycogen. These *Alzheimer type II astrocytes,* however, are not diagnostic of liver failure, but occur in many other metabolic disorders as well.

Oligodendroglia cells respond to injury by multiplying and aggregating around the injured neurons ("satellitosis") (Fig. 19.3). Damaged oligodendroglia cells cease producing myelin, resulting in demyelination, such as in multiple sclerosis or progressive multifocal leukoencephalopathy. Demyelinated areas appear pale in slides stained with special stains for demonstrating myelinated axons.

Oligodendroglia cells can be selectively affected by certain viruses. Infected oligodendroglia cells contain intranuclear viral inclusions, as in progressive multifocal encephalopathy, a disease caused by JC papova virus.

Microglia cells are phagocytic cells that participate in the clean-up of dead and injured cells in the CNS (Fig. 19.4). Microglia cells phagocytize dead neurons (*neuronophagia*) and form glial nodules in response to viral or protozoal infections. Microglia cells found around brain infarcts or abscesses have phagocytized the lipid-rich myelin and therefore have foamy, vacuolated cytoplasm. Such cells are known by the German name "*gitter cells.*"

OVERVIEW OF PATHOLOGY

Infectious Diseases

Brain is prone to many forms of infections, which may present as *meningitis* or *encephalitis*, or more commonly in a combined form—*meningoencephalitis* (Diagram 19.2).

Meningitis may be caused by viruses or bacteria and less often by other pathogens, such as rickettsia, parasites, and fungi. *Viral*

Diagram 19.1. Components of the nervous system. The *neuron* has a large nucleus with a prominent nucleolus. The cytoplasm around the nucleus (*perikaryon*) contains granular endoplasmic reticulum (*Nissl substance*), which is basophilic in routine slides stained with hematoxylin and eosin. The dendrites and axons emanating from the perikaryon are not visible in routine slides but can be demonstrated by silver impregnation. *Astrocytes* have large vesicular nuclei and moderately abundant cytoplasm. *Oligodendroglia* cells have round nuclei surrounded by a clear cytoplasm ("fried egg" appearance). *Microglia* cells have elongated small nuclei with dense chromatin. The cytoplasmic processes of these cells form the neutrophil, which appears as eosinophilic material. The cytoplasmic processes of glia cells can be demonstrated best by silver impregnation. Ependymal cells are cuboidal and form a continuous layer.

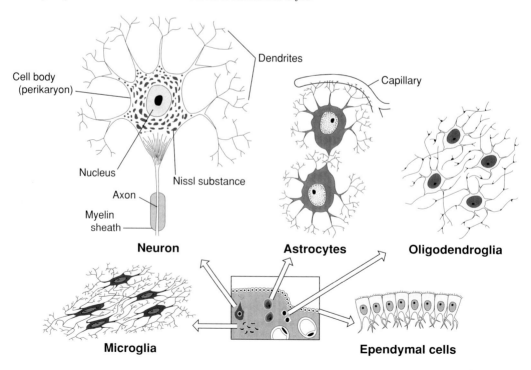

meningitis evokes a lymphocytic reaction (Fig. 19.6), whereas *bacterial meningitis* is marked by an exudate of polymorphonuclear leukocytes (Fig. 19.7). *Tuberculosis* of the meninges is a chronic meningitis characterized by the formation of caseating granulomas in the subarachnoid space. *Syphilitic meningitis*, typical of stage 3 syphilis, is characterized by infiltrates of lymphocytes and plasma cells (Fig. 19.8). Syphilis leads to meningeal fibrosis, which causes compression of axons of afferent sensory nerves where they enter the posterior spinal columns. Such nerves undergo Wallerian degeneration, and the posterior columns of the spinal cord therefore appear demyelinated and devoid of afferent axons of the spinocerebral tract. The intracerebral blood vessels are also affected, which accounts for cerebral ischemia and dementia typical of tertiary syphilis.

Encephalitis is most often caused by viruses, such as herpesvirus, neurotropic viruses such as rabies, or arthropod-borne (arbor) encephalitogenic viruses. Encephalitis due to *arboviruses* is histologically characterized by the accumulation of lymphocytes in the perivascular Virchow-Robin spaces (Fig. 19.9). *Herpesvirus infection*, the most common form of viral encephalitis today, is characterized by cellular infiltrates and focal hemorrhages secondary to the rupture of small cerebral blood vessels. The nuclei of infected neurons contain viral particles and have a ground-glass appearance in histological sections.

Measles virus may cause encephalitis in immunocompromised hosts. This *subacute sclerosing panencephalitis* is histologically recognized by the presence of intranuclear inclusions in the oligodendroglia cells (Fig 19.10).

Progressive multifocal leukoencephalopathy is a form of chronic encephalitis caused by JC papova virus. Viral inclusions can be seen in the nuclei of the infected oligodendroglia cells by electron microscopy. By light microscopy, these nuclei appear enlarged and homogeneously bluish (Fig. 19.11). The disease is associated with foci of demyelination obviously related to oligodendroglial cell injury.

Spongiform encephalopathies are caused by prions, small proteinaceous infectious agents previously known as "slow viruses." Spongiform encephalopathy includes three clinically distinct diseases, *Creutzfeldt-Jakob* disease, *kuru,* and *Gerstmann-Straussler-Sheinker syndrome*, which all show the same pathological features. Histologically, the brain contains numerous microcystic spaces in the cortical gray matter, with no evidence of inflammation (Fig. 19.12).

AIDS affects the brain directly and indirectly predisposes to secondary infection because the immunosuppression of AIDS facilitates the spread of infections to the brain.

AIDS encephalopathy caused by human immunodeficiency virus (HIV) is characterized by mild cerebral atrophy and loss of neurons accompanied by astrogliosis and accumulation of multinucleated phagocytic cells (Fig. 19.13). Secondary infections are caused by bacteria, protozoa, or fungi. Pyogenic bacteria may cause meningitis or brain abscesses (Fig. 19.14).

Toxoplasmosis of the brain is the most common protozoal complication of AIDS. The cysts and trophozoites of *Toxoplasma gondii* provoke an inflammatory reaction and lead to necrosis and hemorrhage of infected brain tissue (Fig. 19.15).

Cryptococcus neoformans is the most common fungal pathogen affecting the brain in AIDS. It usually causes encephalomeningitis. The fungi can be detected in the cerebrospinal fluid (Fig. 19.16).

Demyelinating Diseases

This term encompasses diseases characterized by selective loss of myelin: multiple sclerosis and several congenital disorders such as metachromatic leukodystrophy, Krabbe disease, and adrenoleukodystrophy.

Multiple sclerosis is a chronic demyelinating disorder of unknown etiology and pathogenesis. It is thought to be immune-mediated (Diagram 19.3). Early lesions show infiltrates of lymphocytes and macrophages, which cause the demyelination of white matter in the brain and the spinal cord (Fig. 19.17). Initial foci of demyelination ("plaques") are typically periventricular, but in later stages of the disease, demyelination becomes widespread. The axons remain preserved. Late lesions do not contain lymphocytes.

Krabbe disease, or globoid cell leukodystrophy, is a congenital deficiency of galactocerebroside β-galactosidase that results in massive demyelination of cerebral white matter. The macrophages that ingest the galactocerebroside released in this process have prominent cytoplasm and appear "globoid." These cells accumulate around the blood vessels (Fig. 19.18).

Cerebrovascular Diseases

Disturbances of cerebral circulation present clinically in several acute and chronic forms. *Stroke* is an acute cerebrovascular insufficiency caused by intracerebral hemorrhage or infarction due to vascular occlusion. *Chronic cerebral vascular insufficiency* results in progressive dementia in the elderly and a loss of other neural functions.

Cerebral hemorrhage is a typical complication of hypertension. Bleeding occurs because of rupture of small intracerebral arteries (Fig. 19.19). The extravasated blood and the resultant anoxia cause brain cell necrosis. The hemorrhagic necrotic tissue is phagocytized by microglia cells and blood-derived macrophages, and the area is transformed into a pseudocyst filled with fluid that transudates into the empty space. The surrounding tissue usually shows gliosis and contains hemosiderin-laden macrophages.

Acute brain infarct typically occurs because of the obstruction of an artery by a thrombus overlying a ruptured atheroma or by emboli that have been carried by arterial blood to the brain from the heart or large arteries. Necrosis of the brain occurs quickly because the brain is susceptible to anoxia (Fig. 19.20). Brain infarcts show liquefactive necrosis. Histologically, the infarcts are edematous and contain dead and dying ischemic neurons and cell debris.

Hypotensive cerebral infarcts are multifocal and usually affect the so-called *watershed areas,* the marginal zones supplied by the major branches of both the carotid and basilar arteries. Hypotensive infarcts may present as *laminar necrosis* involving the least perfused, innermost layers of the cortex (Fig. 19.21).

Alzheimer Disease

Alzheimer disease, the most common cause of senile dementia, is a progressive degenerative disease that affects the cerebral cortex. Alzheimer disease is characterized by cortical atrophy that can be seen on gross examination. Histological changes of Alzheimer disease are not specific, but if taken together make the diagnosis of this disease possible (Diagram 19.4). These changes include: loss of neurons, formation of neurofibrillary tangles in the pyramidal neurons, formation of neuritic plaques, and gliosis (Fig. 19.22). In addition to these diffuse changes that involve the cortex in all parts of the brain, the pyramidal neurons of the hippocampus show granulovacuolar degeneration and the formation of glassy eosinophilic cytoplasmic inclusions called Hirano bodies. Amyloid is found in the walls of the small cerebral arteries.

Metabolic, Toxic, and Degenerative Diseases

Organic diseases of the brain and spinal cord may be traced to numerous endogenous, metabolic, and exogenous toxic substances, but are often idiopathic (i.e., of unknown etiology) and are grouped under the nonspecific term of *neurodegenerative disorders*. The clinical symptoms are typical for each neurodegenerative disorders but the pathological findings are rarely unique and almost never pathognomonic. Nevertheless, the typical anatomical distribution and preferential location of lesions to parts of the CNS allow for good clinicopathological correlation (Diagram 19.5).

Alcoholic encephalopathy is partly caused by the direct effects of alcohol on nerve cells and partly related to deficiency of thiamin (vitamin B_1) in the cerebral and cerebellar cortex. The most common pathological finding is atrophy. In addition, patients who have clinical symptoms of *Wernicke syndrome* also show foci of hemorrhage into the mamillary bodies, the hypothalamus, and the periaqueductal portion of the midbrain and the tegmentum of pons (Fig. 19.23). Rapid correction of hyponatremia results in *pontine myelinolysis* in some alcoholics.

Subacute combined degeneration of the spinal cord is a complication of pernicious anemia and the vitamin B_{12} deficiency that typically develops in this disease. Histologically, the spinal cord shows demyelination of posterior and lateral spinal tracts (Fig. 19.24).

Parkinson disease is a neurodegenerative disease of basal ganglia involving primarily the substantia nigra. The disease usually is primary or idiopathic. Secondary Parkinson disease, which is less common, can be traced to pre-existing encephalitis or toxic chemicals and drugs. On gross examination, the brain shows a typical loss of pigmentation of substantia nigra and globus ceruleus. Histologically, these areas show a loss and atrophy of neurons. The neurons that remain are devoid of pigment and often contain round eosinophilic inclusions called "Lewy bodies" (Fig. 19.25).

Huntington disease is a hereditary progressive dementia characterized by neuronal loss in the cerebral cortex and caudate nucleus and putamen. Histologically, these areas of the brain show atrophy, degeneration, and necrosis of neurons (Figure 19.26).

Friedreich ataxia is a neurodegenerative disease of unknown etiology characterized by a loss of cerebral and cerebellar nuclei. The spinal cord shows demyelination and loss of axons in the posterior columns and lateral spinocerebellar tracts (Fig. 19.27).

Neoplasms

The tumors of the CNS are most often derived from glia cells, immature neural cells and their precursors (neuroblasts), neural sheath cells, meninges, or blood vessels. Lymphomas and metastases of solid extracranial tumors may also involve the CNS (Diagram 19.6).

Astrocytic tumors are malignant neoplasms that form a spectrum of histological lesions. At the one end of the spectrum is the well-differentiated astrocytoma; on the other is the highly anaplastic glioblastoma multiforme. The remaining tumors, called anaplastic astrocytomas, fall between these two extremes.

Astrocytoma is a tumor composed of well-differentiated, slow dividing cells resembling fibrillar or protoplasmatic astrocytes of the normal brain (Figure 19.28). Despite the apparently benign appearance of these tumor cells, all astrocytomas grow progressively and ultimately kill the host.

Glioblastoma multiforme, as the name implies, has a variegated gross appearance and shows considerable cellular pleomorphism (Fig. 19.29). This highly malignant tumor is composed of anaplastic astroglial cells that vary in size and shape and grow in many patterns. Despite the marked vascularity of the tumor, areas of ischemic necrosis are common. Necrosis occurs because the tumor outgrows the blood supply and the tumor blood vessels become obliterated by proliferating endothelial cells, which is typical of this brain tumor. Tumor infiltrates the adjacent brain, causing necrosis and destruction.

Oligodendroglioma is a slow-growing tumor composed of oligodendroglia cells (Fig. 19.30). The tumor cells have round nuclei surrounded by clear cytoplasm. The cells appear uniform, and mitoses are rare.

Ependymoma is a tumor composed of ependymal cells. These cells are often arranged around blood vessels in the form of so-called perivascular pseudorosettes (Fig. 19.31). Myxopapillary ependymomas, typically located in the filum terminale of the spinal cord, form papillary structures.

Medulloblastoma is a highly malignant tumor of childhood originating from the cerebellum. It is composed of small cells that have hyperchromatic small oval or round nuclei and very little cytoplasm (Fig. 19.32). The tumor cells form dense sheets and are occasionally arranged into rosettes, reminiscent of those formed by the medulloblasts in the fetal neural tube.

Meningiomas are benign tumors derived from arachnoid cells lining the meninges. Histologically, meningiomas present in several forms. The most common form is the *meningothelial* variant, characterized by whorls of concentrically arranged elongated cells (Fig. 19.33). Some meningiomas are cystic (*microcystic variant*), others have prominent blood vessels (*angioblastic variant*), and some show prominent microcalcification in the form of psammoma bodies (*psammomatous meningioma*). Histological subtyping has no clinical implications since most meningiomas are benign. Malignant meningiomas, recognized by cellular atypia and high mitotic rate, are rare.

Schwannomas are tumors of cranial and spinal nerves composed of Schwann cells (Fig. 19.34). Histologically, these tumors have the same features as the peripheral nerve schwannomas. The tumor cells have uniform spindle-shaped nuclei that often palisade. The myelin sheaths formed from the cytoplasm of neoplastic Schwann cells account for large loose zones of eosinophilic material in parts of the tumor. Only occasionally do these benign tumors evolve into neurogenic sarcoma.

Hemangioblastoma is a benign vascular tumor. Most hemangioblastomas originate from the cerebellum and often in the context of the hereditary *von Hippel–Lindau* syndrome, which includes ocular and urogenital lesions. Histologically, the tumor is composed of thin-walled blood vessels surrounded by clear stromal cells (Fig. 19.35).

Lymphoma of the brain is rare. The incidence of CNS lymphomas has increased in immunosuppressed patients, however, especially those with AIDS. Histologically, the brain is infiltrated with large and/or small atypical lymphoid cells, which usually express B-cell markers (Fig. 19.36).

Metastases to the brain occur in many neoplastic diseases. The most common tumors metastasizing to the brain are carcinomas of the lung, breast, gastrointestinal tract, and kidney and melanoma (Figure 19.37).

NOTES

PLATE 19.1. REACTION OF NEURONS

Figure 19.1.   Normal and injured neurons. A. Normal neuron. The cytoplasm contains aggregates of RNA, the so-called Nissl body. **B.** The injured neuron appears ballooned and is devoid of Nissl substance ("chromatolysis"). **C.** Atrophic neuron adjacent to a normal neuron. The atrophic neuron has less cytoplasm. The nucleus of this cell is not distinct from its amphophilic cytoplasm. **D.** Anoxic neurons have eosinophilic cytoplasm as evidenced by this anoxic Purkinje cell in the cerebellum. **E.** Hurler disease. The cytoplasm of neurons is distended with glucosaminoglycans. **F.** Rabies. Neurons of the brain infected with rabies virus contain intracytoplasmic inclusions resembling red blood cells (Negri body).

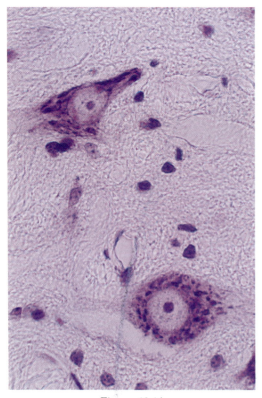

Figure 19.1A

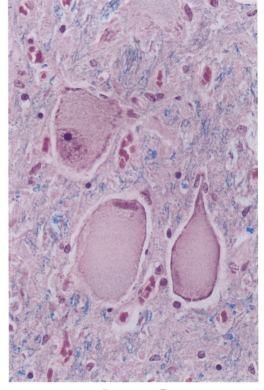

Figure 19.1B

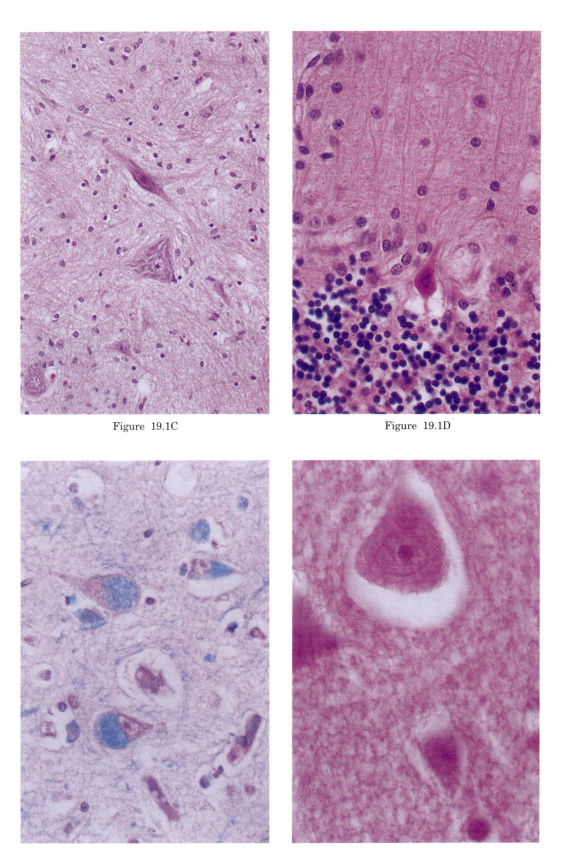

Figure 19.1C

Figure 19.1D

Figure 19.1E

Figure 19.1F

PLATE 19.2. REACTION OF GLIA CELLS TO INJURY

Figure 19.2. **Gliosis. A.** Astrocyte enlarges in response to injury ("gemistocytic transformation"). Gemistocytic astrocytes have prominent eosinophilic cytoplasm. The round nuclei adjacent to astrocytes belong to oligodendroglia cells. Microglia cells with elongated nuclei are not prominent in this field. **B.** Alzheimer type II astrocytes found in chronic liver failure and some other metabolic disorders have vacuolated nuclei with rarefied chromatin, eccentric enlarged nucleoli, and sharply outlined nuclear membrane. The cytoplasm is barely visible.

Figure 19.3. **Reaction of oligodendroglial cells to injury.** The cells surround injured neurons ("*satellitosis*").

Figure 19.4. **Reaction of microglia cells to injury. A.** Focus of neuronophagia. The dead neuron cannot be seen since it has already been phagocytized by the microglia cells. **B.** *Gitter cells* are microglia cells with well-developed vacuolated cytoplasm.

Figure 19.5. **Ependymal cell proliferation.** The pons of a newborn infant shows anastomosing channels lined by ependymal cells. This is a reaction to intrauterine viral infection that has destroyed the normal aqueduct.

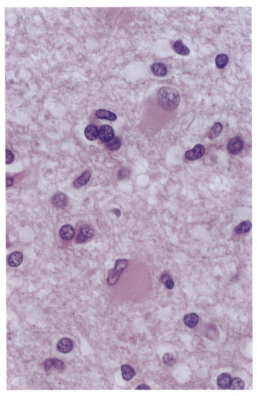

Figure 19.2A

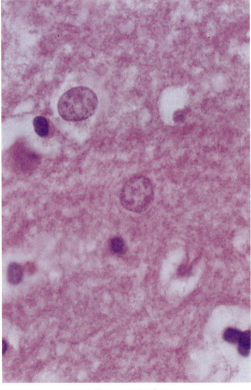

Figure 19.2B

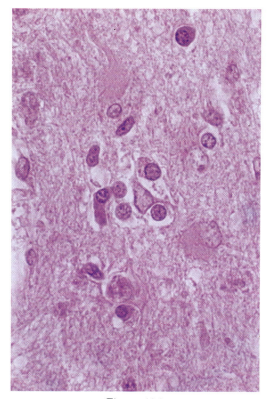

Figure 19.3

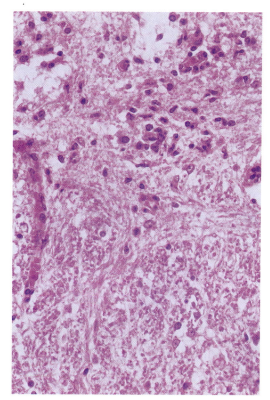

Figure 19.4A

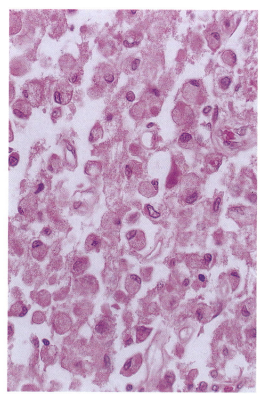

Figure 19.4B

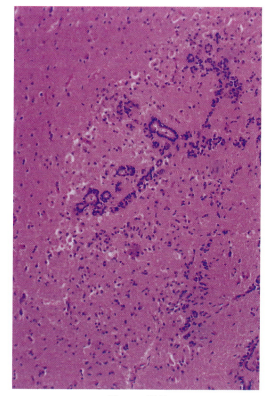

Figure 19.5

PLATE 19.3. INFECTIOUS DISEASES—MENINGITIS

Figure 19.6.   Viral meningitis. The scant exudate on the surface of the brain consists predominantly of lymphocytes.

Figure 19.7.   Bacterial meningitis. In suppurative meningitis, the subarachnoid space contains neutrophils.

Figure 19.8.   Syphilitic meningitis. A. The perivascular meningeal infiltrate consists of lymphocytes and plasma cells. **B.** Loss of posterior columns is a typical complication of syphilitic meningitis, as seen in this silver-impregnated tissue section.

Diagram 19.2.   Important infections of the CNS.

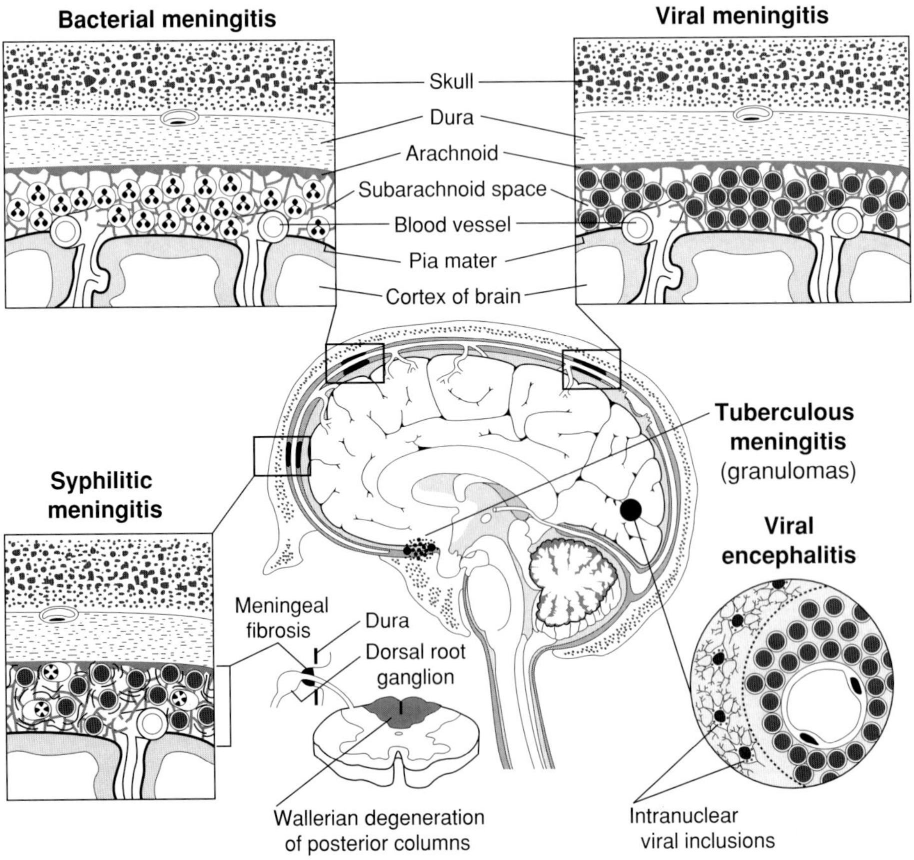

Bacterial meningitis

Viral meningitis

Skull
Dura
Arachnoid
Subarachnoid space
Blood vessel
Pia mater
Cortex of brain

Tuberculous meningitis (granulomas)

Syphilitic meningitis

Viral encephalitis

Meningeal fibrosis
Dura
Dorsal root ganglion

Wallerian degeneration of posterior columns

Intranuclear viral inclusions

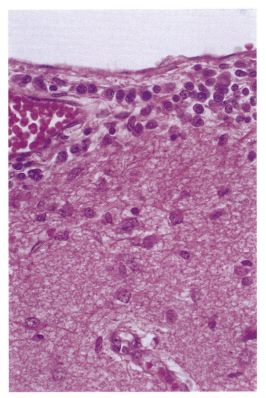

Figure 19.6

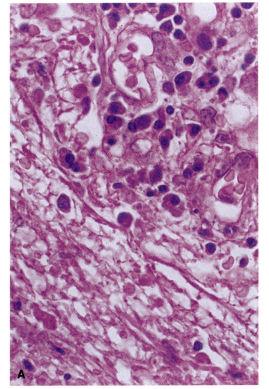

Figure 19.8A

Figure 19.7

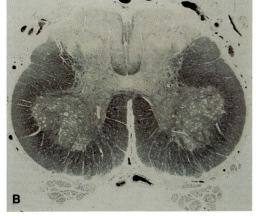

Figure 19.8B

PLATE 19.4. INFECTIOUS DISEASES—ENCEPHALITIS

Figure 19.9. Viral encephalitis. The brain shows lymphocytic infiltrates predominantly in the perivascular Virchow-Robin space. The brain contains an increased number of glial cells.

Figure 19.11. Progressive multifocal leuko-encephalopathy. The nuclei of infected oligodendroglia cells appear enlarged and contain basophilic inclusions that obscure the normal chromatin.

Figure 19.10. Subacute sclerosing panencephalitis. The oligodendroglia cells contain basophilic intranuclear inclusions surrounded by a distinct clear space ("halo"). The astrocytes have undergone gemistocytic transformation.

Figure 19.12. Spongiform encephalopathy (Creutzfeldt-Jakob disease). The cortex contains microcystic spaces, but shows no inflammation.

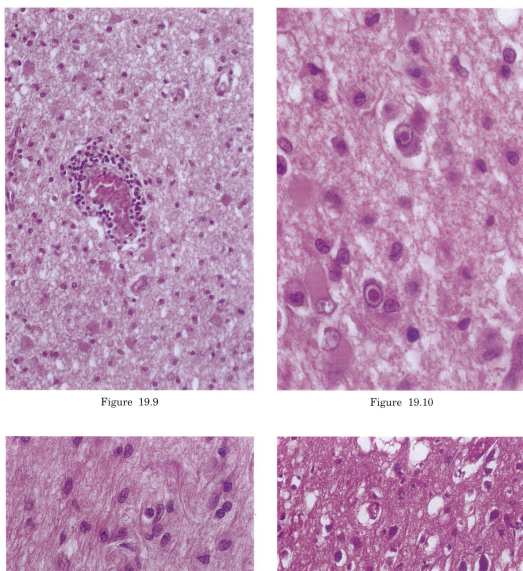

Figure 19.9

Figure 19.10

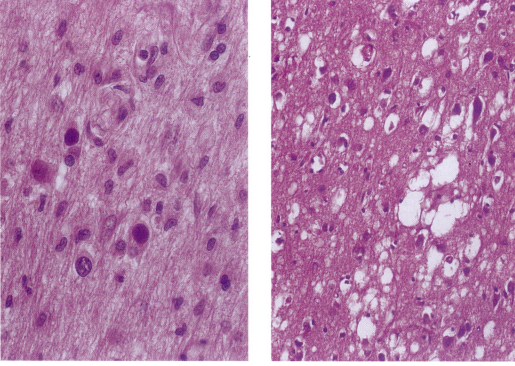

Figure 19.11

Figure 19.12

PLATE 19.5. INFECTIOUS DISEASES—AIDS

Figure 19.13.   AIDS encephalopathy. The brain contains glial nodules composed of mononuclear and multinuclear microglia cells.

Figure 19.14.   Brain abscess. The sharply demarcated space contains pus. The brain surrounding this acute abscess is edematous. A capsule, which is a feature of chronic abscesses, is not evident.

Figure 19.15.   Toxoplasmosis. The brain contains cysts filled with parasites (bradyzoites).

Figure   19.16.   Cryptococcal meningoencephalitis. The subarachnoid space contains budding yeasts (PAS stain).

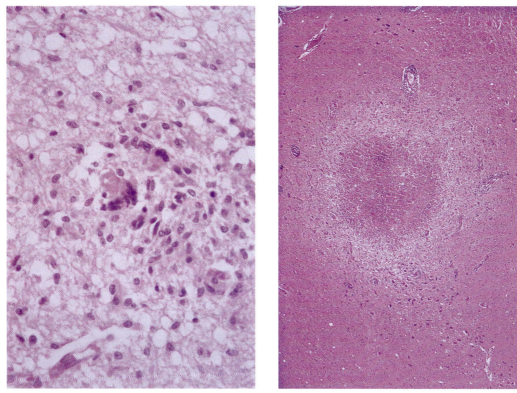

Figure 19.13

Figure 19.14

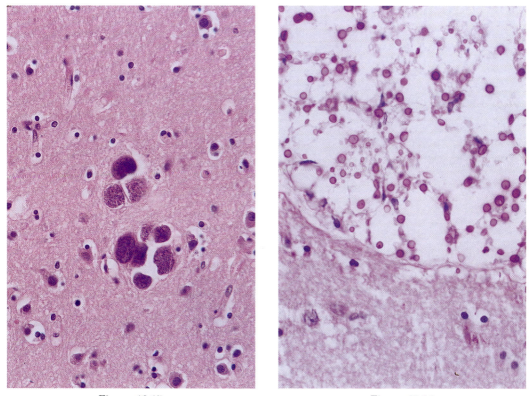

Figure 19.15

Figure 19.16

PLATE 19.6. DEMYELINATING DISEASES

Figure 19.17. Multiple sclerosis. A. Early lesions. The brain shows focal infiltrates of lymphocytes and macrophages. **B.** Periventricular plaques appear as pale areas. **C.** Plaques show demyelination and appear pale and rarefied.

Figure 19.18. Krabbe disease. There is widespread demyelination of cerebral white matter and accumulation of globoid cells. Globoid cells have well-developed cytoplasm and appear rounded.

Diagram 19.3. Multiple sclerosis. Early lesion contains phagocytic cells and lymphocytes. Late lesion shows astrocytosis around demyelinated but preserved axons.

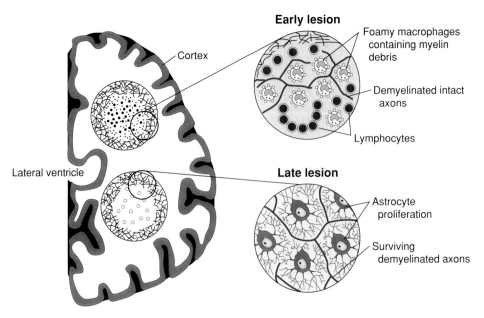

Cortex

Lateral ventricle

Early lesion

Foamy macrophages containing myelin debris

Demyelinated intact axons

Lymphocytes

Late lesion

Astrocyte proliferation

Surviving demyelinated axons

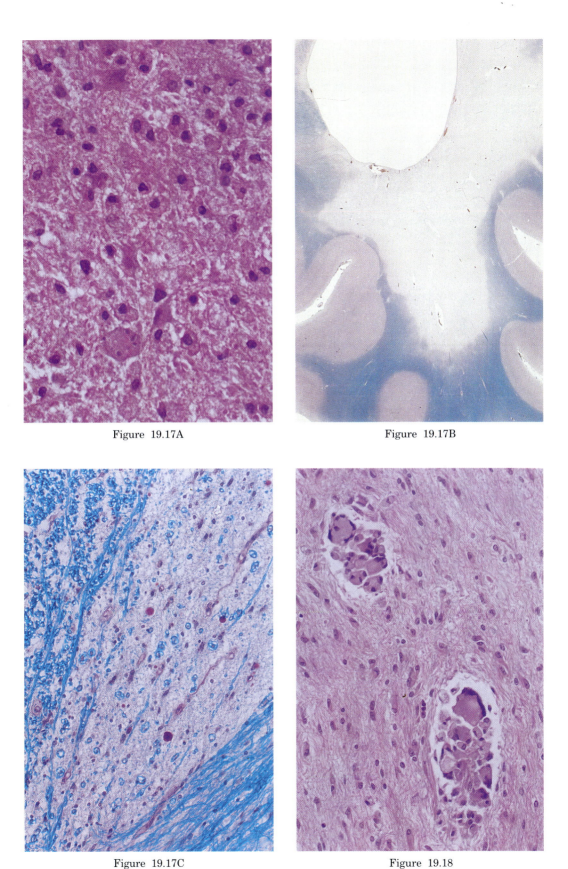

Figure 19.17A

Figure 19.17B

Figure 19.17C

Figure 19.18

PLATE 19.7. CEREBROVASCULAR DISEASES

Figure 19.19.   Intracerebral hemorrhage. A. The brain tissue is permeated with blood. **B.** Edge of an old hemorrhagic focus of brain destruction. Necrotic brain tissue has been replaced by macrophages. There are also gemistocytic astrocytes.

Figure 19.20.   Brain infarct. The area appears edematous and contains cellular debris and eosinophilic ischemic neurons.

Figure 19.21.   Laminar necrosis of the deep cortex of the hippocampus. The necrotic layers appear as pale lines.

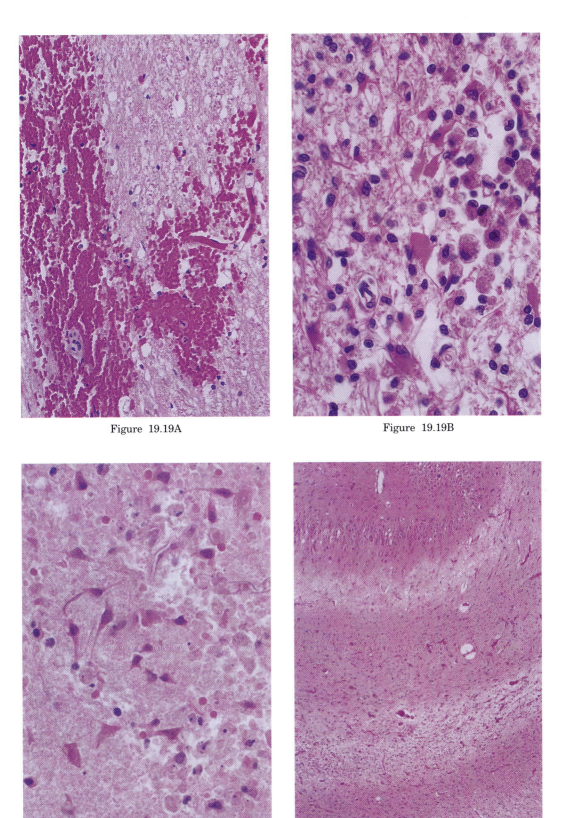

Figure 19.19A

Figure 19.19B

Figure 19.20

Figure 19.21

PLATE 19.8. ALZHEIMER DISEASE

Figure 19.22.   Alzheimer disease. A. Neurons showing neurofibrillary tangles and neuritic plaques, which appear as round filamentous bodies. **B.** Higher-magnification view of neuritic plaques, which consist of entangled glial processes (silver-impregnated tissue sections). **C.** Neurofibrillary tangles in the distended cytoplasm of pyramidal neurons impregnated with silver. **D.** Amyloid in the wall of small arteries. The wall of these vessels appears homogeneously red.

Diagram 19.4.   Alzheimer disease. The neurons show neurofibrillary degeneration or granulovacuolar degeneration. Massive accumulation of condensed neurofibrils in the cytoplasm of neurons results in the formation of neurofibrillary tangles. Neuritic plaques consist of fibrillary processes of degenerated neurons arranged around a central amyloid deposit. Deposits of amyloid are also found in the wall of small blood vessels.

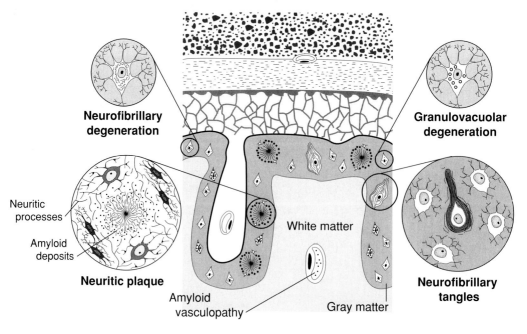

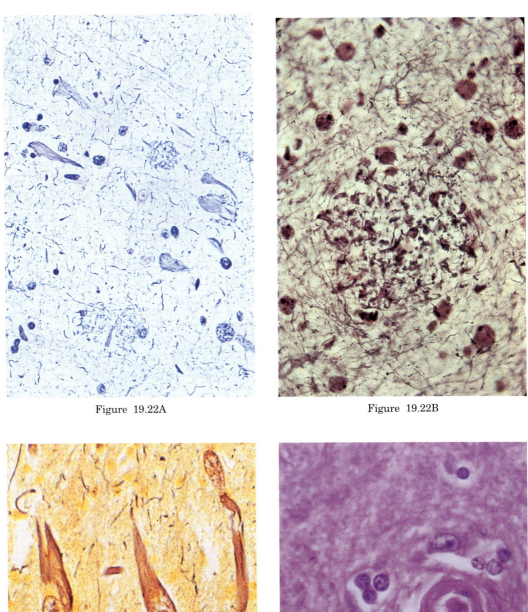

Figure 19.22A

Figure 19.22B

Figure 19.22C

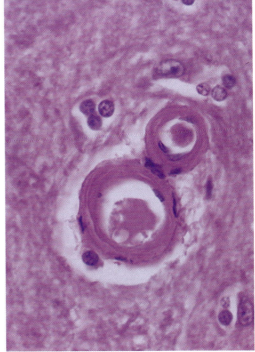

Figure 19.22D

PLATE 19.9. NUTRITIONAL DEFICIENCIES AND TOXIC DISEASES

Figure 19.23. Chronic alcoholism. Hemorrhage into the mamillary bodies typically leads to accumulation of hemosiderin-laden macrophages.

Figure 19.24. Subacute combined degeneration of spinal cord. There is demyelination of posterior, anterior, and lateral columns. The demyelinated columns appear bubbly.

Figure 19.25. Parkinson disease. The depigmented neurons of substantia nigra contain round cytoplasmic inclusions ("Lewy body").

Figure 19.26. Huntington disease. Cortex is devoid of neurons. The remaining neurons are atrophic.

Figure 19.27. Friedreich ataxia. The spinal cord shows demyelination of posterior and lateral columns.

Diagram 19.5. Neurodegenerative nutritional and toxic disorders. Huntington and Alzheimer disease affect the cerebrum. Alcohol abuse combined with nutritional deficiencies affects mammillary bodies and cerebellum. Central pontine myelinolysis is an iatrogenic lesion caused by rapid correction of hyponatremia in chronic alcoholics. Subacute combined degeneration, Friedreich ataxia, and amyotrophic lateral sclerosis affect predominantly the spinal cord and cause demyelination of ascending or descending columns.

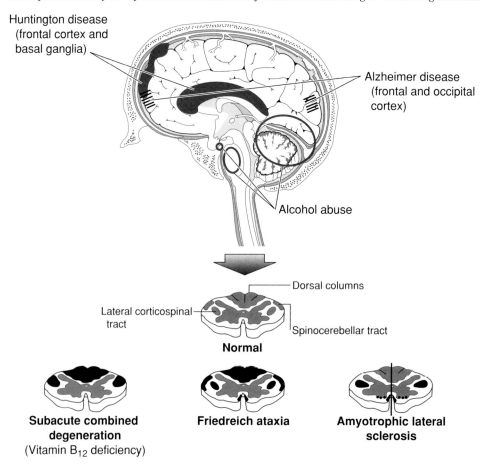

Huntington disease (frontal cortex and basal ganglia)

Alzheimer disease (frontal and occipital cortex)

Alcohol abuse

Dorsal columns

Lateral corticospinal tract

Spinocerebellar tract

Normal

Subacute combined degeneration (Vitamin B$_{12}$ deficiency)

Friedreich ataxia

Amyotrophic lateral sclerosis

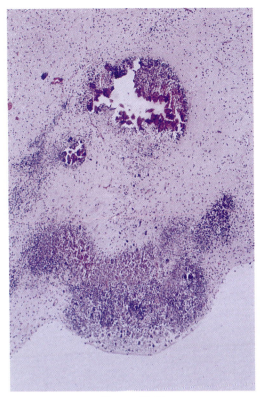

Figure 19.23

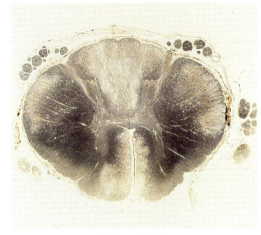

Figure 19.24

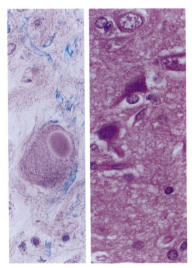

Figure 19.25   Figure 19.26

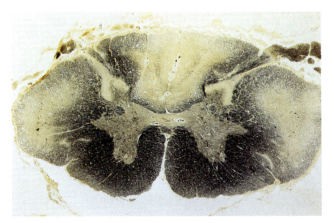

Figure 19.27

PLATE 19.10. NEOPLASMS—ASTROCYTIC TUMORS

Figure 19.28. Astrocytoma. The tumor is composed of well-differentiated astrocytes that show only mild variation in the size and shape of their nuclei.

Figure 19.29. Glioblastoma multiforme. A. Tumor cells show layering "palisading" around areas of necrosis. **B.** Higher-power view of a highly pleomorphic part of the tumor. **C.** The blood vessels in the tumor show luminal narrowing caused by endothelial cell proliferation.

Diagram 19.6. The most common histological features of intracranial tumors. 1. Astrocytoma consists of well-differentiated astrocytes. **2.** Glioblastoma multiforme has a variegated histological appearance and consists of large and small cells. The cells may show palisading around areas of necrosis, which are often prominent. The blood vessels show endothelial cell proliferation. **3.** Oligodendroglioma is composed of a uniform population of oligodendroglia cells. These cells have round nuclei surrounded by a clear cytoplasm. Foci of calcification may be present. **4.** Hemangioblastoma is a cerebellar tumor composed of small blood vessels surrounded by clear stromal cells. **5.** Medulloblastoma is a cerebellar tumor composed of small undifferentiated cells arranged into dense sheets or occasionally forming rosettes. **6.** Schwannoma is composed of whorls of spindle-shaped Schwann cells that often show palisading. The tumor typically originates from the VIII nerve in the cerebellopontine angle. **7.** Ependymoma is composed of small or elongated ependymal cells, which form rosettes or perivascular pseudorosettes. Intracranial tumors originate from the ependymal lining of the ventricles. **8.** Meningioma is composed of meningothelial cells that often form whorls. Calcifications in the form of psammoma bodies may be present. Meningiomas develop from meninges, but are most often located on the convexity of the brain.

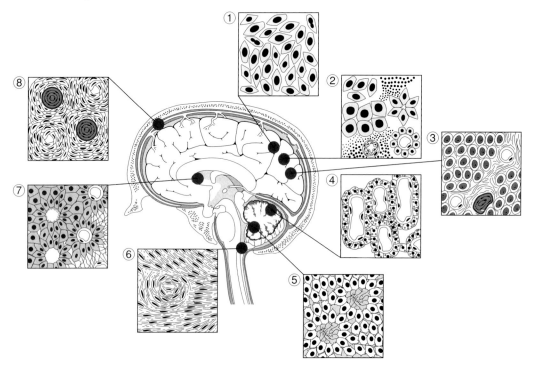

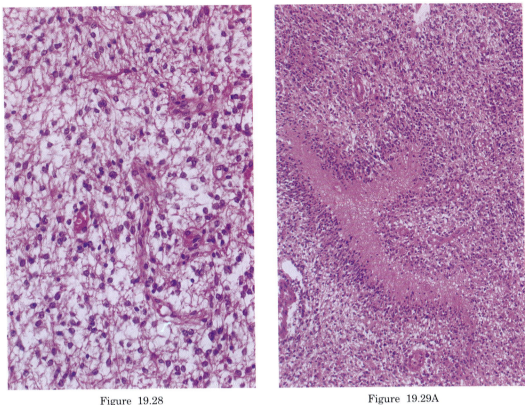

Figure 19.28   Figure 19.29A

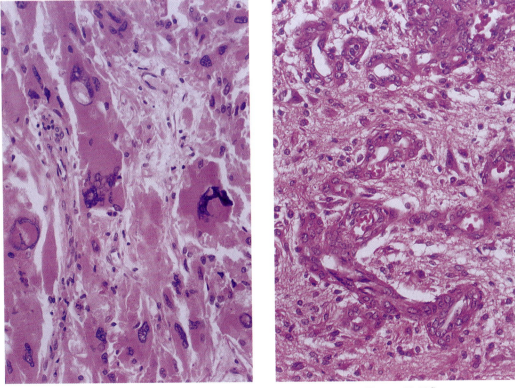

Figure 19.29B   Figure 19.29C

PLATE 19.11. NEOPLASMS—ASTROCYTIC TUMORS

Figure 19.30. Oligodendroglioma. The tumor is composed of a uniform population of cells that have round, centrally located nuclei and clear cytoplasm.

Figure 19.31. Ependymoma. A. The tumor cells have elongated nuclei and form rosettes and perivascular pseudorosettes. **B.** Myxopapillary ependymoma. The tumor cells line tissue cores composed of connective tissue and blood vessels.

Figure 19.32. Medulloblastoma. The tumor is composed of small blue cells.

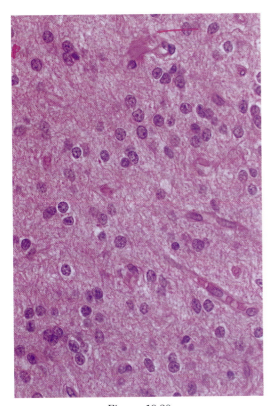

Figure 19.30

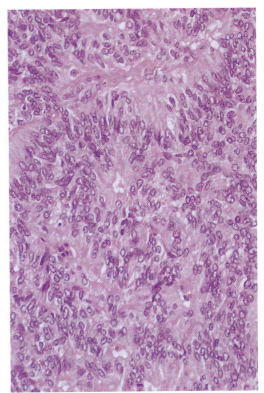

Figure 19.31A

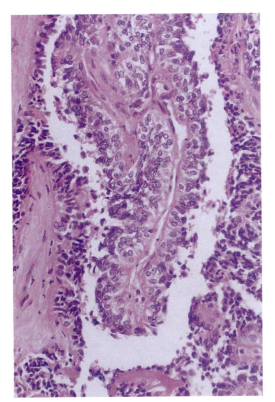

Figure 19.31B

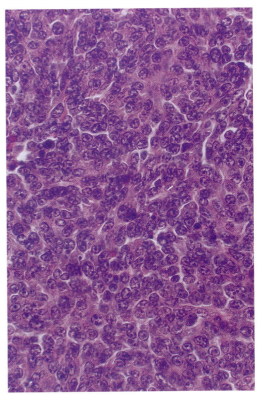

Figure 19.32

PLATE 19.12. MENINGIOMAS, NERVE SHEATH TUMORS, AND MESENCHYMAL TUMORS

Figure 19.33. Meningioma. A. The tumor is located outside of the brain. It contains calcifications. **B.** The tumor is composed of whorls of concentrically layered meningothelial cells.

Figure 19.34. Schwannoma. The tumor is composed of spindle cells forming broad strands and typically arranged in palisades. Cytoplasmic processes of neoplastic Schwann cells form the eosinophilic material between the nuclei.

Figure 19.35. Hemangioblastoma of the cerebellum. The tumor consists of small blood vessels and slit-like capillaries surrounded by clear cells.

Figure 19.36. Lymphoma of the brain. The brain is infiltrated with atypical large lymphoid cells.

Figure 19.37. Metastatic melanoma. The brain is infiltrated with clusters of malignant cells.

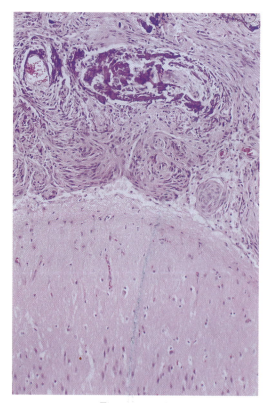

Figure 19.33A

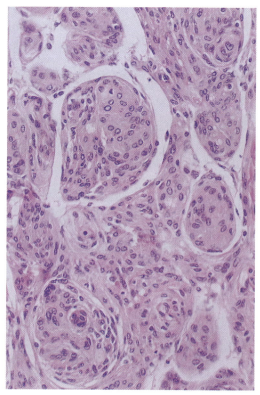

Figure 19.33B

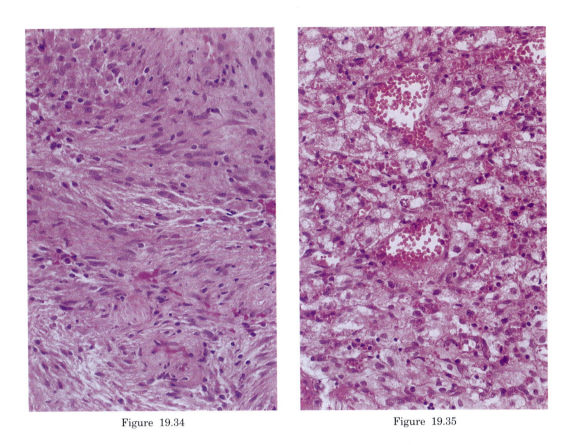

Figure 19.34

Figure 19.35

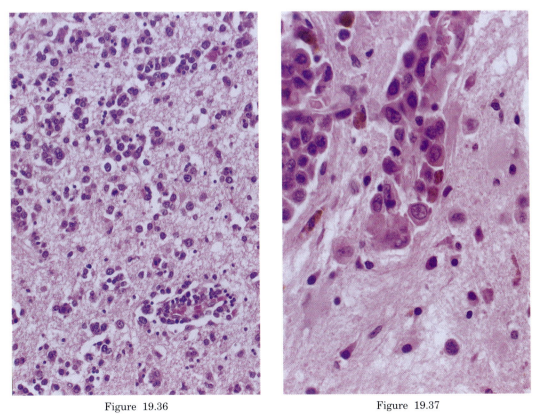

Figure 19.36

Figure 19.37

NOTES

Index

Page numbers in *italic* denote figures; those followed by "t" denote tables.

Pneumonia, 125–128, *132–139*
  interstitial, 127
Polyarteritis nodosa, 96, *118,
  263*
Polycystic kidney diseases, *284*
Polycystic ovary, *338*
Polymorphonuclear granulocytes,
  23
Polymorphonuclear leukocytes,
  26
Polymyositis, 449, *452, 456*
Polyps
  intestinal, 183
  large intestine, 184t
Pompe disease, *108*
Pontine myelinolysis, 462
Postmenopausal endometrial
  atrophy, 322, *334*
Poststreptococcal
    glomerulonephritis, 261,
    272
Preeclampsia, 264
Pregnancy
  ectopic, 325
  pathology of, 325, *348*
Primary testicular infertility,
    297–298
Progressive multifocal
    leukoencephalopathy, 461,
    472
Prolactinoma, pituitary, 370
Prostaglandins, macrophage
    secretion of, 24
Prostate, 297, *298*
  adenocarcinoma, *86*
  carcinoma, 301, *312*
Prostate specific antigen, *86*
Proteinuria, 258
Proteus vulgaris, 299
  pyelonephritis, 265
Protozoa, skin, 399
Pseudomembranous
    inflammation, 25
Pseudomonas aeruginosa,
    pyelonephritis, 265
Psoriasis, 396, *404*
Pulmonary edema, *42*
Pulmonary embolus, *50*
Pulmonary hemorrhage, *44*
Pulmonary scar, ossification of,
    16
Pulmonary system, 123–148
Purpura, 40, *44*
Purulent inflammation, 25, *28*
Pyelonephritis, 265, *288*
Pyknosis, 5, *18*
Pyogenic bacteria, 399

Red blood cells
  deficiency, 151–154, *158–165*
  morphology in anemias, *158,
    160*
Regeneration
  damaged tissues, 23
  healing of inflammation, 25
Renal cell adenoma, 58
Renal cell carcinoma, 265, *290*

Renal failure, 258
Repair and healing, *36*
Resolution, healing of
    inflammation, 25
Respiratory distress syndrome,
    130
Respiratory mucosa, 123
Respiratory system, 123
  normal, *124*
Retinoblastoma, 61, *82*
Rhabdomyolysis, 449, *454*
Rhabdomyoma, 60
  pharynx, *76*
Rhabdomyosarcoma, 60, *78, 88*
  bladder, 267
Rheumatic carditis, 93, *102*
Rheumatic endocarditis, acute
    and subacute, 93
Rheumatic fever, 93, *102*
Rheumatoid arthritis, 427, *442*
Rickets, 424, *430*
Rickettsiae, skin, 399
Riedel thyroiditis, 372, *382*
Rokitansky-Aschoff sinuses, 218
Rosettes, 61
Rotor syndrome, 212

Salivary gland, 179, *180*
  mixed tumors, *80*
  tumors, 181, *188*
Salmonella, 424
Salpingitis, 321, *326, 328*
  acute, *28*
  chronic, *32*
Sarcoidosis, 24, *32,* 126, *140*
  pituitary, *378*
Sarcoma, *66, 86*
  bladder, 267
  endometrial stromal, 322, *336*
Sarcoma botryoides, bladder, 267
Scarring, *36*
  healing of inflammation, 25
Schistocytes, 153
Schistosomiasis, liver, *232*
Schmidt syndrome, 374
Schwannomas, 463, *488*
Scirrhous adenocarcinoma,
    breast, *74*
Scleroderma, *282,* 397, *404*
Sclerosing adenosis, 352
Scrotal edema, *42*
Sebaceous glands, 395
Seborrheic keratosis, 400, *414*
Secondary testicular infertility,
    298
Seminal vesicles, 297
Seminoma, 300, *308*
Septic shock, *54*
Serous inflammation, 25
Serous tumors, ovary, *340*
Sertoli cell tumors, 301, *312*
Sertoli-Leydig cell tumors, 324,
    346
Sex cord cell tumors, *312, 324,
    346*
Sézary syndrome, 154, *168*

Sheehan syndrome, 371
Shock, *39, 41*
  lung, *54*
  pathogenesis of, *54*
Sialadenitis, 179, *186*
Sickle cell anemia, 153, *160, 164*
Sickle cells, 151
Silicone implants, breast, 352,
    356
Silicosis, *142*
Skeletal muscle, neurogenic
    atrophy, *12*
Skin
  basal cell papilloma, *70*
  burns, 25, *34*
  common lesions, 396t
  edema, *42*
  exogenous injury, 398, *406*
  idiopathic diseases, 395, *404*
  immune reactions, 399
  immunological diseases, *412*
  infectious diseases, 398, *410*
  layers, *397*
  neoplasms, 400
  pathology, 395–419
  petechia, *44*
  pustule of, *28*
  sunlight injury, 398
  wounds, 398
Small cell carcinoma, lung, 128,
    148
Solar degeneration, dermis, *406*
Solid adenomas, 58, *70*
Solid carcinomas, 60
Somatotropic adenomas,
    pituitary, 370
Specific granules, 23
Spherocytosis, 151, *160*
Spinal cord, subacute combined
    degeneration, *482*
Spleen, *152*
  hairy cell leukemia, *170*
Spongiform encephalopathy, 461,
    472
Squamous cell carcinoma, 57, 59,
    66, 72, 88, 127, *146,* 181
  cervical, *332*
  gall bladder, 218
  skin, 400, *414*
  tongue, *188*
  urinary tract, 267
  vulvar, 321
Squamous cell papilloma, 58
Squamous epithelium, 4
Squamous hyperplasia, vulva,
    321
Squamous metaplasia,
    endocervical glands, *16*
Staphylococcus, 399
  bacterial endocarditis, 93
Staphylococcus aureus, 125, 424
Stomach, *180*
  carcinoma, *194*
Stomatitis, 179, *186*
Streptococcus, 399
  bacterial endocarditis, 93

COLOR ATLAS OF HISTOPATHOLOGY
